장중경 처방 해설

저자 박병정

·1997년 삼육대학교 약대 졸업
·1997년부터 현재까지 임상약사로 근무
·이메일 : pigdragon1080@hanmail.net

장중경 처방 해설

초판 1쇄 인쇄 2011년 07월 25일
초판 1쇄 발행 2011년 08월 01일

지은이 | 박병정
펴낸이 | 손형국
펴낸곳 | (주)에세이퍼블리싱
출판등록 | 2004. 12. 1(제315-2008-022호)
주소 | 서울특별시 강서구 방화3동 316-3번지 한국계량계측조합 102호
홈페이지 | www.book.co.kr
전화번호 | (02)3159-9638~40
팩스 | (02)3159-9637

ISBN 978-89-6023-645-5 13510

장중경 처방해설

박병정 지음

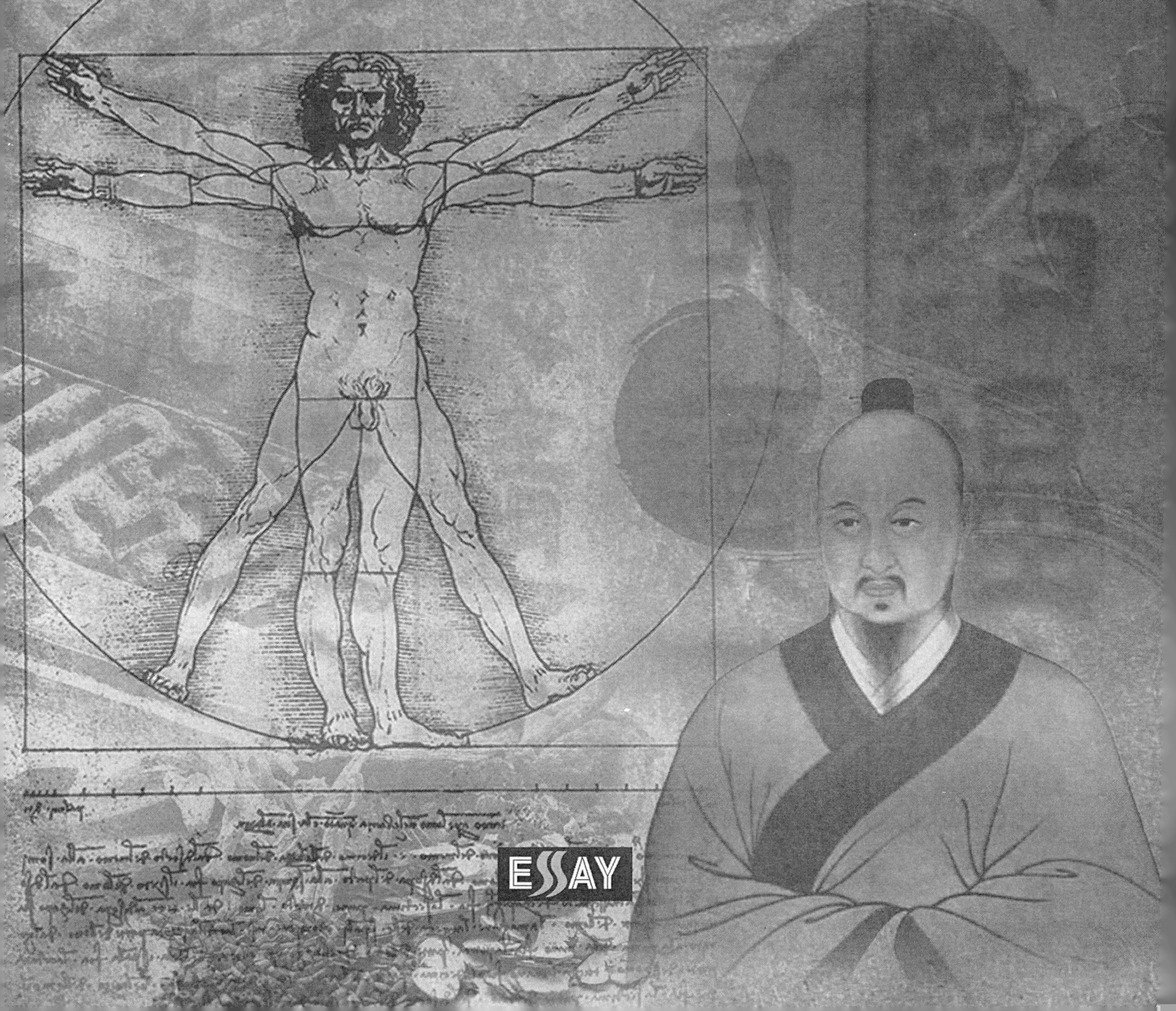

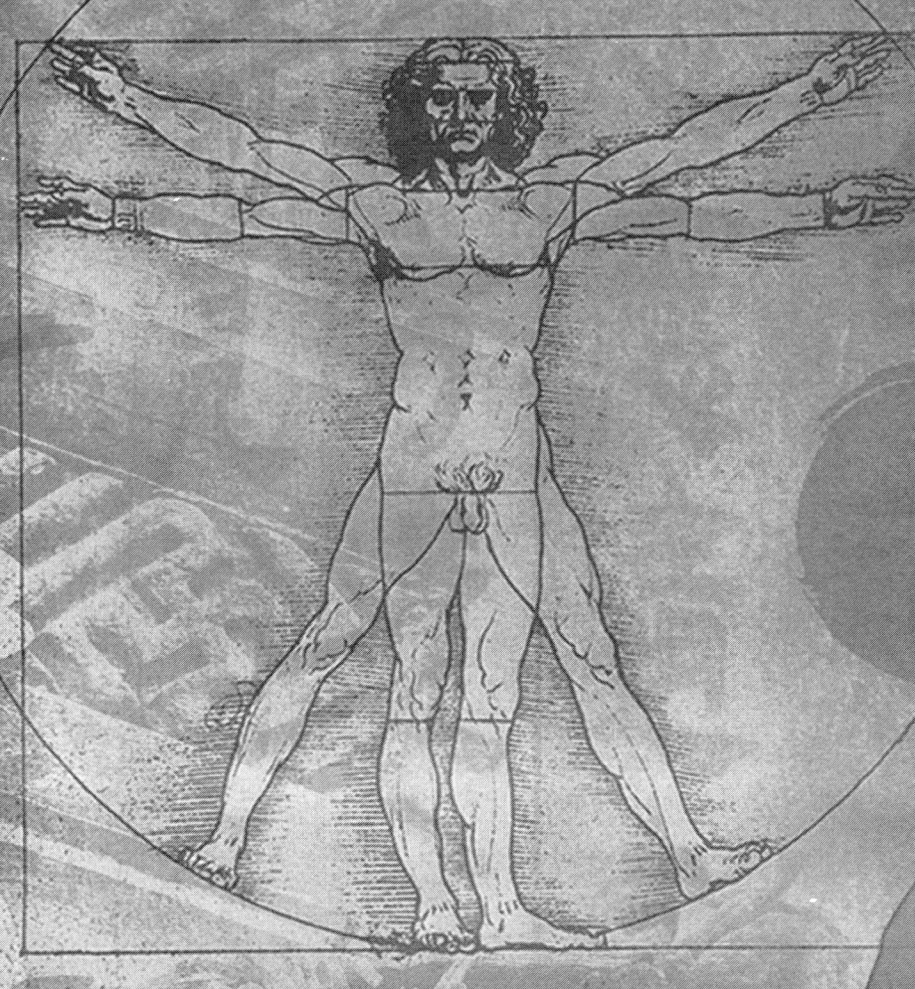

ESSAY

| 프롤로그 |

최근에 "통합의학"이라는 용어가 부각되고 있습니다. "통합의학"에는 다양한 분야의 치료법이 포함되지만, 핵심을 이루는 것은 양-한방의 통합일 것입니다. 완전한 건강의 회복을 위해 의사와 한의사의 소통이 증대하고, 각자 영역의 장점이 교집합을 이뤄가는 것이 "통합의학"의 핵심이 아닐까 생각합니다.

양방은 진단이 명확하나, 만성질환에 대한 완치요법이 과소하고 한방은 완치요법에 대한 근거가 과대하나, 진단은 불명확합니다. 양방은 병명을 명확하게 찾아 주지만, 완치요법이 없는 경우가 많고, 한방은 환자의 건강을 되찾아 주었지만, 어떤 병을 치료했는지가 명확하지 않습니다. 따라서 수많은 만성질환과 종양에 대해, 환자의 고통과 치료비용이 최소화 될 수 있도록 "통합의학"이 활용되어야 하겠습니다.

저는 천연물의 약리를 연구하는 약사입니다. 천연물의 소스는 장 중경님의 "상한론"과 "금궤요략"입니다. 수년간, 수많은 논문과 최신의학 지견을 참고하여 "상한론"과 "금궤요략"을 구성하는 천연물의 약리기전과 처방의 적응증을 정리해 보았습니다.

나름대로 일관성과 합리성을 갖추기 위해 매진하였으나, 오류가 있는 부분도 있을 것입니다. 밝혀 주시면 적극적으로 삭제 또는 수정하겠습니다.

이 책이 "통합의학"이라는 마라톤 레이스에서 중간 중간 만나게 되는 급수대의 물 한 잔이 되었으면 좋겠습니다.

2011년 06월

박병정

| 차례 |

프롤로그

1부 천연물 약리 해설

1. 갈근: genistein ▶ Ionotropic glutamate receptor blocker · 18
2. 감수: tirucallol, 약리 추측 ▶ Aldosterone receptor blocker · 19
3. 감초: glycyrrhetinic acid ▶ 11-beta-hydroxysteroid dehydrogenase1 inhibitor · 20
4. 강랑: ivermectin ▶ Chloride channel blocker · 23
5. 건강: shogaol, 약리 추측 ▶ Intra-neutrophil hydrogen peroxide scavenger · 23
6. 건지황: catalpol, 약리 추측 ▶ CD133+ CFU-GEMM (+) modulator · 25
7. 건칠: urishiol ▶ Fibrosarcoma cell p27 (+) modulator · 26
8. 경미: magnesium ▶ DNA replication cofactor · 27
9. 계지: cinnamic acid ▶ Lactate oxidizer · 28
10. 고삼: trifolirhizin ▶ Protozoa tyrosinase transcription inhibitior · 32
11. 과루근: trichosanthin ▶ Ribosome inactivating protein · 33
12. 과루실: cucurbitacin ▶ Endothelium actin-disrupting agent · 34
13. 과체: elaterin ▶ 최토제 · 36
14. 구감초: 18β-24-Hydroxyglycyrrhetinic acid
    ▶ 11-beta-hydroxysteroid dehydrogenase2 (HSD11B2) inhibitor · 36
15. 구맥: dianoside, 약리 추측 ▶ Plasmodium Falciparum DOXP blocker
    & Plasminogen activator inhibitor-1 (-) modulator · 40
16. 국화: apigenin, 약리 추측 ▶ Phospholipases A2 blocker · 41
17. 규자: palmitic acid ▶ Arachidonic acid-induced platelet aggregation inhibitor · 42
18. 귤피: rutin ▶ Proteolytic activator · 43
19. 길경: platycodin, 약리 추측 ▶ Toll like receptor (+) modulator · 44
20. 난발회: keratin ▶ Oxalator chelater in Urine · 45
21. 당귀: decursin ▶ Erythrocyte PKC inhibitor · 46
22. 대극: euphorin ▶ Diuretic like urethane · 48
23. 대추: cAMP ▶ Protein kinase A acvtivator & Granular organelles inhibitor · 48
24. 대황: emodin ▶ Tyrosine kinase blocker · 50
25. 도인: amygdalin ▶ 4S estrogen receptor (ER):5S estrogen receptor 전환 억제 · 52

26. 동과자: adenine ▶ Diuretic like urea · 53
27. 마자인: α-Linolenic acid(omega-3) ▶ 대장암세포의 세포막 지방산 조성 변화시킴 · 54
28. 마황: ephedrine ▶ Epinephrine receptors agonist · 55
29. 망초: Sodium Sulfate (Na2SO4) ▶ Intraluminal distention pressure 상승시킴 · 57
30. 맥문동:ophiopogonin, 약리 추측 ▶ M. tuberculosis SigF transcription inhibitor · 58
31. 맹충 (등에): anophelin ▶ Thrombin esterase blocker · 59
32. 모려: NaCl ▶ Saline solution · 60
33. 목단피: β-Sitosterol ▶ antioxidant enzyme (+) modulator · 61
34. 목통: hedegeragenin ▶ Diuretic action · 62
35. 반석: KAl(SO4)2·12H2O (Alum) ▶ astringent (수렴제) · 64
36. 반하:triterpenoid (C30H48O7S),약리 추측 ▶ Rho GTPase family (+) modulator · 65
37. 방기: sinomenine ▶ Prostaglandin I2 (+) modulator in venous endothelium · 66
38. 방풍: deltoin ▶ Cyclooxygenase-2 blocker · 68
39. 백두옹: anemonin ▶ NF-kB blocker in small intestine epithelium · 69
40. 백석지: (Al,Mg)2(Si4O10)(OH)2·nH2O ▶ Water absorbent · 70
41. 백엽: tannin ▶ 지혈제 · 71
42. 백전: pregnane glycoside ▶ PXR ligand · 71
43. 백출: atractylon ▶ vascular cell adhesion molecule-1 (VCAM-1) blocker · 72
44. 별갑: chitosan ▶ Lipid absorption inhibitor & Sterol excretion activator · 74
45. 복령: pachymic acid, 약리 추측 ▶ glycoprotein IIb/IIIa (gpIIb/IIIa) blocker · 74
46. 봉밀: xylose & galactose ▶ Heparan sulfate biosynthesis · 76
47. 봉와: rosin ▶ Histidin binder · 77
48. 부소맥: Vitamin B6 (Pyridoxine)
▶ γ-gamma-aminobutyric acid (GABA) & dopamine biosynthesis · 78
49. 부자: hypaconitine, 약리 추측
▶ Macrophage` Voltage-gated proton channels blocker · 78
50. 삭조: cyanidin ▶ Phosphodiesterase C & D inhibitor · 80
51. 산수유: ursolic acid ▶ ERK (extracellular signal-regulated kinases) blocker · 80
52. 산약: diosgenin ▶ Glucose transporters (+) modulator · 82
53. 산조인: jujuboside / sanjoinine
▶ serotonin (+) modulator / norepinephrine (+) modulator · 83
54. 상륙근: KNO3 ▶ Potassium supplements · 84
55. 상백피: α-amyrin ▶ Capsaicin sensitive channel blocker · 85
56. 생강: gingerol ▶ Hydrogen peroxide scavenger · 87
57. 생지황: catalpol, 약리추측
▶ CD133+ circulating endothelial cell progenitor (+) modulator · 89
58. 석고: CaSO4 ▶ Calcium-mediated T cell apoptosis 촉진 · 90
59. 석위: fumaric acid ▶ Plasmodium Falciparum DHODH blocker ·

60. 선복화: taraxasterol ▶ CMV-mediated lipid peroxidation inhibitor · 92
61. 세신: eugenol ▶ Met-hemoglobin reducer · 93
62. 소엽: linoleic acid ▶ Estrogen receptor alpha (ERα) agonist · 95
63. 수질 (거머리): hirudin ▶ Thrombolytic activator · 96
64. 시호:saikosaponin,약리 추측 ▶ Small interfering RNA (siRNA) (+) modulator · 97
65. 신강: alizarin,약리 추측 ▶ Inhibition of Vein smooth muscle cell proliferation · 99
66. 아교: Glycine / Proline / Hydroxyproline / Alanine / 기타 아미노산
▶ Collagen biosynthesis · 101
67. 애엽: cineol ▶ Vasoconstriction · 102
68. 연교: forsythiaside, 약리 추측 ▶ B-cell CD20 blocker · 103
69. 오미자: schizandrin ▶ Acetylcholinesterase inhibitor · 104
70. 오수유: evodiamine ▶ Low-affinity Cholecystokinin (CCK) Rc blocker · 105
71. 왕불류행: vaccaroside, 약리 추측 ▶ Anti-Clostridium tetani · 106
72. 용골: Calcium Carbonate (CaCO3) & Calcium Phosphate (Ca3(PO4)2)
▶ acidosis 교정 · 107
73. 우여량: Fe2O3 ▶ Cytomegalovirus inclusion colitis · 108
74. 운모: sheat silicate ▶ Heat absorber · 109
75. 웅황: 이황화비소 (As2S2) ▶ Flagellated protozoa` pyruvate kinase inhibitor · 110
76. 원화: genkwanin ▶ Type VII collagen (+) modulator · 111
77. 의어 (웃좀): cellulase ▶ calcium oxalate binder ·
78. 의이인: stigmasterol, 약리 추측
▶ Major histocompatibility complex (MHC) (-) modulator · 112
79. 이근백피: potassium citrate
▶ extracellular Ca2+ influx inhibitor
& endoplasmic reticulum (ER) Ca2+ release inhibitor · 113
80. 인삼: panax ginsenoside
▶ Transforming growth factor beta (TGF-β) (+) modulator · 113
81. 인진호: capillarisin ▶ Chenodeoxycholic acid (CDCA) detoxicant · 116
82. 자삼: gallic acid ▶ Mucus astringent · 117
83. 자석영: CaF2 ▶ Phosphate binder · 117
84. 자위 (능소화): campenoside ▶ Plasmodium falciparum Fabl blocker · 118
85. 자충 (흙바퀴): ESW extraction, 약리 추측
▶ Erythrocyte C3b receptor (+) modulator · 119
86. 작약: paeoniflorin ▶ Superoxide scavenger · 18
87. 재백피: β-lapachone ▶ AMPK phosphorylation activator · 121
88. 저령: ergosterol ▶ Mesangial cell proliferation inhibitor · 122
89. 적석지: Al2O3, 2SiO2·4H2O ▶ Cation absorbent · 123
90. 적소두: albumin, 약리추측 ▶ Immunoglobulin Fc region binder · 124
91. 정력자: helveticoside ▶ Cardiac glycoside · 126

92. 제조 (굼벵이): fibrinolytic serine protease ▶ Fibrinolysis · 127
93. 조협: triacanthin ▶ Phosphodiesterase (PDE) blocker · 128
94. 죽여: Tyrosine ▶ Dopamine / Norepinephrine / Epinephrine biosynthesis · 129
95. 죽엽: arundoin, 약리 추측 ▶ β-amyloid gene expression (-) modulator · 130
96. 지모: timosaponin, 약리추측 ▶ nestin (+) modulator · 131
97. 지실: auraptene ▶ Matrix metalloproteinases (MMPs) blocker · 133
98. 진피 (秦皮): aesculetin
▶ NOD2 gene mutation inhibitor (in small intestinal epithelial cell) · 135
99. 창포: asarone ▶ HMG-CoA reductase blocker · 136
100. 천궁: cnidilide ▶ α-adrenergic receptor blocker · 137
101. 초목: xanthoxin ▶ 경련독 · 139
102. 촉초: sanshool ▶ Potassium leak channel blocker · 140
103. 촉칠:dichroine / halofuginone ▶ Vasodilation / Collagen synthesis inhibitor · 141
104. 총백: allicin ▶ Factor VII, IX, X absorbent · 141
105. 치자: crocin ▶ Low-Density Lipoprotein (LDL) antioxidant
& conjugated-bilirubin oxidizer · 143
106. 택사: alisol ▶ Angiotensin II receptor blocker · 144
107. 택칠: quercetin ▶ β-defensin (+) modulator · 146
108. 파두: phorbol ester ▶ Squamous cell PKC activator · 146
109. 패모: verticine ▶ Calcium ATPase blocker · 148
110. 패장 (마타리): oleanolic acid
▶ PPAR (peroxisome proliferator-activated receptors) activator · 149
111. 포부자: aconitine,약리 추측
▶ Neutrophil` Voltage-gated proton channels blocker · 150
112. 해백 (부추): vitamin B1
▶ Pyruvate dehydrogenase & Oxoglutarate dehydrogenase의 coenzymes · 151
113. 행인: benzoic acid ▶ Hydroxyl radical scavenger · 153
114. 향시: L-arginine ▶ Synthesis of nitric oxide · 154
115. 활석: $Mg_3(Si_4O_{10})(OH)_2$ ▶ Nitrogen group & Nucleic acid absorbent · 155
116. 황금: baicalin ▶ Peroxynitrite ($ONOO^-$) scavenger · 157
117. 황기: astragaloside ▶ Tissue plasminogen activator (+) modulator · 159
118. 황련: berberine ▶ Sortase inhibitor · 160
119. 황백: phellodendrine, 약리 추측
▶ Monocyte / Macrophage / Neutrophil CD14 blocker · 162
120. 후박: honokiol ▶ VEGF receptor blocker · 163

2부 적응증 해설

1. 갈근가반하탕: Enterovirus-mediated Meningoencephalitis (장바이러스-매개 뇌수막염) · 166
2. 갈근탕: Mosquito-borne encephalitis virus & Enterovirus-mediated Meningoencephalitis(모기-매개 뇌염바이러스) · 167
3. 갈근황금황련탕: Botulism (보툴리누스 독소증) · 169
4. 감강영출탕: p-ANCA mediated crescentic glomerulonephritis (핵주위 항호중구 세포질 항체-매개 반월상 사구체신염) · 170
5. 감맥대조탕: Bipolar affective disorder (양극성 정동장애) · 172
6. 감초건강탕: Sjogren's syndrom (쇼그렌증후군) · 173
7. 감초마황탕: Type I hypersensitive reaction: first sensitization · 174
8. 감초부자탕: Coxsackie virus-mediated polymyositis & polyarthritis (다발성근염 & 다발성관절염) · 175
9. 감초사심탕: Peptic ulcer-complicated perforation(소화성궤양에 합병된 천공) · 176
10. 감초탕: Viral pharyngitis (바이러스성 인두염) · 178
11. 건강부자탕: Adenovirus infection · 179
12. 건강인삼반하환:Cytomegalovirus-mediated placental villitis(태반융모세포염) · 180
13. 건강황금황련인삼탕: Staphylococcal food poisoning (포도구균 식 중독) · 181
14. 계령오미감초거계가강신하탕 : Chronic left heart failure-mediated alveolar-capillary barrier damage (만성심부전-매개 폐포-모세혈관 장벽 손상) · 183
15. 계령오미감초탕: Pneumonia complications-mediated hypoxemia (폐렴합병증-매개 저산소혈증) · 185
16. 계지가갈근탕: IFN-a mediated Meningoencephalitis (뇌수막염) · 186
17. 계지가계탕:Lipacidemia-mediated Cardiac toxicity(지방산혈증-매개 심장독성) · 187
18. 계지가대황탕: Autoimmune enteropathy & colon cancer (자가면역성 장병증 & 대장암) · 188
19. 계지가부자탕: Acute EBV infection · 190
20. 계지가용골모려탕: Hypernatremia-mediated hypotension (고나트륨혈증) · 192
21. 계지가작약탕: Autoimmune enteropathy (자가면역성 장병증) · 194
22. 계지가황기탕: Eccrine sweat gland capillaritis (에크린분비선 모세혈관염) · 195
23. 계지가후박행자탕:Airway remodeling-mediated Asthma (기도 개형-매개 천식) · 198
24. 계지감초용골모려탕: Rapid hyponatremia (급속 저나트륨혈증) · 198
25. 계지감초탕:Lactacidemia-mediated cardiomyopathy(지방산혈증-매개 심근병증) · 200
26. 계지거계가복령백출탕: Kawasaki disease · 201
27. 계지거작약가마황세신부자탕 : Autoimmune response-mediated Methemoglobinemia · 203
28. 계지거작약가부자탕: IL-1 mediated Cardiac toxicity · 205
29. 계지거작약가촉칠모려용골구역탕: Rapid hypernatremia (급속 고나트륨혈증) · 206

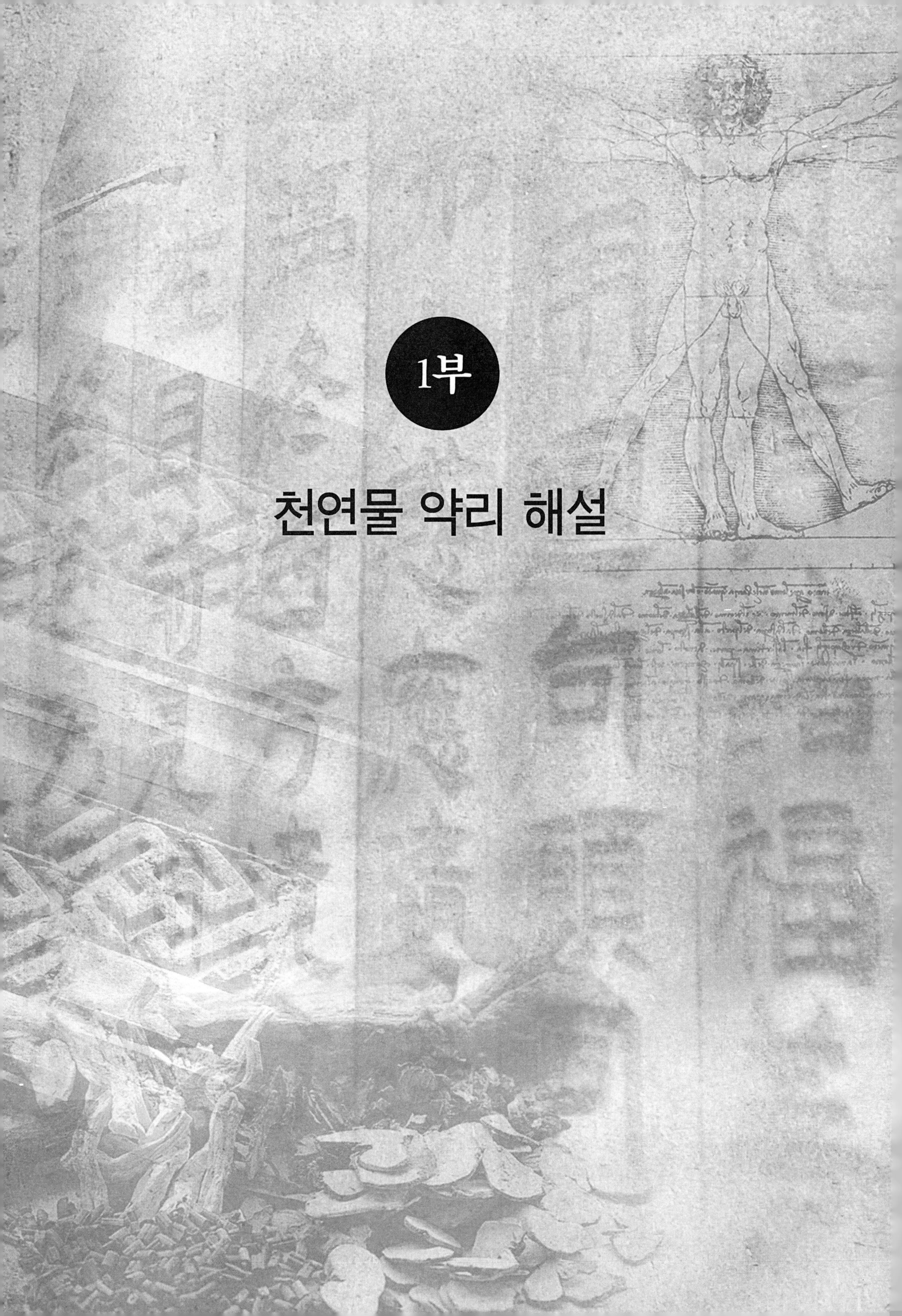

1부

천연물 약리 해설

갈근 (葛根)

생약명 PUERARIAE RADIX

자원 콩과에 속하는 다년생등본인 칡의 뿌리

성분 genistein

약리 Ionotropic glutamate receptor blocker

효능 Inhibition of glutamate-induced postsynaptic cytotoxicity

적응증 Meningoencephalitis / Botulism

적응증예

Mosquito-borne encephalitis virus & Enterovirus-mediated Meningoencephalitis

➡ Mosquito-borne encephalitis virus & Enterovirus
: lymph node & MALT infection
➡ lymph node & MALT: replication
➡ neurotropism target
➡ Astrocyte 감염
➡ IgG mediated cellular response
➡ Microglia 유도: TNF-α 분비
➡ Astrocyte apoptosis ↑
➡ synapse: glutamate 축적
➡ postsynaptic neuron NMDA Rc: glutamate 부착
➡ postsynaptic neuron: glutamate excitotoxicity
➡ encephalitis

처방예

桂枝加葛根湯: IFN-a mediated Meningoencephalitis
葛根湯: Mosquito-borne encephalitis virus & Enterovirus-mediated Meningoencephalitis (모기-매개 뇌염바이러스 & 장바이러스-매개 뇌수막염)
葛根加半夏湯: Enterovirus-mediated Meningoencephalitis (장바이러스-매개 뇌수막염)
葛根黃蓮黃芩湯: Botulism (보툴리누스 독소증)

REFERENCES

1. LI Hong-Chun, ZHANG Guang-Yi[2]. Inhibitory effect of genistein on activation of STAT3 induced by brain ischemia/reperfusion in rat hippocampus[1]. Li HC *et al* / Acta Pharmacol Sin 2003 Nov; 24 (11): 1131-1136.

2. P Charlesworth[2], NH Komiyama[2] and SGN Grant[1]. Homozygous mutation of focal adhesion kinase in embryonic stem cell derived neurons: normal electrophysiologi cal and morphological properties in vitro. BMC Neuroscience 2006, 7:47.

3. V. P. Tsintsadze[1], A. L. Fedorenko[1], T. Sh. Tsintsadze[1], M. Wright[2], J. A. Tanner[2], A. D. Miller[2] and N. A. Lozovaya[1]. Effect of a non-hydrolyzable analog of diad enosine polyphosphates on NMDA-mediated currents in isolated pyramidal neurons of the rat hippocampus. Neurophysiology, Volume 38, Number 3 / 2006, 5: 169-174.

감수 (甘遂)

생약명 EUPHORBIAE KANSUI RADIX

자원 대극과식물인 감수의 뿌리

성분 Tirucallol

약리 추측 aldosterone receptor blocker

효능 원위세뇨관 & 집합관 ➡ Na+ 배설 촉진, K+ 흡수
➡ body fluid volume 감소

적응증 pleural effusion / ascites / ovarian tumor

적응증예

Ovarian cancer

➡ ovulation
➡ ovulation-induced reactive oxidants 생성
➡ ovarian surface epithelium: damage
➡ damage-repair responses 반복
➡ ovarian surface epithelium: DNA damage
➡ ovarian surface epithelium: oncogenesis
➡ EGF autocrine
➡ EGF-Rc & tyrosine kinase domain: 활성화
➡ ovarian cancer: cyst formation

처방예

十棗湯: Pleural effusion (흉막 삼출)
甘遂半夏湯: Ascites (복수)
大黃甘遂湯: Ovarian tumor (난소암)

감초 (甘草)

생약명 GLYCYRRHIZAE RADIX

자원 콩과에 속하는 여러해살이풀인 감초 또는 곧은 감초의 뿌리를 말린 것

성분 glycyrrhetinic acid

약리 11-beta-hydroxysteroid dehydrogenase1 (HSD11B1) inhibitor

약리 해설 11-beta-hydroxysteroid dehydrogenase1
➡ glucocorticoid-selective tissues 존재
➡ HSD11B1 차단
➡ cortisol 분해 억제
➡ glucocorticoid receptors 자극 지속됨

효능 glucocorticoid 작용과 동일
➡ Immune cell: IκBα 생성 증가

➡ NF-κB mediated transcription 억제
➡ B cell 항체 생성 억제 / 백혈구 이동 억제 & cytokine 생성 억제

적응증 Bipolar affective disorder / Type I hypersensitive reaction: first sensitization / Viral pharyngitis / Bacterial pharyngitis / Barrett`s esophagus / 처방예 참고

적응증예

Viral pharyngitis (바이러스성 인두염)

➡ numerous viruses
➡ pharynx: lymph glands infection
➡ B cell: IgM 생성
➡ 보체 유도
➡ 보체의존성 세포용해
➡ virus infected lymph glands: necrosis
➡ swollen lymph glands

처방예

甘麥大棗湯: Bipolar affective disorder (양극성 정동장애)
甘草麻黃湯: Type I hypersensitive reaction: first sensitization
甘草湯: Viral pharyngitis (바이러스성 인두염)
桂枝加龍骨牡蠣湯: Hypernatremia-mediated hypotension (고나트륨혈증-매개 저혈압)
桂枝加黃耆湯: Eccrine sweat gland capillaritis (에크린분비선 모세혈관염)
桂枝芍藥知母湯: Rheumatoid arthritis (류마티스 관절염)
栝蔞桂枝湯: Poliomyelitis (회백수염, 소아마비)
膠艾湯: Uterine bleeding (자궁출혈)
橘皮竹茹湯: Multiple sclerosis (다발성 경화증)
桔梗湯: Bacterial pharyngitis (세균성 인두염)
大黃甘草湯: Barrett`s esophagus (바렛 식도)
大黃蟅蟲丸: Kaposi sarcoma (카포시 육종)
苓甘五味加薑辛半夏杏仁湯: Chronic left heart failure-mediated alveolitis (폐포염)
苓甘五味加薑辛半杏大黃湯: Chronic left heart failure-mediated alveolar carcinoma (만성좌심부전-매개 폐포암)
苓甘五味薑辛湯 : Chronic left heart failure-mediated alveolar-capillary barrier damage (만성좌심부전-매개 폐포-모세혈관 장벽 손상)
麥門冬湯: Pulmonary tuberculosis (폐결핵)
防己茯苓湯: Chronic right heart failure-mediated systemic congestion

(만성우심부전-매개 전신울혈)
防己地黃湯: Cerebral venous sinus thrombosis (뇌 정맥동 혈전증)
防己黃耆湯: Right heart failure-mediated venous congestion (우심부전-매개 정맥울혈)
白頭翁加甘草阿膠湯: Postpartum Crohn's disease (산후 크론병)
白頭翁湯: Crohn's disease (크론병)
茯苓澤瀉湯: Decompensated heart failure (보상기전 실패 심부전)
茯苓杏仁甘草湯: Rheumatic valvulitis (류마티스 판막염)
附子粳米湯: Small intestine stenosis in Behcet's Disease (베체트 소장협착증)
奔豚湯: Epinephrine-mediated encephalopathy (에피네프린-매개 뇌병증)
續命湯: Intracerebral hemorrhage (뇌출혈)
升麻鱉甲湯: Toxoplasmosis (톡소플라즈마증)
溫經湯: Tuberculous endometritis (결핵성 자궁내막염)
王不留行散: Tetanus (파상풍)
越婢湯: Type I hypersensitive reaction: second sensitization
越婢加朮湯: Type I hypersensitive reaction: eosinophil mediated late phase reaction
越婢加半夏湯: Hypersensitivity pneumonitis (과민성 폐렴)
越婢加附子湯: Type I hypersensitive reaction: neutrophil mediated late phase reaction
人參湯: Unstable angina-mediated coronary calcification
(불안정형 협심증-매개 관상동맥 석회화)
調胃承氣湯: Small intestine MALT lymphoma (소장 점막림프조직 림프종)
竹葉湯: Postpartum mononucleosis (산후 단핵구증)
竹皮大丸: Intrapartum Group B streptococcus infection (분만 중 그룹 B 연쇄구균 감염증)
澤漆湯: Respiratory syncytial virus bronchiolitis(호흡기 세포융합 바이러스 세기관지염)
風引湯: Epilepsy (뇌전증)
厚朴七物湯: Gastrointestinal leiomyosarcoma (위장관 평활근육종)

REFERENCE

Yoshihito Shimoyama, Kazuhiro Hirabayashi, Hiroatsu Matsumoto, Toshitsugu Sato, Shoji Shibata, Hideo Inoue. Effects of glycyrrhetinic acid derivatives on hepatic and renal 11beta-hydroxysteroid dehydrogenase activities in rats.
J Pharm Pharmacol, 2003,07, 811-7.

강랑 (蜣蜋)

학명 Gymnopleurus mopsus

자원 쇠똥구리

성분 ivermectin

약리 추측 Chloride channel blocker

적응증 Plasmodium falciparum malaria

적응증예

Plasmodium falciparum malaria

➡ Plasmodium falciparum
➡ hepatocyte entry: sporozoite ▶ schizont 분열
➡ 혈류로 방출
➡ erythrocyte entry
➡ erythrocyte: protein kinase A 생산
➡ protein kinase A: Chloride channel family 활성화
➡ 영양분 출입 통로로 이용됨

처방예

鱉甲煎丸: Plasmodium falciparum malaria (열대열원충 말라리아)

건강 (乾薑)

생약명 Zingiberis siccatum Rhizoma

자원 생강 말린 것

성분 shogaol (oxidized gingerol)

약리 추측 Intra-neutrophil hydrogen peroxide scavenger

효능 Inhibition of neutrophil HClO

적응증 Sjogren's syndrome / 처방예 참고

적응증예

Sjogren's syndrome

➡ exocrine glands cell: endogenous retrovirus 활성화
➡ Anti-SSA/Ro & anti-SSB/La antibodies 출현
➡ neutrophil 유도
➡ neutrophil phagocytosis
➡ HClO 분비 via H2O2
➡ exocrine glands 세포막 손상

처방예

甘草乾薑湯: Sjogren's syndrome (쇼그렌 증후군)
乾薑附子湯: Adenovirus infection
挑花湯: Ulcerative colitis (궤양성대장염)
半夏乾薑散: CMV esophagitis (사이토메가로바이러스 식도염)
茯苓五味乾薑細辛湯: Chronic left heart failure-mediated alveolar-capillary barrier damage (만성좌심부전-매개 폐포-모세혈관 장벽 손상)
六物黃芩湯: Enteropathogenic E. coli
黃連湯: Group A streptococcus (GAS) infection (그룹 A 연쇄상구균감염증)
乾薑黃連黃芩人蔘湯: Staphylococcal food poisoning (포도구균 식 중독)
厚朴麻黃湯: Emphysema (폐기종)
柴胡桂枝乾薑湯: Liver cirrhosis (간경변)
小靑龍湯: Viral pneumonia (바이러스성 폐렴)
半夏瀉心湯: Gastric ulcer (위궤양)
生薑瀉心湯: Duodenal ulcer (십이지장궤양)
甘草瀉心湯: Peptic ulcer-complicated perforation (소화성궤양에 합병된 천공)
乾畺人蔘半夏丸: Cytomegalovirus-mediated placental villitis (태반 융모세포염)

REFERENCE

Arash Khaki[1] D.V.M., Ph.D., Fatemeh Fathiazad[2] Ph.D., Mohammad Nouri[3] Ph.D., Amir Afshin Khaki[4] Ph.D., Chelar C Ozanci[5] D.D.S., Ph.D., Marefat Ghafari-Novin[6] M.D., Ph.D., Mohammad Hamadeh[7] D.V.M., Ph.D. The effects of Ginger on supermat ogenesis and sperm parameters of rat. Iranian Journal of Reproductive Medicine Vol 7. No.1. pp: 7-12, Winter 2009.

건지황 (乾地黃)

생약명 REHMANNIAE RADIX

자원 현삼과에 속하는 다년생 초본인 지황과 회경지황의 건조한 괴경을 말린 것

성분 catalpol

약리 추측 CD133+ CFU-GEMM (+) modulator

효능 hematopoietic stem cell 분화 촉진

적응증 Uterine bleeding / Extra intestinal amoebiasis / Renal failure-mediated anemia

적응증예

Uterine Bleeding

➡ 자궁점막하근종 / 유산후 탈락막 기저층 / 전치태반
➡ 자궁벽 근육 압박
➡ uterin wall: smooth muscle ▶ NF-κB 활성화
➡ uterin wall: smooth muscle ▶ inflammation
➡ intra-uterine artery: 손상
➡ hemorrhage
➡ intra-uterine: erythrocyte 유출

➡ 적혈구 골격단백질 손상
➡ complement 부착
➡ complement cascade: membrane attack complement (MAC) 생성
➡ MAC mediated erythrocyte lysis
➡ hematoma 생성
➡ 조직 허혈: superoxide 생성
➡ 혈관평활근: α-adrenergic Rc Ca channel 자극
➡ vasospasm
➡ severe bleeding

처방예

膠艾湯: Uterine bleeding (자궁출혈)
三物黃芩湯: Extra intestinal amoebiasis (장외 아메바증)
腎氣丸: Endothelin-1 mediated Renal failure

REFERENCE

Ru-Xue Zhang[a], Mao-Xing Li[a] and Zheng-Ping Jia[a]. Rehmannia glutinosa: Review of botany, chemistry and pharmacology. Journal of Ethnopharmacology Volume 117, Issue 2, 8 May 2008, Pages 199-214.

건칠 (乾漆)

생약명 LACCA SINICA EXSICCATA

자원 옻나무과에 속하는 활엽수인 옻나무의 수지를 말린 것

성분 urishiol

약리 추측 fibrosarcoma cell p27 (+) modulator

효능 Apoptosis of fibrosarcoma cell, fibrosarcoma cell ➡ p27 축적
➡ G1 cell cycle 정지
➡ fibrosarcoma cell apoptosis

적응증 Kaposi sarcoma

적응증예

Kaposi sarcoma

➡ HHV8 infected endothelium: IL-6
➡ fibroblast: NF-κB 활성화 ▶ estrogen receptor 발현 ↑
▶ proliferation ↑
▶ fibrosarcoma cell 전환
➡ fibrosarcoma cell: fibroblast growth factor 분비
➡ spindle cell: tyrosine kinase domain 활성화
➡ spindle cell: proliferation & migration
➡ Kaposi's sarcoma 형성

처방예

大黃蟅虫丸: Kaposi sarcoma (카포시 육종)

경미 (硬米)

자원 벼 (Oryza sativa Linne)의 외과피를 벗긴 씨

성분 magnesium

약리 DNA replication cofactor

적응증 pulmonary tuberculosis / secondary tuberculosis / type 1 diabetes / viral thyroiditis / ulcerative colitis / Small intestine stenosis in Behcet's Disease

적응증예

Pulmonary tuberculosis

➡ lung macrophage: M. tuberculosis ▶ persistent infection
➡ starvation & low oxygen pressure
➡ M. tuberculosis: thehalose dimycolate 합성
➡ macrophage fusion 형성
➡ granuloma formation
➡ M. tuberculosis: intracellular growth
➡ M. tuberculosis: hydrolytic enzyme 분비
➡ macrophage necrosis
➡ cavity formation

처방예

麥門冬湯: Pulmonary tuberculosis (폐결핵)
竹葉石膏湯: Secondary tuberculosis (이차성 결핵)
白虎湯: IL-1 mediated Type 1 diabetes
白虎加人蔘湯: Coxsackie B4 virus-mediated Type 1 diabetes
白虎加桂枝湯: viral thyroiditis (바이러스성 갑상선염)
挑花湯: Ulcerative colitis (궤양성대장염)
附子硬米湯: Small intestine stenosis in Behcet's Disease (베체트 소장협착증)

REFERENCE

SHINDO KUMIKO, NAITO SHIGEHIRO, TOYOSHIMA HIDECHIKA. Difference in Mineral Contents of Brown Rice Grains with the Grain Position on the Panicle.-"Nipponbare", "Koshihikari" and "Snow peal". Japanese Journal of Crop Science, VOL.72;NO.4;PAGE.395-408(2003).

계지 (桂枝)

생약명 CINNAMOMI RAMULUS

자원 장나무과의 상록교목식물인 계수나무의 어린 가지

성분 cinnamic acid

약리 lactate oxidizer

약리 해설 lactate ▶ pyruvate 전환

효능 Inhibition of intracellular lactate-mediated cytotoxicity / Activation of Cori-cycle

적응증 Common cold / Lactacidemia-mediated cardiomyopathy / Uterine myoma / Rheumatoid arthritis / 처방예 참고

적응증예

Common cold

➡ skeleton muscle cell
➡ 지속적인 ATP 생산
➡ mitochondrial respiration 반복: superoxide 축적
➡ superoxide dismutase2 고갈
➡ superoxide: Fe^{3+}(ferric ions) ▶ Fe^{2+}(ferrous ion) 환원
➡ ferrous ion-induced lipid peroxidation in mitochondria
➡ mitochondria membrane potential damage
➡ 세포질 pyruvate: mitochondria influx 억제
➡ pyruvate: lactate 환원
➡ high levels of intracellular lactate
➡ 근육내 수소이온 증가: pH 감소
➡ 해당효소 glucose 6-phosphate & phosphofructokinase 활성 감소
➡ ATP 생산 감소
➡ heat 감소
➡ virus infected cell: heat shock protein 발현 ↓
➡ 세포질내 복제된 바이러스 단백질 분해 ↓ & 세포밖에서 바이러스 입자 포획 ↓
➡ 감기 지속

처방예

桂枝湯: Common cold
葛根加半夏湯: Enterovirus-mediated Meningoencephalitis (장바이러스-매개 뇌수막염)
葛根湯: Mosquito-borne encephalitis virus & Enterovirus-mediated Meningoencephalitis (모기-매개 뇌염바이러스 & 장바이러스-매개 뇌수막염)

桂苓五味甘草湯: Pneumonia complications-mediated hypoxemia
(폐렴합병증-매개 저산소혈증)
桂枝加葛根湯: IFN-a mediated Meningoencephalitis (뇌수막염)
桂枝加桂湯: Lipacidemia-mediated Cardiac toxicity (지방산혈증-매개 심장독성)
桂枝加大黃湯: Autoimmune enteropathy & colon cancer (자가면역성 장병증 & 대장암)
桂枝加附子湯: Acute EBV infection
桂枝加龍骨牡蠣湯: Hypernatremia-mediated hypotension (고나트륨혈증-매개 저혈압)
桂枝加芍藥湯: Autoimmune enteropathy (자가면역성 장병증)
桂枝加黃耆湯: Eccrine sweat gland capillaritis (에크린분비선 모세혈관염)
桂枝加厚朴杏子湯: Airway remodeling-mediated Asthma (기도 개형-매개 천식)
桂枝甘草龍骨牡蠣湯: Rapid hyponatremia (급속 저나트륨혈증)
桂枝甘草湯: Lactacidemia-mediated cardiomyopathy (지방산혈증-매개 심근병증)
桂枝去芍藥加麻黃細辛附子湯: Autoimmune response-mediated Methemoglobinemia
桂枝去芍藥加附子湯: IL-1 mediated Cardiac toxicity
桂枝去芍藥加蜀漆牡蠣龍骨救逆湯: Rapid hypernatremia (급속 고나트륨혈증)
桂枝去芍藥湯: IL-1 mediated Cardiac toxicity
桂枝二麻黃一湯: *heat shock protein*-resistant viral infection
桂枝二越婢一湯: *IL-1 deficiency*-mediated viral infection
桂麻各半湯: *IFN-a* resistant viral infection
桂枝茯苓丸: Uterine myoma (자궁근종)
桂枝附子湯: Influenza myositis (인플루엔자 근염)
桂枝人參湯: Rotavirus enteritis (로타바이러스 장염)
桂枝芍藥知母湯: Rheumatoid arthritis (류마티스 관절염)
栝蔞桂枝湯: Poliomyelitis (회백수염, 소아마비)
炙甘草湯: Chagas disease (샤가스 병)
當歸四逆湯: Autoimmune hemolytic anemia (자가면역 용혈성빈혈)
當歸四逆加吳茱萸生薑湯: Autoimmune hemolytic anemia-mediated pancreatitis
(자가면역 용혈성빈혈-매개 췌장염)
大青龍湯: *IFN-γ* resistant viral infection
桃核承氣湯: Cervical cancer (자궁암)
麻黃加朮湯: Immune complexes-mediated vasculitis (면역복합체-매개 혈관염)
麻黃湯: *heat shock protein & IFN-a* resistant viral infection
麻黃升麻湯: Infectious mononucleosis (전염성 단핵구증)
木防己湯: left heart failure-mediated pulmonary venous congestion
(좌심부전-매개 폐정맥 울혈)
木防己湯去石膏加茯苓芒硝湯: Left heart failure-mediated pleural effusion
(좌심부전-매개 흉막삼출)

半夏散及湯: Soft plate ulcer (연구개염)
防己茯苓湯: Chronic right heart failure-mediated systemic congestion
(만성우심부전-매개 전신울혈)
防己地黃湯: Cerebral venous sinus thrombosis (뇌 정맥동 혈전증)
白虎加桂枝湯: Viral thyroiditis (바이러스성 갑상선염)
鱉甲煎丸: Plasmodium falciparum malaria (열대열원충 말라리아)
茯苓甘草湯: Streptococcal rheumatic myocarditis (연쇄구균 류마티스 심근염)
茯苓桂枝甘草大棗湯: Ventricular tachycardia (심실빈맥)
茯苓桂枝白朮甘草湯: Atrial fibrillation (심방세동)
茯苓澤瀉湯: Decompensated heart failure (보상기전 실패 심부전)
薯蕷丸: Malnutrition-mediated disease (영양실조-매개 질병)
小建中湯: Picornavirus infection / Hypoglycemia (저혈당)
小青龍湯: Viral pneumonia (바이러스성 폐렴)
續命湯: Intracerebral hemorrhage (뇌출혈)
柴胡加龍骨牡蠣湯: Viral fulminant hepatitis (바이러스성 전격성간염)
柴胡桂枝乾薑湯: Liver cirrhosis (간경변)
柴胡桂枝湯: Type B hepatitis-mediated immune complex disease
烏頭桂枝湯: Mesenteritis-mediated volvulus (장간막염-매개 장꼬임증)
五苓散: Immune complex-mediated glomerulonephritis (면역복합체-매개 사구체신염)
溫經湯: Tuberculous endometritis (결핵성 자궁내막염)
六物黃芩湯: Pathogenic E. coli infection
茵蔯五苓散: Free bile acids-mediated glomerulonephritis (자유담즙산-매개 사구체신염)
竹皮大丸: Intrapartum Group B streptococcus infection (분만 중 GBS 감염증)
枳實薤白桂枝湯: Unstable angina (불안정형 협심증)
天雄散: bone marrow EBV-mediated neutrophilia (골수 EBV 감염-매개 호중구증가증)
澤漆湯: Respiratory syncytial virus (RSV) bronchiolitis (RSV 세기관지염)
土瓜根散: Endometriosis (자궁내막증식증)
八味腎氣丸: Endothelin-1 mediated Renal failure
風引湯: Epilepsy (뇌전증)
黃耆建中湯: Skeletal smooth muscle capillaritis-mediated disseminated intravascular
coagulation (골격평활근 모세혈관염-매개 파종성 혈관내응고증)
黃耆桂枝五物湯: Axon terminal capillaritis (축삭종말 모세혈관염)
黃耆芍藥桂枝苦酒湯: Chromohidrosis (색깔 땀 분비증)
黃連湯: Group A streptococcus (GAS) infection (그룹 A 연쇄상구균감염증)
厚朴七物湯: Gastrointestinal leiomyosarcoma (위장관 평활근육종)
侯氏黑散: Cerebral infraction (뇌경색)

REFERENCE

1. Saroj P. Mathupala[1], Chaim B. Colen[2], Prahlad Parajuli[2] and Andrew E. Sloan[3].Lactate and malignant tumors: A therapeutic target at the end stage of glyco lysis. Journal of Bioenergetics and Biomembranes, Volume 39, Number1/2007,2, 73-77.

2. S. Wolffram[1], B. Grenacher and E. Scharrer. Sodium-Dependent L-Lactate Uptake by Bovine Intestinal Brush Border Membrane Vesicles. Journal of Dairy Science Vol. 71 No. 12 3267-3273.

3. Jemma L. ELLIOTT, Kevin J. SALIBA and Kiaran KIRK[1]. Transport of lactate and pyruvate in the intraerythrocytic malaria parasite, Plasmodium falciparum. Biochem. J. (2001) 355 (733–739).

고삼 (苦蔘)

생약명 SOPHORAE RADIX

자원 콩과식물인 고삼의 뿌리

성분 trifolirhizin

약리 추측 protozoa tyrosinase transcription inhibitior
효능 Disruption of protozoa`actin cytoskeleton
➡ protozoa 이동 억제

적응증 Extra intestinal amoebiasis / Trichomoniasis

적응증예

Extra intestinal amoebiasis

➡ 장내 정상 기생 원충 amoeba: bacteriophage 감염

➡ amoeba transformation
➡ tyrosinase 생성
➡ 이동에 필요한 actin cytoskeleton 활성화
➡ 장간막 정맥 & 림프관을 통해 장외로 이동
➡ 간 / 뇌 / 흉막 / 폐 / 비장 / 피부
➡ 이동된 조직의 혈관을 통해 영양 섭취
➡ 혈관 손상 & 농양 발생

처방예

三物黃芩湯: Extra intestinal amoebiasis (장외 아메바증)
當歸貝母苦蔘丸: Trichomoniasis in pregnancy (임신부 트리코모나스증)

과루근 (瓜蔞根)

생약명 TRICHOSANTHIS RADIX

자원 박과에 속한 다년생 초목인 하늘타리의 괴근

성분 trichosanthin

약리 ribosome inactivating protein

효능 근섬유아세포 smooth muscle actin 생성 억제 / poliovirus RNA & 단백질 생성 억제

적응증 Liver cirrhosis / Endometriosis / Poliomyelitis

적응증예

Liver cirrhosis

➡ 만성 간손상
➡ 허혈-재관류 반복
➡ 호중구 출현
➡ 간문맥동 내피세포 & 간세포 손상
➡ hepatic stellate cell (HSC) activation

➡ myofibroblast로 변형
➡ ribosome 활성화: collagen 합성
➡ collagen polymerization 생성
➡ liver cirrhosis

Poliomyelitis

➡ motor neuron: poliovirus infection
➡ motor neuron ribosomes: poliovirus RNA & protein 번역
➡ poliovirus replication
➡ motor neuron lysis
➡ Spinal cord myelitis

처방예

柴胡桂枝乾薑湯: Liver cirrhosis (간경변)
土瓜根散: Endometriosis (자궁내막증)
栝蔞桂枝湯: Poliomyelitis (회백수염, 소아마비)

REFERENCE

1. T P Chow, R A Feldman, M Lovett and M Piatak. Isolation and DNA sequence of a gene encoding alpha-trichosanthin, a type I ribosome-inactivating protein. The Journal of Biological Chemistry, 1990, May 25, 265, 8670-8674.

2. Pang-Chui Shaw, Ka-Ming Leeb and Kam-Bo Wong. Recent advances in trichosa nthin, a ribosome-inactivating protein with multiple pharmacological properties. Toxicon, Volume 45, Issue 6, May 2005, Pages 683-689.

과루실 (瓜蔞實)

생약명 PLATYCODI RADIX

자원 박과에 속하는 여러해살이 덩굴풀인 하늘타리의 익은 열매

성분 cucurbitacin

약리 endothelium actin-disrupting agent

효능 endothelium ➡ fibroblast 분화 억제

적응증 Unstable angina / Myocardial infarction / Gastric adenocarcinoma

적응증예

Unstable angina

➡ coronary artery: unstable fibrous cap
➡ 성분: collagen / SMC / proteoglycan / cholesterol monohydrate crystal
➡ smooth muscle cell: VEGF autocrine
➡ smooth muscle cell: proliferation
➡ fibrous cap 내부: 활발한 염증 발생
➡ fibrous cap: expansion
➡ coronary artery: 내강 좁아짐 (완전경색)
➡ myocardiocyte ischemia
➡ unstable angina
➡ 허혈부위 심근세포: 섬유아세포로 분화

처방예

枳實薤白桂枝湯: Unstable angina (불안정형 협심증)
栝蔞薤白白酒湯: Myocardial infarction (심근경색)
栝蔞薤白半夏湯: Myocardial infarction & micro-emboli (심근경색 & 미세혈전)
小陷胸湯: Gastric adenocarcinoma (위암)

REFERENCE

Angela Granessa[a], Valeria Polib and Margarete Goppelt-Struebea[a]. STAT3-independent inhibition of lysophosphatidic acid-mediated upregulation of connective tissue growth factor (CTGF) by cucurbitacin I. Biochemical Pharmacology Volume 72, Issue 1, 28 June 2006, Pages 32-41.

과체 (瓜蔕)

생약명 MELONIS CALYX

자원 박과에 속하는 한해살이 덩굴풀인 참외의 열매꼭지를 말린 것

성분 elaterin

약리 최토제

적응증 Cytomegalovirus infection

적응증예

Cytomegalovirus infection

➡ 인후상피 & 기관지상피 & 식도상피: cytomegalovirus infection
➡ 모세혈관 내피세포: 재감염
➡ 모세혈관 내피세포: 봉입체 세포로 전환
➡ 내피세포 부종
➡ 조직 허혈
➡ 인후부종 / 기도부종 / 식도부종

처방예

瓜蔕散: Cytomegalovirus infection

구감초 (灸甘草)

생약명 GLYCYRRHIZAE RADIX

자원 감초 볶은 것

성분 18β-24-Hydroxyglycyrrhetinic acid

약리 11-beta-hydroxysteroid dehydrogenase2 (HSD11B2) inhibitor

약리 해설 11-beta-hydroxysteroid dehydrogenase2
➡ aldosterone-selective tissues 존재
➡ HSD11B2 차단
➡ cortisol 분해 억제
➡ mineralocorticoid receptors 자극 지속됨

효능 aldosterone 작용과 동일
➡ Na+/ K+ pumps 전사 활성화 & H+ secretion

적응증 Common cold / Asthma / Gastric ulcer / Viral pneumonia / Viral hepatitis / Osteoarthritis / Systemic lupus erythematosis / 처방예 참고

적응증예

Common cold

➡ skeleton muscle cell
➡ 지속적인 ATP 생산
➡ mitochondrial respiration 반복: superoxide 축적
➡ superoxide dismutase2 고갈
➡ superoxide: Fe^{3+}(ferric ions) ▶ Fe^{2+}(ferrous ion) 환원
➡ Ferrous ion-induced lipid peroxidation in mitochondria
➡ mitochondria membrane potential damage
➡ 세포질 pyruvate: mitochondria influx 억제
➡ intracellular hyperlactation
➡ 근육내 수소이온 증가로 pH 감소
➡ 해당효소 glucose 6-phosphate & phosphofructokinase 활성 감소
➡ ATP 생산 감소
➡ Na+/ K+ pump activity 감소
➡ 세포부종 & 세포손상

처방예

桂枝湯: Common cold
葛根加半夏湯: Enterovirus mediated Meningoencephalitis (장바이러스-매개 뇌수막염)
葛根湯: Mosquito-borne encephalitis virus & Enterovirus-mediated Meningoencephalitis
(모기-매개 뇌염바이러스 & 장바이러스-매개 뇌수막염)

葛根黃芩黃連湯: Botulism (보툴리누스 독소증)
甘草乾薑湯: Sjogren's syndrome (쇼그렌 증후군)
甘草附子湯: Coxsackie virus-mediated polymyositis & polyarthritis
(다발성근염 & 다발성관절염)
甘草瀉心湯: Peptic ulcer-complicated perforation (소화성궤양에 합병된 천공)
桂苓五味甘草湯: Pneumonia complications-mediated hypoxemia
(폐렴합병증-매개 저산소혈증)
桂枝加葛根湯: *IFN-a* mediated Meningoencephalitis (*IFN-a* 매개 뇌수막염)
桂枝加桂湯: Lipacidemia-mediated Cardiac toxicity (지방산혈증-매개 심장독성병)
桂枝加大黃湯: Autoimmune enteropathy & colon cancer
(자가면역성 장병증 & 대장암)
桂枝加附子湯: Acute EBV infection
桂枝加芍藥湯: Autoimmune enteropathy (자가면역성 장병증)
桂枝加厚朴杏子湯: Airway remodeling-mediated Asthma (기도 개형-매개 천식)
桂枝甘草龍骨牡蠣湯: Rapid hyponatremia (급속 저나트륨혈증)
桂枝甘草湯: Lactacidemia-mediated cardiomyopathy (지방산혈증-매개 심근병증)
桂枝去桂加茯苓白朮湯: Kawasaki disease
桂枝去芍藥加附子湯: IL-1 mediated Cardiac toxicity
桂枝去芍藥加蜀漆牡蠣龍骨救逆湯: Rapid hypernatremia (급속 고나트륨혈증)
桂枝去芍藥湯: IL-1 mediated Cardiac toxicity
桂枝二麻黃一湯: heat shock protein-resistant viral infection
桂枝二越婢一湯: *IL-1 deficiency*-mediated viral infection
桂麻各半湯: *IFN-a* resistant viral infection
桂枝附子湯: Influenza myositis (인플루엔자 근염)
桂枝人參湯: Rotavirus enteritis (로타바이러스 장염)
炙甘草湯: Chagas disease (샤가스 병)
當歸四逆湯: Autoimmune hemolytic anemia (자가면역 용혈성빈혈)
當歸四逆加吳茱萸生薑湯: Autoimmune hemolytic anemia-mediated pancreatitis
(자가면역 용혈성빈혈-매개 췌장염)
大青龍湯: *IFN-γ* resistant viral infection
麻黃湯: *heat shock protein & IFN-a* resistant viral infection
麻黃加朮湯: Immune complexes-mediated vasculitis (면역복합체-매개 혈관염)
麻黃附子甘草湯: Early autoimmune response for tissue
麻黃升麻湯: Infectious mononucleosis (전염성 단핵구증)
麻黃蓮軺赤小豆湯: Warm autoantibody-mediated hemolytic anemia
(온난자가항체-매개 용혈성빈혈)
麻黃杏仁甘草石膏湯: Asthma (천식)

麻黃杏仁薏苡甘草湯: Reactive arthritis (반응성 관절염)
半夏瀉心湯: Gastric ulcer (위궤양)
半夏散及湯: Soft plate ulcer (연구개염)
白朮附子湯: Myoglobin-mediated renal failure
白虎加桂枝湯: Viral thyroiditis (바이러스성 갑상선염)
白虎加人參湯: Coxsackie B4 virus-mediated Type 1 diabetes
白虎湯: IL-1 mediated Type 1 diabetes
茯苓甘草湯: Streptococcal rheumatic myocarditis (연쇄구균 류마티스 심근염)
茯苓桂枝甘草大棗湯: Ventricular tachycardia (심실빈맥)
茯苓桂枝白朮甘草湯: Atrial fibrillation (심방세동)
茯苓四逆湯: Viral myocarditis (바이러스성 심근염)
四逆加人參湯: Polymyositis-associated gastrointestinal myositis
(다발성근염에 연관된 위장관근염)
四逆散: Hashimoto's thyroiditis (하시모토 갑상선염)
四逆湯: Polymyositis (다발성근염)
生薑瀉心湯: Duodenal ulcer (십이지장궤양)
小建中湯: Picornavirus infection / Hypoglycemia (저혈당)
小柴胡湯: Viral hepatitis (type A,B) (바이러스성 간염)
小青龍湯: Viral pneumonia (바이러스성 폐렴)
柴胡加芒硝湯: Type C hepatitis (C형 간염)
柴胡桂枝乾薑湯: Liver cirrhosis (간경변)
柴胡桂枝湯: Type B hepatitis-mediated immune complex disease
烏頭桂枝湯: Mesenteritis-mediated volvulus (장간막염-매개 장꼬임증)
烏頭湯: Osteoarthritis (퇴행성 관절염)
理中丸: Clostridial necrotic enteritis (클로스트리디움균 괴사성장염)
芍藥甘草附子湯: Human T-Lymphotropic Virus (HTLV) infection
芍藥甘草湯: Inclusion body myositis (봉입체 근염)
竹葉石膏湯: Secondary tuberculosis (이차성 결핵)
梔子甘草豉湯: Coronary arteris spasm & Myocardial ischemia
(관상동맥 경련 & 심근 허혈)
通脈四逆加豬膽汁湯: Systemic lupus erythematosis-associated nervous syetem
dysfunction (전신성 홍반 루푸스에 의한 신경계 손상)
通脈四逆湯: Systemic lupus erythematosis (전신성 홍반 루푸스)
黃芩加半夏生薑湯: Typhoid fever (장티푸스)
黃芩湯: Cholera
黃耆建中湯: Skeletal smooth muscle capillaritis-mediated disseminated intravascular
coagulation (골격근 모세혈관염-매개 파종성 혈관내응고증)

黃連湯: Group A streptococcus (GAS) infection (그룹 A 연쇄상구균감염증)

REFERENCE

Nigel Vickera, Xiangdong Sua, Harshani Lawrencea, Adrian Cruttendenb, Atul Purohitb, Michael J. Reedb and Barry V.L. Pottera. A novel 18β-glycyrrhetin
ic acid analogue as a potent and selective inhibitor of 11β-hydroxysteroid dehydrogenase2. Bioorganic & Medicinal Chemistry Letters, Volume 14, Issu
e 12, 21 June 2004, Pages 3263-3267.

구맥 (瞿麥)

생약명 DIANTHI HERBA

자원 패랭이꽃과에 속하는 여러해살이풀인 패랭이꽃의 전초를 말린 것

성분 dianoside

약리 추측 Plasmodium falciparum DOXP blocker
& plasminogen activator inhibitor-1 (-) modulator

적응증 Plasmodium falciparum malaria / Glomerulosclerosis

적응증예

鱉甲煎丸: Plasmodium falciparum malaria (열대열원충 말라리아)
栝蔞瞿麥丸: Glomerulosclerosis (사구체 경화증)

국화 (菊花)

생약명 CHRYSANTHEMI FLOS

자원 엉거시과 국화속의 다년초 식물로 여러해살이 풀인 국화의 꽃

성분 apigenin

약리 추측 Phospholipases A2 blocker

효능 arachidonic acid 대사 억제

적응증 Cerebral infarction

적응증예

Cerebral infarction

➡ brain blood vessel: atherothrombotic or embolic
➡ 허혈 주변부 뇌세포: calcium influx ↑
- ▶ Phospholipases A2 activation
- ▶ arachidonic acid 대사 증가
- ▶ cyclooxygenase-2 mediated prostaglandins 생성
- ▶ neutrophil 유도
- ▶ neutrophil degranulation
- ▶ extracellular H2O2 ↑
- ▶ neuroinflammation

처방예

候氏黑散: Cerebral infarction (뇌경색)

REFERENCE

Xiaoman Hong, Rukiyah Van Dross, Diane F. Birt and Jill C. Pelling. The chemoprev entive bioflavonoid apigenin inhibits TPA-induced COX-2 expression in human HaCA T keratinocytes. Proc Amer Assoc Cancer Res, Volume 45, 2004: 2231.

규자 (葵子)

생약명 MALVAE SEMEN

자원 아욱과에 속한 일년생초본인 아욱의 성숙한 종자

성분 palmitic acid

약리 추측 Arachidonic acid-induced platelet aggregation inhibitor

적응증 Deep venous thrombosis in pregnancy

적응증예

Deep venous thrombosis in pregnancy

➡ 임신 first trimester: 자궁 커짐
➡ 장골 정맥 압박
➡ vein endothelium damage
➡ IL-6: platelet activation
➡ platelet: arachidonic acid metabolism ↑
➡ platelet aggregation
➡ deep venous thrombosis

처방예

葵子茯苓散: Deep venous thrombosis in pregnancy (임신부 심부정맥혈전증)

REFERENCE

Packham MA, Guccione MA, Bryant NL, Livne A. Palmitic acid-labeled lipids selectively incorporated into platelet cytoskeleton during aggregation. Lipids. 1990 Jul;25(7):371-8.

귤피 (橘皮)

생약명 CITRI RETICULATAE VIRIDE PERICARPIUM

자원 운향과에 속하는 귤나무의 익지 않은 열매의 껍질을 말린 것

성분 rutin

약리 proteolytic activator
효능 Degradation of pathogenic protein complex

적응증 Myelitis / Multiple sclerosis / Chylothorax

적응증예

Myelitis

➡ myelin basic protein & EBV capsid, papilloma virus L2, etc
➡ molecular mimicry response
➡ spinal cord: myelin basic protein ▶ IgG & complement 부착
➡ spinal cord myelitis
➡ myelin plaque 생성
➡ nerve conduction disorders

처방예

橘皮湯: Myelitis (척수염)
橘皮竹茹湯: Multiple sclerosis (다발성 경화증)
橘皮枳實生薑湯: Chylothorax (유미 흉증)

REFERENCE

N. Kamalakkannan, P. Stanely Mainzen Prince. The influence of rutin on the extracellular matrix in streptozotocin-induced diabetic rat kidney. Journal of Pharmacy and Pharmacology. Volume 58, Issue 8, pages 1091–1098, August 2006

길경 (桔梗)

생약명 PLATYCODI RADIX

자원 도라지과에 속하는 여러해살이 풀인 도라지의 뿌리

성분 platycodin

약리 추측 Toll like receptor (+) modulator

약리 해설 공생세균 ▶ 내피세포 TLR 부착
▶ TLR signal 작동
▶ IL-1 & TNF-a 분비
▶ 공생세균 병원성 억제

효능 Activation of TLR-mediated innate immunity

적응증 Bacterial pharyngitis / Impetigo / Ecthyma / Epiglottitis / Cerebral infraction / Postpartum EBV activation-mediated mononucleosis / Haemophilus pneumonia / Alzheimer's disease

적응증예

Bacterial pharyngitis

➡ pharynx: commensal bacteria
➡ staphylococcus aureus / streptococcus pyrogen: transformation
➡ MyD88 (TLR adaptor protein) 억제 단백질 분비
➡ 내피세포의 TLR signal 차단
➡ IL-1 & TNF-a 분비 감소
➡ staphylococcus aureus / streptococcus pyrogen: activation
➡ pharynx infection
➡ B cell: IgM 생성
➡ 보체 유도
➡ 보체의존성 세포용해
➡ pharyngitis

Cerebral infraction

➡ 완전 뇌세포 허혈: 세포질 lactate ↑ ▶ 세포내 산증 ▶ ATP 고갈
▶ β-amyloid 분비
▶ β-amyloid plaque 생성
▶ 신경 퇴행

➡ microglia: TLR 활성화

➡ β-Amyloid 식균 촉진

처방예

桔梗湯: Bacterial pharyngitis (세균성 인두염)
排膿散: Impetigo (농가진)
排膿湯: Ecthyma (단독)
竹葉湯: Postpartum EBV activation-mediated mononucleosis
(산후 EBV 활성화-매개 단핵구증)
候氏黑散: Cerebral infarction (뇌경색)
三物小白散: Epiglottitis (후두개염)

난발회 (亂髮灰)

자원 사람 머리카락을 불에 태워 만든 재

성분 keratin

약리 Oxalator chelater in Urine

효능 Urolithiasis

처방예

滑石白魚湯: Urolithiasis (요로돌증)

REFERENCE

W. F. Coello and M. A. Q. Khan. Protection against heavy metal toxicity by mucus and scales in fish. Archives of Environmental Contamination and Toxicology Volume 30, Number 3, 319-326, DOI: 10.1007/BF00212289

당귀 (當歸)

생약명 ANGELICAE GIGANTIS RADIX

자원 산형과에 속하는 여러해살이 풀인 참당귀의 뿌리를 말린 것

성분 decursin

약리 erythrocyte PKC inhibitor

약리 해설 Iron deficiency / complement / toxoplasma, etc
➡ adducin+spectrin+actin complex 분리
➡ deformity erythrocyte 생성
➡ intravascular & extravascular hemolysis

효능 Inhibition of intravascular & extravascular hemolysis

적응증 Pregnancy hypertention / Pregnancy trichomonasis / Postpartum hypotension / Autoimmune hemolytic anemia / Polyclonal IgM cold agglutinins - mediated hemolytic anemia / Spherocytosis / Toxoplasmosis

적응증예

Autoimmune hemolytic anemia

➡ erythrocyte: autoantibody 생성
➡ complement 유도
➡ erythrocyte: protein kinase C 활성화
➡ adducin phosphorylation
➡ adducin-spectrin-actin complex: 분리됨
➡ deformity erythrocyte
➡ Met hemoglobin 형성
➡ Methemoglobinemia
➡ tissue hypoxia

Pregnancy essential supplements

➡ pregnancy
➡ 혈액량 & 적혈구 증가

➡ Iron deficiency & vitB 12 deficiency
➡ 적혈구 골격단백질 결함
➡ deformity erythrocyte 생성
➡ 산소포화도 감소
➡ 조직 허혈

처방예

當歸芍藥散: Pregnancy hypertention (임신고혈압)
當歸散: Pregnancy essential supplements (임신 필수보충제)
當歸貝母苦蔘丸: Pregnancy trichomoniasis (임신부 트리코모나스증)
當歸建中湯: Postpartum hypotension (산후저혈압)
當歸四逆湯: Autoimmune hemolytic anemia (자가면역 용혈성빈혈)
當歸四逆加吳茱萸生薑湯: Autoimmune hemolytic anemia-mediated pancreatitis (자가면역 용혈성빈혈-매개 췌장염)
赤豆當歸散: Polyclonal IgM cold agglutinins - mediated hemolytic anemia (다클론IgM 한냉응집소-매개 용혈성빈혈)
當歸生薑羊肉湯: Spherocytosis (원형적혈구증)
升摩鱉甲湯: Toxoplasmosis (톡소플라즈마증)

REFERENCE

1. Barbara A. Klarl, Philipp A. Lang, Daniela S. Kempe, Olivier M. Niemoeller, Ahmad Akel, Malgorzata Sobiesiak, Kerstin Eisele, Marlis Podolski, Stephan M. Huber, Thomas Wieder, and Florian Lang. Protein kinase C mediates erythrocyte "programmed cell death" following glucose depletion. Am J Physiol Cell Physiol 290: C244-C253, 2006.

2. Jeong Hun Kim,1 Jin Hyoung Kim,1 You Mie Lee,2 Eun-Mi Ahn,3 Kyu-Won Kim,4 Young Suk Yu1. Decursin inhibits retinal neovascularization via suppression of VEGFR-2 activation. Molecular Vision 2009; 15:1868-1875.

대극 (大戟)

생약명 EUPHORBIAE PEKINENSIS RADIX

자원 대극과의 다년생 초본식물인 대극이나 꼭두서니과의 다년생 초본식물인 홍아대극의 뿌리

성분 euphorin

약리 Diuretic like urethane

적응증 Severe pleural effusion

처방예

十棗湯: Severe pleural effusion (흉막 삼출)

REFERENCE

S. E. Dicker. The renal effects of urethane and colchicine in adult rats. Br J Pharmacol Chemother. 1951 June; 6(2): 169-181.

대추 (大棗)

생약명 JUJUBAE FRUCTUS

자원 갈매나무과에 속하는 잎이 지는 키나무인 대추나무의 익은 열매를 말린 것

성분 cAMP (Cyclic adenosine monophosphate)

약리 Protein kinase A acvtivator / Granular organelles inhibitor

효능 Activation of glycogenolysis / Activation of DNA replication / Inhibition of granular organelles phosphorylation

적응증 Common cold / Hypersensitive reaction

적응증예

Type I hypersensitive reaction

➡ allergen 침입
➡ B cell allergen specific IgE Rc: allergen binding
➡ CD4+ Th cell: CD4+ Rc ▶ allergen binding
➡ CD4+ Th cell: IL-4 분비
➡ B cell: allergen specific IgE 생산 ↑
➡ mast cell FcR γ: IgE binding
➡ Phospholipase C activation
➡ diacylglycerol & Inositol trisphosphate 생성
➡ Inositol trisphosphate -> endoplasmic reticulum: calcium 분비
➡ 세포질: granule-bound adenylate cyclase 활성화
➡ cAMP ↑
➡ cAMP-dependent protein kinase 활성화
➡ cAMP ↓
➡ 세포질 granule-membrane protein: phospholylation
➡ 세포질 granule swelling
➡ vasoactive amines degranulation : histamine / serine proteases / serotonin / heparin

처방예

桂枝湯: Common cold
麥門冬湯: Pulmonary tuberculosis (폐결핵)
半夏瀉心湯: Gastric ulcer (위궤양)
小柴胡湯: Viral hepatitis (type A, B) (바이러스성 간염)
越婢湯: Type I hypersensitive reaction

REFERENCE

Y.M. Chang, J.J. Du. EXTRACTION AND SEPARATION OF CAMP FROM ZIZYPHUS JUJUBA FRUIT. ISHS Acta Horticulturae 840: I International Jujube Symposium.

대황 (大黃)

생약명 RHEI RADIX ET RHIZOMA

자원 마디풀과의 여러해살이 식물인 장엽대황의 줄기

성분 emodin

약리 tyrosine kinase blocker

효능 Inhibition of cancer cell proliferation

적응증 Cervical cancer / Ovarian cancer / Endometrioma / Placenta accreta / 처방예 참고

적응증예

Cervical cancer

➡ cervical squamous epithelium: human papillomavirus (HPV) infection
➡ cervical squamous epithelium: oncogenic change
➡ EGF autocrine
➡ EGF-Rc & tyrosine kinase domain: 활성화
➡ squamous epithelium: hyperplasia
➡ squamous cell carcinoma

처방예

桃核承氣湯: Cervical cancer (자궁암)
大黃甘遂湯: Ovarian cancer (난소암)
抵當湯: Endometrioma (자궁내막종)
抵當丸: Endometrial adenocarcinoma (자궁내막선종)
下瘀血湯: Placenta accreta (태반유착)
大黃甘草湯: Barrett`s esophagus (바렛 식도)
瀉心湯: H. pylori-mediated stomach bleeding
大黃黃連瀉心湯: Gastric MALT lymphoma (위장 점막림프조직 림프종)
小承氣湯: Diffuse large B cell lymphoma of gastric MALT
(위장 점막림프조직의 미만성 B세포 림프종)
調胃承氣湯: Small intestine MALT lymphoma (소장 점막림프조직 림프종)

大承氣湯: Diffuse large B cell lymphoma of small intestine MALT
(소장 점막림프조직의 미만성 B세포 림프종)
己椒藶黃丸: Mesenteric lymphoma (장간막 림프종)
大陷胸湯: Intestine MALT lymphoma-complicated perforation
(소장 점막림프종에 합병된 천공)
大陷胸丸: Post-perforation peritonitis (천공후 복막염)
附子瀉心湯: Cholecystitis (담낭염)
大黃硝石湯: Klatskin tumor (간문부 담관암)
大黃附子湯: Distal extrahepatic cholangiocarcinoma (원위부 간외담관암)
大柴胡湯: Hepatocellular carcinoma (간암)
三物備急丸: Esophageal adenocarcinoma & Small cell lung carcinoma
& Gastrointestinal stromal tumor (식도암 & 소세포폐암 & 위장관 간질 종양)
茯苓甘草五味薑辛半夏杏仁大黃湯: Chronic left heart failure-mediated alveolar
carcinoma (만성 좌심부전-매개 폐포암)
厚朴七物湯: Gastrointestinal leiomyosarcoma (위장관 평활근육종)
厚朴三物湯: Adenomatous polyp (선종성 용종)
麻子仁丸: Colon cancer (대장암)
大黃牧丹皮湯: Diverticulitis (게실염)
枳實梔子大黃豉湯: Fibrous cap formation in Abdominal arteries
(복부동맥 섬유덮개 형성)
厚朴大黃湯: Lung adenocarcinoma & Large cell lung carcinoma (폐선암 & 대세포폐암)
大黃䗪虫丸: Kaposis sarcoma (카포시 육종)

REFERENCE

1. Hiranthi Jayasuriya, Nuphavan M. Koonchanok, Robert L. Geahlen, Jerry L. McLaughlin, Ching-Jer Chang. Emodin, a Protein Tyrosine Kinase Inhibitor from Polygonum cuspidatum. J. Nat. Prod., 1992, 55 (5), pp 696−698
2. Michael B. Sporn& Anita B. Roberts. Autocrine growth factors and cancer. Nature313, 28 February 1985, 745 - 747

도인 (桃仁)

생약명 PERSICAE SEMEN

자원 복숭아나무의 익은 열매의 씨를 말린 것

성분 amygdalin,

체내 활성 성분 amygdalin metabolite ➡ thiocyanate

약리 4S estrogen receptor (ER) ➡ 5S estrogen receptor 전환 억제

약리 해설 ER 평소 상태, 4S monomer 형태 (estrogen 저친화성)
➡ 5S dimer 전환 (estrogen 고친화성)
➡ DNA 복제 촉진

효능 Inhibition of estrogen-mediated cell proliferation

적응증 Cervical cancer / Placenta accreta / Endometrioma / Uterine myoma / Diverticulitis / Kaposi sarcoma

적응증예

Uterine myoma

➡ normal myocyte
➡ tumor initiator: genetic factor (?)
➡ somatic mutation
➡ mutated myocyte
➡ estrogen & progesterone
➡ mitogenesis
➡ clonal expansion
➡ myoma
➡ myoma: estrogen receptor-mediated rapidly growth

처방예

挑核承氣湯: Cervical cancer (자궁암)

下瘀血湯: Placenta accreta (태반유착)
抵當湯: Endometrioma (자궁내막종)
桂枝茯苓丸: Uterine myoma (자궁근종)
大黃牧丹皮湯: Diverticulitis (게실염)
大黃蟅虫丸: Kaposi`s sarcoma (카포시 육종)

REFERENCE

BARRY M. WEICHMAN AND ANGELO C. NOTIDES. Estradiol-binding Kinetics of the Activated and Nonactivated Estrogen Receptor*. THE JOURNAL OF BIOLOGI CAL CHEMISTRY, Vol. 252, No. 24, Issue of December 25, pp. 8856-8862, 1977.

동과자 (冬瓜子)

생약명 BENINCASAE SEMEN

자원 박과에 속한 동아의 여문 씨를 말린 것

성분 urea

약리 알카리환경의 G- bacteria의 세포막 파괴

처방예

大黃牧丹皮湯: Diverticulitis (게실염)

REFERENCE

J. H. Kang-Meznarich and G. A. Broderick. Effects of Incremental Urea Supplementation on Ruminal Ammonia Concentration and Bacterial Protein Formation1,2. J. Anim Sci. 1980. 51:422-431.

마자인 (麻子仁)

생약명 CANNABIS FRUCTUS

자원 뽕나무과의 일년생 초본인 삼의 성숙된 열매

성분 α-Linolenic acid (omega-3)

약리 대장암 세포의 세포막 지방산 조성 변화시킴

약리 해설 colon cancer 세포막 지방산 형태: α-Linoleic acid (omega-6)

➡ omega-3 diet
➡ colon cancer 세포막 지방산: omega-3 전환
➡ diacyl glycerol ↓
➡ arachidonic acid ↓
➡ cell proliferation 억제

적응증 Colon cancer

적응증예

Colon cancer

➡ 세포막 지방산 α-Linoleic acid (omega-6)
➡ diacyl glycerol ↑
➡ arachidonic acid ↑
➡ cell proliferation 촉진

처방예

麻子仁丸: Colon cancer (대장암)

REFERENCE

1. Tomio Narisawa, [1, 4 4] Masahiro Takahashi, [1] Hitoshi Kotanagi, [1] Hisashi Kusaka, [1] Yoshihiko Yamazaki, [1] Hirofumi Koyama, [1] Yoko Fukaura, [1] Yukio Nishizawa, [2] Mieko Kotsugai, [2] Yoshihiro Isoda, [2] Jiro Hirano [2] Noritoshi Noritoshi [3]. Inhibitory

Effect of Dietary Perilla Oil Rich in the n-3 Polyunsaturated Fatty Acid α-Linolenic Acid on Colon Carcinogenesis in Rats. Jpn. J. Cancer Res. 82, 1089- -1096, October 1991.

2. Bin Liang, Shan Wang, Ying-Jiang Ye, Xiao-Dong Yang, You-Li Wang, Jun Qu, Qi-Wei Xie, and Mu-Jun Yin. Impact of postoperative omega-3 fatty acid-supplemented parenteral nutrition on clinical outcomes and immunomodulations in colorectal cancer patients. World J Gastroenterol. 2008 April 21; 14(15): 2334-2439.

마황 (麻黃)

생약명 EPHEDRAE HERBA

자원 마황과의 다년생 관목양 초본식물

성분 ephedrine

약리 Epinephrine receptors agonist

약리 해설 natural killer cell & mast cell & basophil & eosinophil
➡ epinephrine Rc 자극
➡ adenylate cyclase 활성화
➡ cAMP ↑
➡ granule-membrane protein: phospholylation 억제
➡ degranulation / secretion 억제

적응증 heat shock protein-resistant viral infection / *heat shock protein & IFN-a* resistant viral infection / Viral pneumonia / Type I hypersensitive reaction / Asthma / 처방예 참고

적응증예

heat shock protein & IFN-a resistant viral infection

➡ lymph node immune cell: virus infection

➡ lymph node immune cell: virus infection ▶ IL-1 분비 ▶ 발열 유도
➡ lymph node immune cell: heat shock protein 활성화 ▶ virus replication 억제
➡ *heat shock protein & IFN-a: 회피 바이러스인 경우*
➡ IL-1 지속
➡ B cell: proliferation
➡ 중화 항체 최고조 ▶ virus activity ↓
➡ virus infected cell: antibody 부착-〉 mature NKc 유도
➡ mature NKc: secretion & degranulation
➡ TRAIL / granule / TNF-α ↑
➡ antibody coated virus-infected cell: TRAIL & FAS & granule 작동
▶ 당대사 급격한 증가
▶ lactate ↑
▶ mitochondria ROS ↑
▶ mitochondria dysfunction
▶ apoptosis

처방예

甘草麻黃湯: Type I hypersensitive reaction: first sensitization
桂枝二麻黃一湯: *heat shock protein*-resistant viral infection
桂枝二越婢一湯: *IL-1 deficiency*-mediated viral infection
桂麻各半湯: *IFN-a* resistant viral infection
桂枝去芍藥加麻黃細辛附子湯: Autoimmune response mediated Methemoglobinemia
大青龍湯: *IFN-γ* resistant viral infection
麻黃湯: *heat shock protein & IFN-a* resistant viral infection
麻黃加朮湯: Immune complexes-mediated vasculitis (면역복합체-매개 혈관염)
麻黃升麻湯: Infectious mononucleosis (전염성 단핵구증)
麻黃蓮軺赤小豆湯: Warm autoantibody-mediated hemolytic anemia
(온난자가항체-매개 용혈성빈혈)
麻黃杏仁甘草石膏湯: Asthma (천식)
麻黃杏仁薏苡甘草湯: Reactive arthritis (반응성 관절염)
麻黃附子甘草湯: Early autoimmune response for tissue
麻黃附子細辛湯: Early autoimmune response for erythrocyte
小青龍湯: Viral pneumonia (바이러스성 폐렴)
烏頭湯: Osteoarthritis (퇴행성 관절염)
越婢湯: Type I hypersensitive reaction: second sensitization
越婢加朮湯: Type I hypersensitive reaction: eosinophil-mediated late phase reaction

越婢加半夏湯: Hypersensitivity pneumonitis (과민성 폐렴)
越婢加附子湯: Type I hypersensitive reaction: neutrophil-mediated late phase reaction
厚朴麻黄湯: Emphysema (폐기종)

망초 (芒硝)

자원 테날드석 (thenardite, Na_2SO_4) 또는 미라빌석 (mirabilite, $Na_2SO_4 \cdot 10H_2O$)

성분 Sodium Sulfate (Na_2SO_4)

약리 Intraluminal distention pressure (장관 팽창압력) 상승시킴

약리 해설 Na_2SO_4 diet
➡ osmotic pressure ↑
➡ intraluminal distention pressure ↑
➡ leacked out of submucosa
➡ submucosa lymphatic leaking
➡ lymph fluid ▶ 장관 배출

적응증 MALT lymphoma / Diverticulitis / Cervical cancer / Pleural effusion / Type C hepatitis / Klatskin tumor

적응증예

Small intestine MALT lymphoma

➡ 주로 ileum: pathogenic microorganisms ▶ persistent infection
➡ B cell infiltration
➡ Peyer`s patch: B cell clones formation
➡ pathogenic microorganisms: persistent antigenic stimulation
➡ B cell: genetic alteration
➡ B cell: neoplastic transformation

처방예

調胃承氣湯: Small intestine MALT lymphoma (소장 점막림프조직 림프종)

大承氣湯: Diffuse large B cell lymphoma of small intestine MALT
(소장 점막림프조직의 미만성 B세포 림프종)
大黃牧丹皮湯: Diverticulitis (게실염)
桃核承氣湯: Cervical cancer (자궁암)
木防己去石膏加茯苓芒硝湯: Left heart failure-mediated pleural effusion
(좌심부전-매개 흉막삼출)
柴胡加芒硝湯: Type C hepatitis (C형 간염)
大黃硝石湯: Klatskin tumor (간문부 담관암)

REFERENCE

J S Lee. Intraluminal distension pressure on intestinal lymph flow, serosal transudati on and fluid transport in the rat. J Physiol. 1984 October ; 355: 399−409.

맥문동 (麥門冬)

생약명 LIRIOPIS TUBER

자원 백합과에 속한 다년생 초본인 맥문동이나 소엽 맥문동의 괴근

성분 ophiopogonin

약리 추측 M. tuberculosis SigF transcription inhibitor

효능 Inhibition of M. tuberculosis growth

적응증 Pulmonary tuberculosis / Secondary tuberculosis / Tuberculous endometritis / Chagas disease

적응증예

Pulmonary tuberculosis

➡ lung macrophage: M. tuberculosis -> persistent infection

➡ starvation & low oxygen pressure
➡ M. tuberculosis: thehalose dimycolate 합성
➡ macrophage: focal adhesion kinase 활성화
➡ macrophage fusion 형성
➡ blood macrophage 유도됨
➡ macrophage fusion 증가
➡ granuloma formation
➡ M. tuberculosis: SigF overexpression
➡ M. tuberculosis: intracellular growth
➡ M. tuberculosis: hydrolytic enzyme 분비
➡ macrophage necrosis
➡ cavity formation
➡ 심한 기침이 유발되고 몸 밖으로 M. tuberculosis 전파됨

처방예

麥門冬湯: pulmonary tuberculosis (폐결핵)
竹葉石膏湯: secondary tuberculosis (이차성 결핵)
溫經湯: Tuberculous endometritis (결핵성 자궁내막염)
炙甘草湯: Chagas disease (샤가스 병)

맹충 (䖟虫)

학명 Tabanus bivittatus Matsumura

자원 등에과에 속하는 등에를 말린 것

성분 anophelin

약리 Thrombin esterase blocker

효능 Inhibition of fibrin formation

적응증 Kaposis sarcoma / Endometrioma / Endometrial adenocarcinoma

처방예

大黃蟅虫丸: Kaposi sarcoma (카포시 육종)
抵當湯: Endometrioma (자궁내막종)
抵當丸: Endometrial adenocarcinoma (자궁내막선종)

REFERENCE

L. L. Zavalova[1], A. V. Basanova[2] and I. P. Baskova[2]. Fibrinogen−Fibrin System Regulators from Bloodsuckers. Biochemistry (Moscow), Volume 67, Number 1 / 2002, 1, p135-142.

모려 (牡蠣)

학명 Ostrea gigas

자원 굴껍데기를 곱게 갈은 것

성분 NaCl

효능 Saline solution

적응증 Rapid hyponatremia / Rapid hypernatremia / Hyponatremia mediated hypotension / Lymphedema / Bornavirus interneuron infection

적응증예

Rapid hyponatremia

➡ IL-1 mediated fever
➡ 땀: water loss
➡ 물 섭취 않으면: 고장성 탈수 / 물 섭취하면: 등장성 탈수
➡ hyponatremia: 세포외액이 세포내부로 이동됨
➡ 뇌세포: 세포내의 유기성 삼투질(organic osmolytes)을 감소시킴
▶ 뇌세포부종을 교정함

➡ Rapid hyponatremia 경우
➡ 유기성 삼투질을 통한 뇌세포부종의 교정 실패
➡ neuron: Na+ & water accumulation
➡ Na+/ K+ pump: dysfunction
➡ 뇌세포 부종
➡ 두개내압 ↑
➡ 신경학적 증상 발생

처방예

桂枝甘草龍骨牡蠣湯: Rapid hyponatremia (급속 저나트륨혈증)
桂枝去芍藥加蜀漆牡蠣救逆湯: Rapid hypernatremia (급속 고나트륨혈증)
桂枝加龍骨牡蠣湯: Hyponatremia-mediated hypotension (저나트륨혈증-매개 저혈압)
牡蠣澤瀉湯: Lymphedema (림프부종)
栝蔞牡蠣散: Bornavirus interneuron infection

목단피 (牧丹皮)

생약명 MOUTAN CORTEX

자원 미나리아재비과의 다년생 낙엽성 소관목인 목단의 뿌리껍질

성분 β-Sitosterol

약리 antioxidant enzyme (+) modulator

효능 Production of manganese superoxide dismutase & glutathione peroxidase

적응증 Uterine myoma / Diverticulitis / Endothelin-1 mediated Renal failure

적응증예

Uterine myoma

➡ normal myocyte
➡ tumor initiator: genetic factor (?)
➡ somatic mutation

➡ mutated myocyte
➡ estrogen & progesterone
➡ mitogenesis
➡ myoma: estrogen receptor-mediated rapidly growth
➡ myoma tissue: ischemic-reperfusion
➡ lactate 축적 & superoxide 증가
➡ manganese superoxide dismutase & glutathione peroxidase 고갈
➡ myoma tissue: oxidant stress
➡ necrosis

처방예

桂枝茯苓丸: Uterine myoma (자궁근종)
大黃牧丹皮湯: Diverticulitis (게실염)
八味腎氣丸: Endothelin-1 mediated Renal failure

REFERENCE

1. Marta Vivancos, Juan J. Moreno. β-Sitosterol modulates antioxidant enzymeresponse in RAW 264.7 macrophages. Free Radical Biology and Medicine, Volume 39, Issue 1, 1 July 2005, Pages 91-97.

2. G. Cipriani, E. Rapizzi, A. Vannacci, R. Rizzuto, F. Moroni, and A. Chiarugi. Nuclear Poly(ADP-ribose) Polymerase-1 Rapidly Triggers Mitochondrial Dysfunction. J. Biol. Chem, 2005, 280: 17227-17234.

목통 (木通)

생약명 AKEBIAE CAULIS

자원 으름덩굴과에 속한 으름의 목질 줄기를 건조한 것

성분 hedegeragenin

약리 Diuretic action

효능 신사구체에 축적된 dimer hemoglobin 배출

적응증 Autoimmune hemolytic anemia / Autoimmune hemolytic anemia-mediated pancreatis

적응증예

Autoimmune hemolytic anemia

➡ erythrocyte: autoantibody 생성
➡ complement 유도
➡ erythrocyte: protein kinase C 활성화
➡ adducin phosphorylation
➡ adducin-spectrin-actin complex: 분리됨
➡ erythrocyte membrane: 불안정해짐
➡ deformity erythrocyte
➡ 삼투압에 취약해짐
➡ intravascular hemolysis
➡ dimer hemoglobin 형성
➡ dimer hemoglobin: heptoglobin 결합 ▶ 비장&간 운반 & 분해
➡ heptoglobin 부족: dimer hemoglobin ▶ 신사구체 축적 ▶ 핍뇨성 신부전 발생

처방예

當歸瀉逆湯: Autoimmune hemolytic anemia (자가면역 용혈성빈혈)
當歸瀉逆加吳茱萸生薑湯: Autoimmune hemolytic anemia-mediated pancreatis (자가면역 용혈성빈혈-매개 췌장염)

REFERENCE

Kazunori Hashimotoa, *, Masami Higuchia, Bunsho Makinoa, Iwao Sakakibaraa, Masayoshi Kuboa, Yasuhiro Komatsua, Masao Marunoa, b and Minoru Okadaa. Quantitative analysis of aristolochic acids, toxic compounds, contained in some medicinal plants. Journal of Ethnopharmacology Volume 64, Issue 2, 1 February 1999, Pages 185-189.

반석 (礬石)

학명 Alunitum

자원 황산염류 광물인 명반을 가공 결정한 것

성분 $KAl(SO_4)_2 \cdot 12H_2O$ (aluminium potassium sulfate = Alum)

약리 astringent (수렴제)

약리 해설 뇌경색 & beriberi ➡ 뇌세포에 Na 유입 ➡ 삼투압 상승
➡ 수분 유입 ➡ 뇌세포 부종 발생
➡ Alum: 세포내 수분 수렴

적응증 Cerebral infarction / Beriberi

적응증예

Cerebral infarction

➡ brain blood vessel: atherothrombotic or embolic
➡ 폐색 부위: 속목동맥 / 앞대뇌동맥 / 중간대뇌동맥 / 후대뇌동맥 (후두 뇌경색, 시상 뇌경색) / 기저동맥 (중뇌 뇌경색, 뇌교 경색) / 소뇌 뇌경색 / 측부 연수 뇌경색
➡ 완전 뇌세포 허혈: 세포질 lactate ↑ ▶ 세포내 산증 ▶ ATP 고갈
▶ ion pump 손상 ▶ 세포외액 유입 ▶ 뇌세포부종

처방예

候氏黑散: Cerebral infarction (뇌경색)
礬石湯: Beriberi (각기병)

REFERENCE

Hanna Peleg1, Keith K. Bodine2 and Ann C. Noble3. The Influence of Acid on Astringency of Alum and Phenolic Compounds. Oxford Journals Life Sciences & Medicine Chemical Senses Volume23, Issue3 Pp. 371-378.

반하 (半夏)

생약명 PINELLIAE RHIZOMA

자원 천남성과에 속하는 여러해살이풀인 끼무릇의 덩이줄기를 말린 것

성분 triterpenoid ($C30H48O7S$)

약리 추측 Rho GTPase family (+) modulator

약리 해설 Rho GTPase family 활성화
➡ focal adhesion 생성 / heparan sulfate 합성 촉진

효능 Activation of cell restitution / Activation of cell adhesion / heparin 유사 작용

효능 해설 상피 & 점막세포 손상
➡ 인근 정상세포: focal kinase 활성화
➡ 손상부위로 이동 (restitution)

적응증 Gastric ulcer / Gastric adenocarcinoma / Viral hepatitis / 처방예 참고

적응증예

Gastric ulcer

➡ Helicobacter pylori in Stomach body & antrum
➡ Helicobacter pylori: 병원성 균으로 형질전환
➡ peptidoglycan: macrophage 유도
➡ extracellular peroxynitrite ($ONOO^-$): 상피세포 손상
➡ Helicobacter pylori: CagE gene
➡ neutrophil 유도 ▶ neutrophil: phagocytosis & degranulation
➡ 점막세포 손상

처방예

半夏散及湯: Soft plate ulcer (연구개염)
半夏苦酒湯: Laryngitis (후두염)
半夏厚朴湯: Inferior pharyngeal stenosis in Behcet's Disease (베체트 하인두 협착증)

小半夏湯: Esophagitis in Behcet's Disease (베체트 식도염)
小半夏加茯笭湯: Superior vena cava thrombosis in Behcet's Disease (베체트 상대정맥 혈전증)
小陷胸湯: Gastric adenocarcinoma (위암)
附子硬米湯: Small intestine stenosis in Behcet's Disease (베체트 소장협착증)
半夏乾薑散: CMV esophagitis (사이토메가로바이러스 식도염)
生薑半夏湯: Herpesvirus vagus neuritis (헤르페스 미주신경염)
旋覆花代赭石湯: CMV esophageal hiatal hernia(사이토메가로바이러스 식도열공헤르니아)
半夏瀉心湯: Gastric ulcer (위궤양)
生薑瀉心湯: Duodenal ulcer (십이지장궤양)
甘草瀉心湯: Peptic ulcer complicated perforation (소화성궤양에 합병된 천공)
大半夏湯: Pyloric stenosis in Behcet's Disease (베체트 유문협착증)
小柴胡湯: Viral hepatitis (type A, B) (바이러스성 간염)
越婢加半夏湯: Hypersensitivity pneumonitis (과민성 폐렴)
小靑龍湯: Viral pneumonitis (바이러스성 폐렴)
茯笭甘草五味乾薑細辛半夏湯: Chronic left heart failure-mediated alveolitis (만성심부전-매개 폐포염)
厚朴麻黃湯: Emphysema (폐기종)
澤漆湯: RSV bronchiotitis (호흡기 세포융합 바이러스 세기관지염)
栝蔞薤白半夏湯: Myocardial Infarction & micro-emboli (심근경색 & 미세혈전)
厚朴生薑半夏甘草人蔘湯: Pancreatic ductal adenocarcinoma (췌장암)
射干麻黃湯: Pharynx diphtheria (디프테리아 인두염)
麥門冬湯: Pulmonay tuberculosis (폐결핵)
黃芩加半夏生薑湯: Salmonella typhi (장티푸스)
六物黃芩湯: Pathogenic E. coli infection
乾薑人蔘半夏丸: CMV-mediated placental villitis (사이토메가바이러스-매개 태반 융모세포염)

방기 (防己)

생약명 STEPHANIAE TETRANDRAE RADIX

자원 방기과 식물인 목방기의 뿌리

성분 sinomenine

약리 prostaglandin I2 (+) modulator in venous endothelium

효능 venous vasodilation (정맥혈관 확장)

적응증 Left heart failure-mediated pleural effusion / Left heart failure-mediated pulmonary venous congestion / Right heart failure-mediated venous congestion / Mesenteric lymphoma

적응증예

Right heart failure-mediated venous congestion

➡ venous congestion: ankles / legs / abdomen / liver / lung / heart
➡ tissue hypoxia
➡ capillary endothelium: VCAM-1 발현
➡ monocyte adhesion
➡ monocyte ROS burst
➡ capillaritis
➡ fibrin clot 형성

처방예

木防己去石膏加茯苓芒硝湯: Left heart failure-mediated pleural effusion (좌심부전-매개 흉막삼출)

木防己湯: Left heart failure-mediated pulmonary venous congestion (좌심부전-매개 폐정맥 울혈)

防己茯苓湯: Chronic right heart failure-mediated systemic congestion (만성우심부전-매개 전신울혈)

防己黃耆湯: Right heart failure-mediated venous congestion (우심부전-매개 정맥울혈)

己椒藶黃丸: Mesenteric lymphoma (장간막 림프종)

REFERENCE

Seiichiro Nishidaa and Hiroyasu Satoha. In vitro pharmacological actions of sinomenine on the smooth muscle and the endothelial cell activity in rat aorta. Life Sciences, Volume 79, Issue 12, 15 August 2006, Pages 1203-1206

방풍 (防風)

생약명 LEDEBOURIELLAE RADIX

자원 산형과에 속한 다년생초본인 방풍의 뿌리

성분 deltoin

약리 cyclooxygenase-2 blocker

적응증 Cerebral infarction / Rheumatoid arthritis

적응증예

Rheumatoid arthritis

➡ synovitis: IL-8 분비
➡ neutrophil 유도
➡ neutrophil elastase: hyaluronate destruction ▶ synovitis
➡ neutrophil: IL-1 분비
➡ synovial fibroblast 활성화
➡ synovial fibroblast: prostaglandin E2 분비
➡ chodrocyte: copper-zinc superoxide dismutase 소진
➡ superoxide ↑
➡ chondrocytis
➡ cartilage muscle: 대사 항진
➡ lactate ↑
➡ cartilage muscle inflammation

처방예

候氏黑散: Cerebral infarction (뇌경색)
桂枝芍藥知母湯: Rheumatoid arthritis (류마티스 관절염)

REFERENCE

Ban HS, Lim SS, Suzuki K, Jung SH, Lee S, Lee YS, Shin KH, Ohuchi K. Inhibitory effects of furanocoumarins isolated from the roots of Angelica dahurica on prostaglandin E2 production. Planta Med. 2003 May;69(5):408-12

백두옹 (白頭翁)

생약명 PULSATILLAE RADIX

자원 미나리아재비과 여러해살이 풀인 할미꽃의 뿌리

성분 anemonin

약리 NF-kB blocker in small intestine epithelium

적응증 Crohn's disease

적응증예

Crohn's disease

➡ small intestine epithelial cell: Mycobacterium, other pathogenic bacteria 융합
➡ Mycobacterium, other pathogenic bacteria: unusual peptidoglycan 생성
➡ 상피세포 NOD2 gene mutation
➡ Mycobacterium, other pathogenic bacteria: 면역반응 시작됨
➡ 상피세포 NF-kB pathway
➡ IL-32 발현
➡ macrophage 침착: TNF-α 분비
➡ 소장상피세포 & 술잔세포 & 근육층 & Mycobacterium, other pathogenic bacteria : apoptosis
➡ granulomatous colitis

처방예

白頭翁湯: Crohn's disease (크론병)
白頭翁加甘草阿膠湯: Postpartum Crohn's disease (산후 크론병)

REFERENCE

1. Hampe J, Cuthbert A, Crouchr PJ, Mirza MM, Mascheretti S, Fisher S, Frenzel H, King K, Hasselmeyer A, MacPherson AJ, Bridger S, van Deventer S, Forbes A, Nikolaus S, Lennard-Jones JE, Foelsch UR, Krawczak M, Lewis C, Schreiber S,

Mathew CG. Association between insertion mutation in NOD2 gene and Crohn's disease in German and British populations. Lancet. 2001 Jun16;357(9272):1925-8.

2. Huiqin Duana, Yongdong Zhangb, Jianqin Xub, Jian Qiaob, Zhanwei Suoa, Ge Hua and Xiang Mua. Effect of anemonin on NO, ET-1 and ICAM-1 production in ratintestinal microvascular endothelial cells. Journal of Ethnopharmacology, Volume 104, Issue 3, 6 April 2006, Pages 362-366.

백석지 (白石脂)

학명 Halloysite

자원 Fe2O3를 제거한 고령토

성분 $(Al,Mg)_2(Si_4O_{10})(OH)_2 \cdot nH_2O$

약리 Water absorbent

적응증 Cerebral edema (뇌부종)

처방예

風引湯: Epilepsy (뇌전증)

REFERENCE

Jihuai Wu, Jianming Lin, Meng Zhou, Congrong Wei. Synthesis and properties of starch-graft-polyacrylamide/clay superabsorbent composite. Macromolecular Rapid Communications Volume 21, Issue 15, pages 1032−1034, October 2000.

백엽 (柏葉)

생약명 BIOTAE CACUMEN

자원 측백나무의 가지와 잎을 말린 것

성분 tannin

약리 지혈제

약리 해설 tannin hydroxyl group
➡ 혈관 콜라겐의 아미노기와 결합
➡ 파열된 콜라겐층 고정화

처방예

柏葉湯: Esophageal varices bleeding (식도 정맥류 출혈)

REFERENCE

Margarita Naish1,*, Michael N Clifford2, Gordon G Birch1. Sensory astringency of 5-O-affeoylquinic acid, tannic acid and grape-seed tannin by a time-intensity procedure. Journal of the Science of Food and Agriculture Volume 61, Issue 1,pages 57–64, 1993

백전 (白前)

생약명 CYNANCHI ATRATI RADIX

자원 박주가리과의 여러해살이 풀인 백미꽃의 뿌리

성분 pregnane glycoside

약리 PXR ligand (PXR: pregnane X receptor)

약리 해설 PXR ligand ➡ detoxification protein 전사 촉진
➡ immune response 활성화

처방예

澤漆湯: RSV (respiratory syncytial virus) bronchiolitis (호흡기 세포융합 바이러스 세기관지염)

백출 (白朮)

생약명 ATRACTYLODIS MACROCEPHALAE RHIZOMA

자원 국화과에 속하는 다년생 초본인 백출의 건조한 뿌리

성분 atractylon

약리 vascular cell adhesion molecule-1 (VCAM-1) blocker

효능 Inhibition of leukocyte adhesion

적응증 Immune complex-mediated glomerulonephritis / Atrial fibrillation / 처방예 참고

적응증예

Atrial fibrillation

➡ 관상동맥 질환 / 류머티스성 판막 질환 / 갑상선 항진증 / 고혈압 / 기타 원인
➡ atrial myocardiocyte: ischemia
➡ 심방 세동
➡ atrial endocardial endothelial cell: blood velocities ↓
➡ endocardial endothelial cell: nitric oxide 생성
➡ NADPH oxidase ↑
➡ oxidative stress
➡ endocardial endothelial cell: VCAM-1 발현
➡ monocyte 부착

➡ thrombus formation

처방예

五苓散: Immune complex-mediated glomerulonephritis (면역복합체-매개 사구체신염)
茵蔯五苓散: Free bile acids-mediated glomerulonephritis(자유담즙산-매개 사구체신염)
豬苓散: IgA nephropathy (IgA 신병증)
茯苓戎鹽湯: Immune complex-mediated rapidly progressive glomerulonephritis (면역복합체-매개 급속진행성 사구체신염)
茯苓桂枝白朮甘草湯: Atrial fibrillation (심방세동)
甘草乾薑苓朮湯: p-ANCA mediated crescentic glomerulonephritis (핵주위 항호중구 세포질 항체-매개 반월상 사구체신염)
茯苓澤瀉湯: Decompensated heart failure (보상기전 실패 심부전)
茯苓飮方: Aortic aneurysm in Behcet's Disease (베체트 대동맥류)
防己黃耆湯: Right heart failure-mediated venous congestion (우심부전-매개 정맥울혈)
眞武湯: c-ANCA associated vasculitis (항호중구 세포질항체-매개 혈관염)
附子湯: p-ANCA associated vasculitis (핵주위 항호중구 세포질항체-매개 혈관염)
桂枝去桂茯苓白朮湯: Kawasaki disease
薯蕷丸: Malnutrition-mediated disease (영양실조-매개 질병)
當歸散: Pregnancy essential supplements (임신 필수보충제)
當歸芍藥散: Pregnancy hypertention (임신고혈압)
澤瀉湯: Hypertension
越婢加朮湯: Type I hypersensitive reaction: eosinophil mediated late phase reaction
白朮附子湯: Myoglobin-mediated renal failure
桂枝芍藥知母湯: Rheumatoid arthritis (류마티스 관절염)

REFERENCE

DAVID G. CORLEY. INFLANNATORY MEDIATION OBTAINED FROM ATRACTYLODES LANCEA. Patent Application Publication, Jul, 5, 2001, US2001/0006686 A1.

별갑 (鱉甲)

학명 AMYDAE CARAPAX

자원 자라의 등껍질

성분 chitosan

약리 Lipid absorption inhibitor & Sterol excretion activator

적응증 Plasmodium falciparum malaria / Toxoplasmosis

처방예

鱉甲煎丸: Plasmodium falciparum malaria (열대열원충 말라리아)
升麻鱉甲湯: Toxoplasmosis (톡소플라즈마증)

REFERENCE

Ikuo. Ikeda, Michihiro. Sugano, Katsuko. Yoshida, Eiji. Sasaki, Yasushi. Iwamoto, Kouta. Hatano. Effects of chitosan hydrolyzates on lipid absorption and on serum and liver lipid concentration in rats. J. Agric. Food Chem., 1993, 41 (3), pp 431–435.

복령 (茯苓)

생약명 PORIA

자원 구멍쟁이버섯과에 속한 진균인 복령의 균핵

성분 pachymic acid

약리 추측 glycoprotein IIb/IIIa (gpIIb/IIIa) blocker

효능 Inhibition of thrombus formation

적응증 Vasculitis (혈관염) / Thrombosis (혈전증)

적응증예

vasculitis

➡ 혈관내피세포: 손상
➡ 내피세포: Von Willebrand factor (vWF) 분비
➡ platelet GPIb: vWF 부착
➡ platelet 고정
➡ platelet 1차 응집
➡ ADP / serotonin / thromboxane A2 분비
➡ platelet 활성화
➡ glycoprotein IIb/IIIa 발현
➡ fibrinogen 부착
➡ platelet 2차 응집
➡ thrombus formation

처방예

桂枝茯苓丸: Uterine myoma (자궁근종)
桂枝去桂茯苓白朮湯: Kawasaki disease
桂苓五味甘草湯: Pneumonia complications-mediated hypoxemia (폐렴합병증-매개 저산소혈증)
眞武湯: c-ANCA associated vasculitis (항호중구 세포질항체-매개 혈관염)
附子湯: p-ANCA associated vasculitis (핵주위 항호중구 세포질항체-매개 혈관염)
茯苓四逆湯: Viral myocarditis (바이러스성 심근염)
小半夏可茯苓湯: Superior vena cava thrombosis in Behcet's Disease (베체트 상대정맥 혈전증)
茯苓飮方: Aortic aneurysm in Behcet's Disease (베체트 대동맥류)
防己茯苓湯: Chronic right heart failure-mediated systemic congestion (만성우심부전-매개 전신울혈)
茯苓五味乾薑細辛湯: Chronic left heart failure-mediated alveolar-capillary barrier damage (만성좌심부전-매개 폐포-모세혈관 장벽 손상)
茯苓甘草湯: Streptococcal rheumatic myocarditis (연쇄구균 류마티스 심근염)
茯苓杏仁甘草湯: Rheumatic valvulitis (류마티스 판막염)
木防己去石膏加茯苓芒硝湯: Left heart failure-mediated pleural effusion

(좌심부전-매개 흉막삼출)
茯苓桂枝甘草大棗湯: Ventricular tachycardia (심실빈맥)
茯苓桂枝白朮甘草湯: Atrial fibrillation (심방세동)
茯苓澤瀉湯: Decompensated heart failure (보상기전 실패 심부전)
茯苓戎鹽湯: Immune complex-mediated rapidly progressive glomerulonephritis
(면역복합체-매개 급속진행성 사구체신염)
甘草乾薑苓朮湯: p-ANCA mediated crescentic glomerulonephritis
(핵주위 항호중구 세포질 항체-매개 반월상 사구체신염)
五苓散: Immune complex-mediated glomerulonephritis (면역복합체-매개 사구체신염)
茵蔯五苓散: Free bile acids-mediated glomerulonephritis(자유담즙산-매개 사구체신염)
豬苓湯: Anti-GBM glomerulonephritis (항-기저막 사구체신염)
豬苓散: IgA nephropathy (IgA 신병증)
八味腎氣丸: Endothelin-1 mediated renal failure
薯蕷丸: Malnutrition-mediated disease (영양실조-매개 질병)
當歸芍藥散: Pregnancy hypertention (임신고혈압)
柴胡加龍骨牡蠣湯: Viral fulminant hepatitis (바이러스성 전격성간염)

봉밀 (蜂蜜, 꿀)

학명 Apis cerana Fabricius.

자원 꿀벌이 식물의 꽃꿀이나 다른 당단물을 날라다가 가공하여 벌방에 저장한 진한 단맛 액체

성분 xylose & galactose

약리 Heparan sulfate biosynthesis

효능 Intestinal adhesion 방지 / hyaluronate & glucosaminoglycan & chondroitin 합성 촉진

적응증 Pyloric stenosis in Behcet's Disease / Osteoarthritis / Mesenteritis-mediated volvulus / Volvulus

처방예

大半夏湯: Pyloric stenosis in Behcet's Disease (베체트 유문협착증)

烏頭湯: Osteoarthritis (퇴행성 관절염)
烏頭桂枝湯: Mesenteritis-mediated volvulus (장간막염-매개 장꼬임증)
大烏頭煎: Volvulus (장꼬임증)

봉와 (蜂窩)

자원 벌집

성분 rosin

약리 Histidin binder

약리 해설 Plasmodium falciparum, pfHRP1단백질 (Histidine-rich protein)
➡ erythrocyte entry
➡ rosin: pfHRP1 부착
➡ P. falciparum: 적혈구 침입 실패

적응증 Plasmodium falciparum malaria

처방예

鱉甲煎丸: Plasmodium falciparum malaria (열대열원충 말라리아)

REFERENCE

E. Hochulia, H. Döbelia and A. Schachera. New metal chelate adsorbent selective for proteins and peptides containing neighbouring histidine residues. Journal of Chromatography A Volume 411, 1987, Pages 177-184.

부소맥 (浮小麥)

생약명 TRITICI IMMATRI SEMEN

자원 벼과에 속한 일년생 또는 이년생 초본인 밀의 익지 않은 종자

성분 Vitamin B_6 (Pyridoxine)

효능 Biosynthesis of γ-gamma-aminobutyric acid (GABA) & dopamine

적응증 Biopolar affective disorder

적응증예

Bipolar affective disorder

➡ Vitamin B6 부족
➡ Pyridoxal phosphate ↓
➡ γ-aminobutyric acid (GABA) & dopamine 생성 ↓
➡ GABA 부족 ▶ 신경 흥분 & dopamine 부족 ▶ 슬픔

처방예

甘草小麥大棗湯: Biopolar affective disorder (양극성 정동장애)

부자 (附子)

생약명 ACONITI IATERALIS PREPARATA RADIX

자원 미나리아재비과에 속하는 다년생 초본인 부자의 건조한 자근

성분 hypaconitine

약리 추측 macrophage` Voltage-gated proton channels blocker

약리 해설 Voltage-gated proton channels

➡ 식균작용에 의해 증가된 세포내 H+을 세포외로 방출시키는 채널
➡ Voltage-gated proton channels 차단
➡ H+ 방출 억제
➡ 세포내 pH ↓
➡ 세포대사 정지됨

효능 Inhibition of macrophage metabolism

적응증 Polymyositis / Systemic lupus erythematosis / Viral myocarditis / Osteoarthritis / 처방예 참고

적응증예

Systemic lupus erythematosis

➡ Type IV & V collagen autoantibody
➡ basement membrane & interstitial tissue: autoantibody 부착
➡ antibody-dependent cell-mediated cytotoxicity (ADCC)
➡ macrophage 유도
➡ macrophage phagocytosis
➡ connective tissue disease & collagen vascular disease 발생
➡ 모세혈관 퇴행 및 소실 / 피부괴사 / 위장관 허혈 / 폐간질 염증 / 신경계 손상

처방예

四逆湯: Polymyositis (다발성근염)
四逆加人蔘湯: Polymyositis-associated gastrointestinal myositis (다발성근염에 연관된 위장관근염)
白通湯: Henoch−Schönlein purpura-associated colitis (헤노호-쉐라인 자반증에 연관된 대장염)
白通四逆加猪膽汁湯: Henoch−Schönlein purpura-associated colitis & paralytic ileus (헤노호-쉐라인 자반증에 연관된 대장염 & 장마비)
通脈四逆湯: Systemic lupus erythematosis (전신성 홍반 루푸스)
茯苓四逆湯: Viral myocarditis (바이러스성 심근염)
烏頭湯: Osteoarthritis (퇴행성 관절염)
烏頭桂枝湯: Mesenteritis-mediated volvulus (장간막염-매개 장꼬임증)
乾薑附子湯: Adenovirus infection
薏苡附子敗醬散: Appendicitis (충수염)

삭조 (蒴藋)

학명 Euscaphis japonica (Thunb.) Kanitz

자원 고추나무과 말오줌 때의 열매와 종자

성분 cyanidin

약리 추측 Phosphodiesterase C & D inhibitor

약리 해설 Tetanospasmin이 신경세포에 부착할 때 경세포의 Phosphodiesterase C & D을 이용함

효능 Tetany

처방예

王不留行散: Tetany (파상풍)

REFERENCE

Hitoshi Matsumoto,*† Yuko Nakamura,† Shuji Tachibanaki,‡ Satoru Kawamura, ‡ and Masao Hirayama†. Stimulatory Effect of Cyanidin 3-Glycosides on the Regeneration of Rhodopsin. J. Agric. Food Chem., 2003, 51 (12), pp 3560−3563.

산수유 (山茱萸)

생약명 CORNI FRUCTUS

자원 산수유과(층층나무과)에 속한 낙엽소교목인 산수유나무의 성숙한 과실

성분 ursolic acid

약리 ERK (extracellular signal-regulated kinases) blocker

효능 Inhibition of tubular cell apoptosis (콩팥 세뇨관세포 세포자멸사 억제)

적응증 Endothelin-1 mediated Renal failure

적응증예

Endothelin-1 mediated Renal failure

➡ overwork
➡ cortisol ↑
➡ angiotensin II ↑
➡ renal artery endothelium: angiotensin II type 1 Rc 자극
➡ renal artery endothelium: endothelin-1 생산
➡ renal artery: strong, long-lasting constriction
➡ monocyte: endothelin receptor subtype A
➡ monocyte 활성화: ROS burst
➡ renal artery: vasculitis
➡ tubular endothelium: ischemia
➡ ERK (extracellular signal-regulated kinases) 1/2 phosphorylation
➡ caspase 3 활성화
➡ tubular endothelium: apoptosis

처방예

八味腎氣丸: Endothelin-1 mediated renal failure

REFERENCE

1. Jianzhong Wanga, Chun Ouyanga, b, Xiangmei Chena, Bo Fua, Yang Lua, Quan Honga. STAT3 Inhibits Apoptosis of Human Renal Tubular Epithelial Cells Induced by ATP Depletion/Recovery. Nephron Exp Nephrol 2008;108:e11-e18.

2. Su-Ui Leea, c, Sang-Joon Parkb, Han Bok Kwakd, Jaemin Ohd, Yong Ki Mina and Seong Hwan Kima. Anabolic activity of ursolic acid in bone: Stimulating osteoblast differentiation in vitro and inducing new bone formation in vivo. Pharmacological Research Volume 58, Issues 5-6, November-December 2008, Pages 290-296.

3. Jian-zhen SHAN1, Yan-yan XUAN2, Shu ZHENG2, Qi DONG2, Su-zhan ZHANG†‡2. Ursolic acid inhibits proliferation and induces apoptosis of HT-29 colon cancer cells by inhibiting the EGFR/MAPK pathway. Journal of Zhejiang University SCIENCE B 2009 Vol. 10 No. 9 p. 668~674.

산약 (山藥)

생약명 DIOSCOREAE RHIZOMA

자원 서여과(마과)에 속하는 다년생 초본인 참마 또는 마의 건조한 근경

성분 diosgenin

약리 Glucose transporters (+) modulator

효능 Inhibition of tubular cell apoptosis

적응증 Endothelin-1 mediated Renal failure

적응증예

Endothelin-1 mediated Renal failure

➡ overwork
➡ cortisol ↑
➡ angiotensin II ↑
➡ renal artery endothelium: angiotensin II type 1 Rc 자극
➡ renal artery endothelium: endothelin-1 생산
➡ renal artery: strong, long-lasting constriction
➡ monocyte: endothelin receptor subtype A
➡ monocyte 활성화: ROS burst
➡ renal artery: vasculitis
➡ tubular endothelium: ischemia
➡ tubular endothelium: lactate ↑ ▶ ATP ↓

➡ tubular endothelium: reperfusion

➡ tubular endothelium: reactive oxygen species ↑

➡ ERK (extracellular signal-regulated kinases) 1/2 phosphorylation

➡ caspase 3 활성화

➡ tubular endothelium: apoptosis

처방예

八味腎氣丸: Endothelin-1 mediated renal failure

REFERENCE

Alexander Weidemann*,, Wanja M. Bernhardt*, Bernd Klanke*, Christoph Daniel* Björn Buchholz*, Valentina Câmpean, Kerstin Amann, Christina Warnecke*, Michael S. Wiesener, Kai-Uwe Eckardt* and Carsten Willam*. HIF Activation Protects From Acute Kidney Injury. J Am Soc Nephrol 19: 2008. 486-494

산조인 (酸棗仁)

생약명 ZIZYPHI SPINOSAE SEMEN

자원 갈매나무과의 낙엽교목 멧대추나무의 여문씨의 핵

성분 jujuboside / sanjoinine

약리 추측 serotonin (+) modulator / norepinephrine (+) modulator

적응증 Basilar artery hemorrhage-mediated Insomnia

적응증예

Basilar artery hemorrhage-mediated Insomnia

➡ overwork

➡ cortisol ↑
➡ basilar artery (뇌바닥동맥) endothelium: endothelin-1 발현
➡ basilar artery endothelium: leukocyte 침윤
➡ leukocyte cytokine
➡ basilar artery: arteriovenous malformation
➡ basilar artery: hemorrhage
➡ thrombus 형성
➡ basilar artery: smaller branches ▶ ischemia
➡ smaller branches: vasospasm
➡ brain stem: ischemia & apoptosis
➡ locus coeruleus (청반핵) 손상 & raphe nucleus (솔기핵) 손상
➡ raphe nucleus: serotonin-mediated NREM sleep 유도: 실패
& locus coeruleus: norepinephrine-mediated REM sleep 유도: 실패
➡ 수면 생리작용 깨짐

처방예

酸棗仁湯: Basilar artery hemorrhage-mediated Insomnia
(뇌저동맥 출혈에 의한 불면증)

REFERENCE

Zi-li Youa,, Qing Xiaa, Fan-rong Liangb, Yi-jun Tanga, Cong-lun Xua, Jian Huanga, Ling Zhaob, Wen-zheng Zhangc and Jia-jia Hec. Effects on the expression of GABAA receptor subunits by jujuboside A treatment in rat hippocampal neurons. Journal of Ethnopharmacology Volume 128, Issue 2, 24 March 2010, Pages 419-423.

상륙근 (商陸根)

생약명— Phytolaccae Radix

자원 쌍떡잎식물 중심자목 자리공과의 여러해살이풀의 뿌리

성분 KNO3

효능 hypokalemia (저칼륨혈증)

적응증 Lymphedema

적응증예

Lymphatic filariasis (림프 사상충증)

➡ severe disease
➡ malnutrition
➡ protein breakdown
➡ antibody 감소
➡ filarial parasite infection: *Brugia malayi, Wuchereria bancrofti, Brugia timori*
➡ adult filaria: microfilaria 생산
➡ adult filaria: collagen encoding gene 발현
▶ collagen synthesis
▶ sheath 생성
➡ sheathed microfilaria 출현
➡ 이동: lymphatic vessels
➡ lymphatic vessels: obstruction
➡ tissue: accumulation of protein-rich fluid
➡ fibroblast 활성화: collagen 분비
➡ fibrosclerosis
➡ edema tissue: water accumulation
➡ hyponatremia
➡ 세포외액이 세포내부로 이동
➡ lymphedema ↑

처방예

牡蠣澤瀉湯: Lymphedema (림프부종)

상백피 (桑白皮)

생약명 MORI CORTEX

자원 뽕나무과에 속하는 낙엽교목인 뽕나무 및 동속 근연식물의 건조한 근피

성분 α-amyrin

약리 Capsaicin sensitive channel blocker

약리 해설 muscle cell, capsaicin-sensitive channel 자극
➡ 척수로 구심성 신호 전달
➡ capsaicin-sensitive channel 차단
➡ 근육세포에서 척수로의 구심성신호 차단됨

적응증 Tetany
➡ rusty metal: wound ▶ Clostridium tetani infection
➡ Clostridium tetani: tetanospasmin 분비
➡ peripheral motor neurons: tetanospasmin infection
➡ motor neuron membrane disialoganglioside: tetanospasmin B chain 부착
➡ retro-axonal transport
➡ spinal cord interneuron: infection
▶ tetanospasmin A chain: proteolytic activity
▶ synaptobrevin degrading
▶ GABA & glycine 분비 차단
▶ inhibitory impulse 중단
▶ neuromuscler junction: acethycholine 지속
▶ muscle cell: potassium channel open ▶ K 배출
▶ 근수축 지속
▶ spastic paralysis

처방예

王不留行散: Tetany (파상풍)

REFERENCE

R. C. P. Lima-Júnior, D. I. M. Sousa, G. A. C. Brito, G. M. Cunha, M. H. Chaves, V. S. N. Rao and F. A. Santos. Modulation of acute visceral nociception and bladder inflammation by plant triterpene, α, β-amyrin in a mouse model of cystitis: role of tachykinin NK1-receptors, and K+ATP channels. Inflammation Research Volume 56, Number 12, 487-494, DOI: 10.1007/s00011-007-7023-4

생강 (生薑)

생약명 ZINGIBERIS RHIZOMA RECENS

자원 생강과에 속한 다년생 초본인 생강의 근경

성분 gingerol

약리 hydrogen peroxide scavenger

효능 Inhibition of hydrogen peroxide-mediated cytotoxicity / Activation of cell migration

효능 해설 상피 & 점막세포 손상

➡ 인근 정상세포: focal kinase 활성화
➡ 손상부위로 이동 (restitution)
➡ intracellular hydrogen peroxide 축적
➡ actin cytoskeleton 수축력 저하
➡ cell migration 저하

적응증 Common cold / Viral pneumonitis / 처방에 참고

적응증예

Common cold

➡ skeleton muscle cell
➡ 지속적인 ATP생산
➡ mitochondrial respiration 반복: superoxide 발생
➡ superoxide dismutase 작용: hydrogen peroxide 생성
➡ Catalase, GSH-Px 작용: H2O & O2 전환
➡ Catalase, GSH-Px 고갈
➡ hydrogen peroxide 축적
➡ 저농도 hydrogen peroxide: PKC 자극 ▶ PKC mediated signal 활성화
➡ 고농도 hydrogen peroxide: PKC 억제 ▶ 근수축 감소

Viral pneumonia

➡ main cause: influenza virus
➡ bronchial cell infection

➡ CC chemokine 분비
➡ eosinophil 유도
➡ bronchitis
➡ alveolar epithelial cell infection
➡ neutrophil 유도
➡ alveolar-capillary barrier 손상
➡ 폐포 간질: erythrocyte 유입 & 수분 축적
➡ Met hemoglobin 형성
➡ alveolar epithelium: ischemia
➡ alveolitis

처방예

桂枝湯: Common cold
桂枝二麻黃一湯: *heat shock protein*-resistant viral infection
桂麻各半湯: *IFN-a* resistant viral infection
大青龍湯: *IFN-γ* resistant viral infection
桂枝二越婢一湯: *IL-1 deficiency*-mediated viral infection
桂枝去桂茯苓白朮湯: Kawasaki disease
桂枝去芍藥加麻黃細辛附子湯: Autoimmune response mediated Methemoglobinemia
生薑半夏湯: Herpesvirus vagus neuritis (헤르페스 미주신경염)
生薑瀉心湯: Duodenal ulcer (십이지장궤양)
甘草瀉心湯: Peptic ulcer complicated perforation (소화성궤양에 합병된 천공)
生薑甘草湯: Mycoplasma pneumonia
半夏厚朴湯:Inferior pharyngeal stenosis in Behcet's Disease (베체트병 하인두 협착증)
小半夏湯: Esophagitis in Behcet's Disease (베체트 식도염)
小半夏加茯笭湯: Superior vena cava thrombosis in Behcet's Disease (베체트 상대정맥 혈전증)
小柴胡湯: Viral hepatitis (type A, B) (바이러스성 간염)
越婢湯: Type I hypersensitive reaction: second sensitization
越婢加朮湯:Type I hypersensitive reaction: eosinophil mediated late phase reaction
越婢加半夏湯: Hypersensitivity pneumonitis (과민성 폐렴)
越婢加附子湯: Type I hypersensitive reaction: neutrophil mediated late phase reaction
小青龍湯: Viral pneumonitis (바이러스성 폐렴)
桂枝去芍藥加附子湯: IL-1 mediated Cardiac toxicity
桂枝去芍藥加蜀漆牡蠣龍骨救逆湯: Rapid hypernatremia (급속 고나트륨혈증)

REFERENCE

Amar Bahadur Singh1, Akanksha2, Nilendra Singh3, Rakesh Maurya2 and Arvind Kumar Srivastava1. Anti-hyperglycaemic, lipid lowering and anti-oxidant properties of [6]-gingerol in db/db mice. International Journal of Medicine and Medical Sciences. Vol. 1(12), pp. 536-544, December, 2009.

생지황 (生地黃)

생약명 REHMANNIAE RADIX

자원 현삼과에 속하는 다년생 초본인 지황과 회경지황의 건조한 괴경

성분 catalpol

약리 추측 CD133+ circulating endothelial progenitor cell (+) modulator

효능 vessel bud formation (혈관싹 형성)

적응증 Chagas disease

적응증예

Chagas disease

➡ heart parasympathetic neuron: Trypanosoma cruzi 부착
➡ lysosome: 세포 표면으로 이동하여 T. cruzi 융합
➡ lysosome disruption
➡ 세포질: T. cruzi replication
➡ T. cruzi: Trypomastigotes 형태로 전환
➡ 세포밖 전파
➡ heart parasympathetic neuron 파괴 & myocardial fiber 손상
➡ 심장 전기전도계 손상
➡ 심실 수축 ↓

➡ 관상동맥 혈류 감소
➡ myocardium ischemia
➡ myogenesis & angiogenesis: 불충분하면 급사

처방예

炙甘草湯: Chagas disease (샤가스 병)

REFERENCE

Ru-Xue Zhang[a], Mao-Xing Li[a] and Zheng-Ping Jia[a]. Rehmannia glutinosa: Review of botany, chemistry and pharmacology. Journal of Ethnopharmacology Volume 117, Issue 2, 8 May 2008, Pages 199-214.

석고 (石膏)

학명 GYPSUM 규산염류에 속한 천연함수 황산칼슘

자원 규산염류에 속한 천연함수 황산칼슘

성분 $CaSO_4$

약리 Calcium-mediated T cell apoptosis 촉진

약리 해설

T-cell apoptosis 생리

➡ antigen: T-Cell activation
➡ tyrosine kinases 활성화
➡ PLC-Gamma1 phosphorylation
➡ PIP2 (Phosphatidylinositol 4,5-bisphosphate) 분해
➡ Protein Kinase C and IP3 (Inositol 1,4,5-trisphosphate) 활성화
➡ extracellular space Ca^{2+}: influx ↑ & Endoplasmic Reticulum Ca^{2+}: efflux ↑

➡ transcription activation
➡ T-Cell: maturation
➡ TCR stimulation: apoptosis induction
➡ extracellular space Ca2+: influx ↑ & Endoplasmic Reticulum Ca2+: efflux ↑
➡ calcineurin activation
➡ NFATP (Nuclear Factor of Activated T-Cells Pre-existing Component) 활성화
➡ Nur77 transcription
➡ T-Cell apoptosis
➡ 세포내 Ca2+부족: T-Cell apoptosis 실패

적응증 IL-1 mediated Type 1 diabetes / Viral thyroiditis / Coxsackie B4 virus-mediated Type 1 diabetes / Left heart failure-mediated pulmonary venous congestion / Astma / Emphysema / Secondary tuberculos / Type I hypersensitive reaction

적응증예

Coxsackie B4 virus-mediated Type 1 diabetes

➡ β-cell: coxsackie B4 virus infection
➡ β-cell: HLA-DR expression
➡ HLA-DR: glutamic acid decarboxylase (GAD) 제시
➡ coxsackie B4 virus: 2C protein & β-cell: GAD
➡ molecular mimicry
➡ GAD specific CD8+ T cell 출현
➡ CD8+ T cell: β-cell 공격
➡ β-cell loss ↑
➡ Type 1 diabetes

처방예

白虎湯: IL-1 mediated Type 1 diabetes
白虎加人蔘湯: Coxsackie B4 virus-mediated Type 1 diabetes
白虎加桂枝湯: Viral thyroiditis (바이러스성 갑상선염)
桂枝二越婢一湯: *IL-1 deficiency*-mediated viral infection
大青龍湯: *IFN-γ* resistant viral infection
木防己湯: Left heart failure-mediated pulmonary venous congestion
(좌심부전-매개 폐정맥 울혈)
文蛤湯: Chronic obstructive pulmonary disease (COPD)-mediated hyponatremia
麻杏甘石湯: Astma (천식)

厚朴麻黃湯: Emphysema (폐기종)
竹葉石膏湯: Secondary tuberculosis (이차성결핵)
越婢湯: Type I hypersensitive reaction: second sensitization
越婢加朮湯:Type I hypersensitive reaction: eosinophil-mediated late phase reaction
越婢加半夏湯: Hypersensitivity pneumonitis (과민성 폐렴)
越婢加附子湯: Type I hypersensitive reaction: neutrophil-mediated late phase reaction

REFERENCE

C.W. Distelhorst*[1] and H.L. Roderick†. Ins(1,4,5)P3-mediated calcium signals and apoptosis: is there a role for Bcl-2?. Biochemical Society Transactions (2003) Volume 31, part 5.

선복화 (旋覆花)

생약명 INULAE FLOS

자원 국화과에 속하는 다년생 초본인 금불초 및 동속 근연식물의 두상화서

성분 taraxasterol

약리 추측 Cu2+ induced lipid peroxidation inhibitor

적응증 Portal vein thrombosis / CMV esophageal hiatal hernia

적응증예

Portal vein thrombosis

➡ portal vein endothelium: cytomegalovirus infection
➡ cytomegalovirus replication: superoxide ↑
➡ portal vein endothelium: Cu2+ induced lopid peroxidation
➡ portal vein endothelium: apoptosis

처방예

旋覆花湯: Portal vein thrombosis (간문맥 혈전증)
旋覆花代赭石湯: CMV esophageal hiatal hernia (사이토메가로바이러스 식도열공헤르니아)

REFERENCE

1. Roberto Can-Aké,1 Gilda Erosa-Rejón,[1] Filogonio May-Pat,2 Luis M. Peña-Rodríguez,[1] and Sergio R. Peraza-Sánchez[1*]. Bioactive Terpenoids from Roots and Leaves of Jatropha gaumeri. Rev. Soc. Quím. Méx. 2004, 48, 11-14.

2. Soo Jung Kim a,b, Thomas K. Varghese a,b, Zheng Zhang a,b, Lee C. Zh aob, Gail Thomas a,b, Mary Hummel a,b,c,† and Michael Abecassis a,b,c,*,†. Renal Ischem ia/ Reperfusion Injury Activates the Enhancer Domain of the Human Cytomegalovirus major Immediate Early Promoter. American Journal of Transplantation, Volume 5 Issue 7, Pages 1606 - 1613.

세신 (細辛)

생약명 ASARI HERBA CUM RADICE

자원 마두령과 (쥐방울덩굴과)에 속한 다년생 초본인 족도리 또는 북세신, 한성세신의 전초와 뿌리

성분 eugenol

약리 met-hemoglobin reducer

약리 해설 erythrocyte membrane: complement fixation & osmotic pressure
➡ erythrocyte membrane injury
➡ met-hemoglobin reductase ↓
➡ hemoglobin ferrous (Fe^{2+}) ▶ ferric (Fe^{3+})

➡ met-hemoglobin 형성

효능 met-hemoglobinaemia

적응증 Autoimmune hemolytic anemia / 처방예 참고

처방예

當歸四逆湯: Autoimmune hemolytic anemia (자가면역 용혈성빈혈)
當歸四逆加吳茱萸生薑湯: Autoimmune hemolytic anemia-mediated pancreatitis (자가면역 용혈성빈혈-매개 췌장염)
麻黃附子細辛湯: Early autoimmune response for erythrocyte
茯苓五味乾薑細辛湯 : Chronic left heart failure-mediated alveolar-capillary barrier damage (만성좌심부전-매개 폐포-모세혈관 장벽 손상)

REFERENCE

1. Benevolent Orighomisan Atolaiye[1*], Matthew Ayorinde Adebayo[2], Ogo-Oluwa Oluwatoyin Jagha[3], Adebisi Olonisakin[1] and Comfort Ogenyi Agbo[1]. Evaluation of the potency of certain substances as antioxidants in the assessment of red cell viability. Journal of Medicinal Plants Research Vol. 3(6), pp. 485-4 92, June,2009

2. K. A. Naidu. Eugenol — an inhibitor of lipoxygenase-dependent lipid peroxidation Prostaglandins, Leukotrienes and Essential Fatty Acids, Volume 53, Issue 5, November 1995, Pages 381-383.

3. Xin G.; Kumaravelu P.; Subramaniyam S.; Dakshinamoorthy D.P.; Devaraj N.S.1. . The antioxidant effect of eugenol on CCl4-induced erythrocyte damage in rats. Journal of Nutritional Biochemistry, Volume 7, Number 1, January 1996,pp 23-28

소엽 (蘇葉)

생약명 PERILLAE FOLIUM

자원 순형과의 일년초인 차조기나 주름차조기의 잎

성분 linoleic acid

약리 추측 estrogen receptor alpha (ERα) agonist

효능 Activation of squamous cell division

적응증 Inferior pharyngeal stenosis in Behcet's Disease (베체트 하인두 협착증)

➡ streptococcus infection
➡ streptococcus surface protein & 하인두 정맥 epithelium
➡ molecular mimicry
➡ antibody-dependent cell-mediated cytotoxicity: macrophage 유도
➡ 하인두 정맥 epithelium: vasculitis
➡ vein occlusion
➡ angiogenesis
➡ 신생혈관 출혈
➡ inferior pharynx squamous cell: necrosis
➡ inferior pharyngeal stenosis

처방예

半夏厚朴湯: Inferior pharyngeal stenosis in Behcet's Disease (베체트 하인두 협착증)

REFERENCE

Rémy Le Guévela, †, ‡, Frédérik Ogera, ‡, Aurélien Lecorgneb, Zuzana Dudasovac, Soizic Chevanceb, Arnaud Bondond, Peter Barathc, Gérard Simonneauxb and Gilles Salberta,. Identification of small molecule regulators of the nuclear receptor HNF4α based on naphthofuran scaffolds. Bioorganic & Medicinal Chemistry Volume 17, Issu e 19, 1 October 2009, Pages 7021-7030.

수질 (水蛭)

학명 Hirudo nipponica Whitman

자원 거머리 말린 것

성분 hirudin

약리 Thrombolytic activator

약리 해설 hirudin C-terminus ➡ thrombin 부착 ➡ thrombolysis

효능 Lysis of Thrombi-fibrin complex

적응증 Kaposis sarcoma / Endometrioma / Endometrial adenocarcinoma

적응증예

Kaposis sarcoma

➡ lymphatic endothelium: Human herpesvirus 8 (HHV8) infection
➡ HHV8 infected endothelium: hyperplasia
➡ peritumoral & intratumoral angiogenesis
➡ hyperplasia endothelium: erythrocyte 유입
➡ spindle cell 형성
➡ spindle cell: tyrosine kinase domain 활성화
➡ spindle cell: proliferation
➡ Kaposi's sarcoma 형성
➡ migration
➡ 이동 조직: skin / mouth / respiratory tract / gastrointestinal tract
➡ Kaposi's sarcoma: lysis
➡ hemorrhagic patches
➡ 합병증: obstruction / organ perforation / sepsis

처방예

大黃䗪虫丸: Kaposis sarcoma (카포시 육종)
抵當湯: Endometrioma (자궁내막종)

抵當丸: Endometrial adenocarcinoma (자궁내막선종)

REFERENCE

1. XIUDONG WANG [1]; GUANGMAN ZHANG [2]; LISHENGWANG [1]; QINGLIN ZHANG [1]; YIDE QIN [2]; CHUTSE WU [1]; AIPING YU [1];. A fusion protein with improved thrombolytic effect and low bleeding risk. Thrombosis and haemostasis, 2009, vol. 102, no6, pp. 1194-1203.

2. K. Rübsamen, V. Eschenfelder. Effect of Recombinant Hirudin (LU 52369) on Reocclusion Rates after Thrombolysis in Rabbits. Haemostasis 1991;21 (Suppl. 1):93-98.

3. Andreas Greinacher, MD; Norbert Lubenow, MD. Recombinant Hirudin in Clinical Practice. Circulation. 2001;103:1479.

시호 (柴胡)

생약명 BUPLEURI RADIX

자원 산형과에 속하는 다년생 초본인 시호의 건조한 뿌리

성분 saikosaponin

약리 추측 small interfering RNA (siRNA) (+) modulator

효능 Inhibition of Hepatitis virus RNA replication

효능 해설 hepatitis A virus ▶ RNA polymerase / hepatitis B virus ▶ RNA Polymerase II / hepatitis C virus ▶ RNA-dependent RNA polymerase ▶ virus replicon RNAs 생성
➡ small interfering RNAs (siRNA)

➡ virus replicon RNAs: cleavage

적응증 Viral hepatitis (type A,B) / Type B hepatitis-mediated immune complex disease / Type C hepatitis / Cirrhosis / Hepatocellular carcinoma / Hashimoto's thyroiditis

적응증예

Viral hepatitis (type A,B)

Type A hepatitis

➡ contaminated water & food: digestion
➡ intestinal endothelium : hepatitis A virus (HAV) infection
➡ HAV virion 성숙
➡ intestinal lumen: 방출
➡ portal vein endothelium: 침투
➡ Kupffer cells: HAV infection
➡ phagocytosis & respiratory burst
➡ extracellular: peroxynitrite ($ONOO^-$) ↑
➡ hepatitis &
➡ hepatocyte: HAV infection
➡ RNA polymerase
➡ virus replicon RNAs 생성
➡ hepatocyte: viral antigen 발현
➡ cytotoxic T cell 유도
➡ hepatitis

Type B hepatitis

➡ blood & body fluid: transmission
➡ Kupffer cells: HBV infection
➡ phagocytosis & respiratory burst
➡ extracellular: peroxynitrite ($ONOO^-$) ↑
➡ hepatitis &
➡ hepatocyte: hepatitis B virus (HBV) infection
➡ RNA Polymerase II
➡ virus replicon RNAs 생성
➡ hepatocyte: viral antigen 발현
➡ cytotoxic T cell 유도
➡ hepatitis

처방예

小柴胡湯: Viral hepatitis (type A, B) (바이러스성 간염)
柴胡桂枝湯: Type B hepatitis-mediated immune complex disease
柴胡加芒硝湯: Type C hepatitis (C형 간염)
柴胡加龍骨牡蠣湯: Viral fulminant hepatitis (바이러스성 전격성간염)
柴胡桂枝乾薑湯: Liver cirrhosis (간경변)
大柴胡湯: Hepatocellular carcinoma (간암)
四逆散: Hashimoto's thyroiditis (하시모토 갑상선염)

REFERENCE

1. Kusov Y, Kanda T, Palmenberg A, Sgro JY, Gauss-Müller V. Silencing of hepatitis A virus infection by small interfering RNAs. J Virol. 2006 Jun;80(11): 5599-610.

2. McCaffrey, Anton P.[1] RNA Interference Inhibitors of Hepatitis B Virus. Annals of the New York Academy of Sciences, Volume 1175, Number 1, September 2009, pp. 15-23(9).

3. Kapadia, Sharookh B,; Brideau-Andersen, Amy; Chisari, Francis V. Interference of hepatitis C virus RNA replication by short interfering RNAs. Proceedings of the National Academy of Science, vol. 100, Issue 4, p.2014-2018.

신강 (新絳)

생약명 RUBIAE RADIX

자원 꼭두서니과에 속하는 꼭두서니 및 동속 근록식물의 뿌리 = 茜根

성분 alizarin

약리 추측 Inhibition of Vein smooth muscle cell proliferation

적응증 Portal vein thrombosis

적응증예

Portal vein thrombosis

➡ portal vein endothelium: cytomegalovirus infection
➡ cytomegalovirus replication: superoxide ↑
➡ portal vein endothelium: Cu2+ induced peroxidation
➡ portal vein endothelium: apoptosis
➡ tissue factor 분비
➡ thrombin formation
➡ fibrin formation
➡ fibrin: smooth muscle cell 이동 & 증식
➡ vein wall: stiffness
➡ portal vein: outflow block

처방예

旋覆花湯: Portal vein thrombosis (간문맥 혈전증)

REFERENCE

Susie A. Steitz, Mei Y. Speer, Gabrielle Curinga, Hsueh-Ying Yang, Paul Haynes, Ruedi Aebersold, Thorsten Schinke, Gerard Karsenty, Cecilia M. Giachelli. Smooth Muscle Cell Phenotypic Transition Associated With Calcification: Upregulation of Cbfa1 and Downregulation of Smooth Muscle Lineage Markers. Circulation Research. 2001;89:1147.

아교 (阿膠)

생약명 ASINI GELATINUM

자원 말과에 속하는 동물인 당나귀의 가죽껍질을 끓여서 가공한 농축물질
성분 Glycine / Proline / Hydroxyproline / Alanine / 기타 아미노산

약리 Collagen biosynthesis

적응증 Uterine Bleeding / Postpartum Crohn's disease / Bacterial endocarditis

적응증예

Bacterial endocarditis

➡ bacteria infection: Streptococci / Staphylococci
➡ bacteremia
➡ heart endocardium valve: Streptococci / Staphylococci infection
➡ heart valve (주로, mitral valve): bacteria colony 형성
➡ Streptococci / Staphylococci 대사 ↑: superoxide ↑
➡ macrophage: Streptococci / Staphylococci 식균 ▶ NO 증가
➡ extracellular peroxynitrite ($ONOO^-$) 생성
➡ valve collagen: destruction
➡ valvulitis

처방예

膠艾湯: Uterine Bleeding (자궁출혈)
白頭翁加甘草阿膠湯: Postpartum Crohn's disease (산후 크론병)
黃連阿膠湯: Bacterial endocarditis (세균성 심내막염)

REFERENCE

W. A. Schroeder, Lois M. Kay, Joann LeGette, Lewis Honnen, F. Charlotte Green. The Constitution of Gelatin. Separation and Estimation of Peptides in Partial Hydrolysates. J. Am. Chem. Soc., 1954, 76 (13), pp 3556-3564.

애엽 (艾葉)

생약명 ARTEMISIAE ARGI FOLIUM

자원 국화과에 속하는 다년생 초본인 황해쑥 및 들쑥을 건조한 것

성분 cineol

약리 vasoconstriction

적응증 Uterine bleeding / Esophageal varices bleeding

적응증예

Esophageal varices bleeding

➡ liver cirrhosis
➡ portal hypertension
➡ esophageal veins: congestion
➡ 식도 모세혈관 내피: 허혈
➡ 식도 모세혈관 내피: selectin 발현
➡ neutrophil 유도
➡ neutrophil degranulation
➡ esophageal varices bleeding

처방예

膠艾湯: Uterine bleeding (자궁출혈)
栢葉湯: Esophageal varices bleeding (식도 정맥류 출혈)

REFERENCE

Lee, T. H., G. J. Wang, C. K. Lee, Y. H. Kuo and *Chou. C. H. 2002. Inhibitory effects of glycosides from the leaves of Melaleuca quinquenervia on vas cular contraction of rats. Planta Medica 68: 492-496.

연교 (連翹)

생약명 FORSYTHIAE FRUCTUS

자원 목서과에 속하는 낙엽관목인 개나리와 의성개나리 및 당개나리의 과실

성분 forsythiaside

약리 추측 B-cell CD20 blocker

적응증 Warm autoantibody-mediated hemolytic anemia
➡ bone marrow B-cell: Epstein-Barr virus infection
➡ Myeloid DCs: IL-12 분비
➡ natural killer cell 유도
➡ natural killer cell: IFN-γ 분비
➡ B-cell proliferation
➡ NKc-generated hydroxyl radical 유출
➡ B-cell: mutation
➡ B-cell: malignant proliferation
➡ B-cell lymphoproliferative disorders
➡ bone marrow: acidity ↓ ▶ bone marrow injury
➡ B-cell CD20: antigen binding
➡ warm & cold autoantibody 분비
➡ erythrocyte: warm autoantibody (IgG) 부착
➡ spleen macrophage FcR: IgG Fc region 부착
➡ IgG coated erythrocyte: macrophage phagocytosis
➡ hemolysis ↑

처방예

麻黃連翹赤小豆湯: Warm autoantibody-mediated hemolytic anemia
(온난자가항체-매개 용혈성빈혈)

오미자 (五味子)

생약명 SCHIZANDRAE FRUCTUS

자원 목련과에 속한 낙엽 목질등목인 오미자 또는 화 중오미자의 성숙한 과실

성분 schizandrin

약리 acetylcholinesterase inhibitor

효능 Inhibition of muscle fiber acetylcholinesterase
➡ acetylcholine 작용 지속
➡ 근수축 강화

적응증 Viral pneumonia / Emphysema / 처방예

적응증예

Emphysema

➡ lobule (폐소엽) bronchiol epithelium: chronic infection
➡ dendritic cell: antigen 제시
➡ immature T cell: T-helper type 2 (Th2) cells 분화
➡ Th2 cells: chemokine 분비
➡ eosinophil 유도
➡ bronchiolitis
➡ Th2 cells: CXCR3 분비
➡ neutrophil 유도
➡ neutrophil degranulation
➡ 폐포 간질: chronic inflammation
➡ alveolitis
➡ emphysema
➡ alveolar-capillary gas exchange ↓

처방예

小青龍湯: Viral pneumonia (바이러스성 폐렴)
桂苓五味甘草湯: Pneumonia-mediated hypoxemia (폐렴합병증-매개 저산소혈증)

桂苓五味甘草去桂加薑辛夏湯: Chronic left heart failure-mediated alveolar-capillary barrier damage (만성좌심부전-매개 폐포-모세혈관 장벽 손상)

苓甘五味加薑辛半夏杏仁湯: Chronic left heart failure-mediated alveolitis (만성좌심부전-매개 폐포염))

苓甘五味加薑辛半杏大黃湯: Chronic left heart failure-mediated alveolar carcinoma (만성좌심부전-매개 폐포암)

厚朴麻黃湯: Emphysema (폐기종)

REFERENCE

1. EMOTO MASATAKA, TOGO HIDEYUKI, MIYAZAWA MITSUO. Inhibition of acetylcholinesterase(AChE) activity by Schisandra chinensis. Nippon Kagakkai Koen Yokoshu, VOL.78th;NO.2;PAGE.1327(2000).

2. Hung TM, Na M, Min BS, Ngoc TM, Lee I, Zhang X, Bae K. Acetylcholinesterase inhibitory effect of lignans isolated from Schizandra chinensis. Arch Pharm Res. 2007; 30(6):685-90

오수유 (吳茱萸)

생약명 Evodia rutaecarpa (Juss) Benth

자원 운향과(Rutaceae)식물인 오수유의 미성숙 과실

성분 evodiamine

약리 low-affinity Cholecystokinin (CCK) Rc blocker

적응증 Pancreatitis / Autoimmune hemolytic anemia-mediated pancreatitis / Tuberculous endometritis

적응증예

Pancreatitis

➡ gallstone / autoimmune pancreatitis / virus infection
➡ 췌장 선방세포의 직접적 손상 또는 췌관 손상
➡ 췌장 선방세포내 산성화
➡ low-affinity Cholecystokinine (CCK) receptor 자극
➡ protein kinase C 활성화
➡ 선방세포 vacuole: pro-enzyme 활성화
➡ 산성화 조건: 췌장 선방세포내 공포 깨짐
➡ pro-enzyme: 세포질로 방출
➡ 선방세포 자가분해됨
➡ pancreatitis

처방예

吳茱萸湯: Pancreatitis (췌장염)
當歸四逆加吳茱萸生薑湯: Autoimmune hemolytic anemia-mediated pancreatitis (자가면역 용혈성빈혈-매개 췌장염)
溫經湯: Tuberculous endometritis (결핵성 자궁내막염)

REFERENCE

Wu CL, Hung CR, Chang FY, Lin LC, Pau KY, Wang PS. Effects of evodiamine on gastrointestinal motility in male rats. Eur J Pharmacol. 2002 Dec20;457(2-3):169-76.

왕불류행 (王不留行)

생약명 VACCARIAE SEMEN

자원 석죽과(패랭이꽃과)에 속하는 일년생 혹은 이년생 초본인 맥람채의 성숙한 종자

성분 vaccaroside

약리 추측 Anti-Clostridium tetani

적응증 Tetanus

➡ rusty metal: wound
➡ Clostridium tetani infection
➡ lymphatic system & blood 재배치
➡ Clostridium tetani: tetanospasmin 분비
➡ peripheral motor neurons: tetanospasmin infection
➡ retro-axonal transport
➡ spinal cord interneuron: infection
➡ tetanospasmin A chain: proteolytic activity
➡ synaptobrevin degrading
➡ GABA & glycine 분비 차단
➡ inhibitory impulse 중단
➡ neuromuscler junction: acethycholine 지속
➡ 근수축 지속
➡ spastic paralysis

처방예

王不留行散: Tetany (파상풍)

용골 (龍骨)

학명 Fossilia Ossis Mastodi

자원 큰 포유동물의 화석화된 뼈

성분 Calcium Carbonate (CaCO3) & Calcium Phosphate (Ca3(PO4)2)

효능 acidosis

적응증 Rapid hyponatremia / Rapid hypernatremia / Hyponatremia-mediated hypotension / Viral fulminant hepatitis

적응증예

Hyponatremia mediated hypotension

➡ 체액 손실: 위장관 / 피부 / 기관지 / 요로 / 생식기 / 출혈
➡ hypovolemic hypernatremia
➡ hypotension
➡ tissue ischemia
➡ ischemia cell
➡ NF-κB 활성화
➡ ischemia cell: inflammation
➡ lactatemia
➡ acidosis

처방예

桂枝甘草龍骨牡蠣湯: Rapid hyponatremia (급속 저나트륨혈증)
桂枝去芍藥加蜀漆牡蠣救逆湯: Rapid hypernatremia (급속 고나트륨혈증)
桂枝加龍骨牡蠣湯: Hyponatremia-mediated hypotension (저나트륨혈증-매개 저혈압)
柴胡加龍骨牡蠣湯: Viral fulminant hepatitis (바이러스성 전격성간염)

우여량 (禹餘粮)

학명 Limonite

자원 갈철광

성분 Fe_2O_3, 체내 활성 성분은 위액에 분해된 $FeCl_2$

효능 봉입체 형성한 대장 모세혈관 내피세포 apoptosis 유도

효능 해설 $FeCl_2$

➡ 소장에서 흡수되지 않고 대장으로 이동
➡ 저산소 상태의 점막하 모세혈관 내피: $FeCl_2$ 흡수 증가됨
➡ 모세혈관 내피 세포막 침착
➡ Fe^{2+}: Haber-Weiss 반응

➡ hydroxyl radicals (•OH) 생성
➡ 세포막 지질 과산화
➡ 봉입체 형성한 대장 모세혈관 내피세포: apoptosis
➡ 점막상피 허혈 개선

적응증 Cytomegalovirus inclusion colitis
➡ colon mucosa: capillary endothelial cells
➡ cytomegalovirus (CMV) replication
➡ inclusion body 형성
➡ capillary endothelial cells: giant cell
➡ 모세혈관 내강 좁아져서 점막상피에 혈류량 감소됨
➡ mucosa cell: necrosis
➡ dead mucosa cell: protein-rich fluid
➡ pus 생성
➡ 수분 흡수 ↓

처방예

赤石脂禹餘粮湯: Cytomegalovirus inclusion colitis (사이토메가로바이러스 봉입체 대장염)

운모 (雲母)

학명 MICA

자원 X2Y4~6Z8O2(OH,F)4의 화학식을 가진 층상 규산염광물, 광물 중에서 가장 쪼개짐이 완전하며 돌비늘이라고도 함

성분 sheat silicate

효능 Heat absorber

적응증 Plasmodium malariae & vivas & ovale malaria
➡ liver stage: sporozoite
➡ bloodstream stage: merozoite
➡ erythrocyte stage: ring trophozoite

➡ monocyte CD36: ring collagen 부착
➡ monocyte phagocytosis: ring-stage-infected erythrocyte
➡ ring-stage-infected erythrocyte: schizont 증식 (48~72 hours)
➡ monocyte: TNF-α 분비
➡ severe fever: 39-41℃
➡ excessive sweating: 알카리 소실
➡ 대사성 산중

처방예

蜀漆散: Plasmodium malariae & vivas & ovale malaria (사일열원충 & 삼일열원충 & 난형열원충)

REFERENCE

V. G. Zil'berberg[1], A. M. Vyal'tsev[1], N. I. Kirkun[1], V. I. Pavlenko[1] and B. V. Glebovskii[1]. Aluminum oxide electrical insulation plasma coatings for heat sinks of electronic equipment. Powder Metallurgy and Metal Ceramics, Volume 31, Number 3 / 1992:3, page 230-232.

웅황 (雄黃)

학명 Realgar

기원 단사정계(單斜晶系)에 속하는 귤홍색의 반투명한 광석

성분 이황화비소 (As2S2)

약리 toxoplasma gondii ` pyruvate kinase inhibitor

약리 해설 pyruvate kinase SH group
➡ As2S2 binding
➡ pyruvate kinase 불활성화
➡ mitochondria dysfunction

➡ toxoplasma gondii: death

적응증 Toxoplasmosis

➡ cyst 섭취: toxoplasma gondii infection

➡ tachyzoites: erythrocyte 침입

➡ erythrocyte: calcium influx ↑ ▶ protein kinase C 활성화

▶ mitochondria respiration ↑

▶ tachyzoites multiplication

처방예

升麻鱉甲湯: Toxoplasmosis (톡소플라즈마증)

REFERENCE

Carol M. Schiller, Bruce A. Fowler and James S. Woods. Pyruvate metabolism after invivo exposure to oral arsenic*1. Chemico-Biological Interactions Volume 22, Issue 1, July 1978, Pages 25-33.

원화 (芫花)

생약명 Daphnis Genkwa Flos

자원 팥꽃나무의 잎 피기 전 꽃봉오리를 따다가 말린 것

성분 genkwanin

약리 추측 Type VII collagen (+) modulator

적응증 Pleurisy (늑막염)

처방예

十棗湯: Pleural effusion (흉막 삼출)

의이인 (薏苡仁)

생약명 COICIS SEMEN

자원 벼과에 속한 일년생 또는 다년생 초본인 율무의 성숙한 종인

성분 stigmasterol

약리 추측 major histocompatibility complex (MHC) (-) modulator

적응증 Reactive arthritis / Postherpetic neuralgia / Appendix

적응증예

Reactive arthritis

➡ genital, urinary, gastrointestinal tract: bacterial infection
➡ Chlamydia trachomotis / Ureaoplasma urealyticum / Salmonella spp / Shigella spp / Yersinia spp / Campylobacter spp
➡ bacteria antibody 출현
➡ joint synoviocyte: HLA-B27 (MHC class I allele) 발현
➡ molecular mimic response
➡ HLA-B27: bacteria antibody 부착
➡ antibody-dependent cellular cytotoxicity
➡ Natural killer cell (NKc) 유도
➡ NKc: TRAIL-dependent secretion
➡ synovitis

처방예

麻杏薏甘湯: Reactive arthritis (반응성 관절염)
薏苡附子散: Postherpetic neuralgia (대상포진후 신경통)
薏苡附子敗將散: Appendicitis (충수염)

이근백피 (李根白皮)

생약명 Pruni Radicii Cortex

자원 자두나무 뿌리의 백피

성분 potassium citrate

약리 extracellular Ca2+ influx inhibitor

적응증 Epinephrine-mediated encephalopathy

처방예

奔豚湯: Epinephrine-mediated encephalopathy (에피네프린-매개 뇌병증)

REFERENCE

M Bonilla, KW Cunningham. Calcium release and influx in yeast: TRPC and VGCC rule another kingdom. Sci STKE (2002) 2002: PE17.

인삼 (人蔘)

생약명 GINSENG RADIX

자원 두릅나무과에 속하는 여러해살이풀인 인삼의 뿌리

성분 panax ginsenoside

약리 Transforming growth factor beta (TGF-β) (+) modulator

효능 Activation of cell proliferation & development / Antiproliferation of oncogenesis cell

적응증 Gastric ulcer / Duodenal ulcer / pulmonary tuberculosis / Left heart failure-mediated pleural effusion / Coxsackie B4 virus mediated Type 1 diabetes / Viral hepatitis (type A, B) / Type C hepatitis / Viral fulminant hepatitis / Pancreatitis / Multiple sclerosis / Pancreatic ductal adenocarcinoma / 처방예 참고

적응증예

Duodenal ulcer

➡ Chronic gastric ulcer
➡ 유문부 D cell 손상
➡ somatostatin ↓
➡ gastrin ↑ : 위산 분비 ↑
➡ 십이지장: 위산에 노출됨
➡ 십이지장 상피: 위산 & 펩신 자극
➡ 십이지장 상피세포의 위상피화
➡ 십이지장: Helicobacter pylori 정착
➡ Helicobacter pylori: 병원성 균으로 형질전환
➡ H. pylori peptidoglycan: type IV secretion system 형성
➡ peptidoglycan: macrophage 유도
➡ extracellular peroxynitrite ($ONOO^-$): 상피세포 손상
➡ Helicobacter pylori: CagE gene
➡ epithelial cell: IL-8 분비
➡ neutrophil 유도
➡ neutrophil degranulation
➡ 점막세포 손상
➡ duodenal ulcer

처방예

半夏瀉心湯: Gastric ulcer (위궤양)
生薑瀉心湯: Duodenal ulcer (십이지장궤양)
甘草瀉心湯: Peptic ulcer-complicated perforation (소화성궤양에 합병된 천공)
大半夏湯: Pyloric stenosis in Behcet's Disease (베체트 유문협착증)
茯苓飮方: Aortic aneurysm in Behcet's Disease (베체트 대동맥류)
麥門冬湯: Pulmonary tuberculosis (폐결핵)
竹葉石膏湯: Secondary tuberculosis (이차성결핵)
溫經湯: Tuberculous endometritis (결핵성 자궁내막염)
木防己去石膏加茯苓芒硝湯: Left heart failure-mediated pleural effusion

(좌심부전-매개 흉막삼출)

木防己湯: Left heart failure-mediated pulmonary venous congestion
(좌심부전-매개 폐정맥 울혈)

白虎加人蔘湯: Coxsackie B4 virus mediated Type 1 diabetes

小柴胡湯: Viral hepatitis (type A,B) (바이러스성 간염)

柴胡桂枝湯: Type B hepatitis-mediated immune complex disease

柴胡加芒硝湯: Type C hepatitis (C형 간염)

柴胡加龍骨牡蠣湯: Viral fulminant hepatitis (바이러스성 전격성간염)

黃連湯: Group A streptococcus (GAS) infection (그룹 A 연쇄상구균감염증)

乾薑黃連黃芩人蔘湯: Staphylococcal food poisoning (포도구균 식 중독)

六物黃芩湯: Pathogenic E. coli infection

大健中湯: Intussusception (장 중첩)

乾薑人蔘半夏丸: Cytomegalovirus-mediated placental villitis (태반 융모세포염)

吳茱萸湯: Pancreatitis (췌장염)

當歸四逆加吳茱萸生薑湯: Autoimmune hemolytic anemia-mediated pancreatitis
(자가면역 용혈성빈혈-매개 췌장염)

橘皮竹茹湯: Multiple sclerosis (다발성경화증)

附子湯: p-ANCA associated vasculitis (핵주위 항호중구 세포질 항체-매개 혈관염)

茯苓四逆湯: Viral myocarditis (바이러스성 심근염)

四逆加人蔘湯: Polymyositis-associated gastrointestinal myositis
(다발성근염에 연관된 위장관근염)

厚朴生薑半夏甘草人參湯: Pancreatic ductal adenocarcinoma (췌장암)

REFERENCE

1. 김성우, 정지헌, 조병기. 인삼유래 Ginsenoside Rg3에 의한 항-주름 효과. 대한화장품학회, 제30권 제2호, 2004, 221-225.

2. Hao Y, Wang P, Wu J, Qiu QY. Effects of ginsenoside and berberine on secretion of immunosuppressive cytokines in lung carcinoma cell line PG. J Chin Integr Med / Zhong Xi Yi Jie He Xue Bao. 2008; 6(3): 278-282.

3. TetsutoKanzaki[1], NobuhiroMorisaki[1], RitsukoShiina[1] & YasushiSaito[1]. Role of transforming growth factor-β pathway in the mechanism of wound healing by saponin from Ginseng Radix rubra. British Journal of Pharmacology, (1998) 125, 255−262.

4. Tascilar M, Skinner HG, Rosty C, Sohn T, Wilentz RE, Offerhaus GJ, Adsay V, Abrams RA, Cameron JL, Kern SE, Yeo CJ, Hruban RH, Goggins M. The SMAD4 protein and prognosis of pancreatic ductal adenocarcinoma. Clin Cancer Res, 2001 Dec;(12):3853-6.

5. I Abiatari, J Kleeff, J Li, K Felix, M W Büchler, H Friess. Hsulf-1 regulates growth and invasion of pancreatic cancer cells. J Clin Pathol2006;59:1052-1058.

인진호 (茵蔯蒿)

생약명 ARTEMISIAE CAPILLARIS HERBA

자원 국화과에 속하는 여러해살이 풀인 생당쑥의 전초를 말린 것

성분 capillarisin

약리 추측 Chenodeoxycholic acid (CDCA) detoxicant

효능 Inhibition of CDCA-mediated hepatocyte apoptosis

적응증 Intrahepatic cholangiocarcinoma / Free bile acids-mediated glomerulonephritis

적응증예

Intrahepatic cholangiocarcinoma

➡ HBV, HCV: chronic cholangiocyte infection
➡ intrahepatic cholangitis
➡ cholangiocyte: adenomatous hyperplasia
➡ chlangiocarcinoma
➡ intrahepatic bile duct: obstruction
➡ hepatocyte: chenodeoxycholic acid (CDCA) 축적
➡ CDCA: hydrophilic group 독성
➡ ROS 발생

➡ GSH 고갈
➡ mitochondria dysfunction
➡ hepatocyte apoptosis

처방예

茵蔯蒿湯: Intrahepatic cholangiocarcinoma (간내담도암)
茵蔯五苓散: Free bile acids-mediated glomerulonephritis (자유담즙산-매개 신사구체신염)

자삼 (紫參)

학명 Porygonum bistorta L.

자원 마디풀과에 속하는 범꼬리의 뿌리 줄기

성분 gallic acid

약리 Mucus astringent

적응증 RSV (respiratory syncytial virus) bronchiolitis

처방예

澤漆湯: RSV (respiratory syncytial virus) bronchiolitis (호흡기 세포융합 바이러스 세기관지염)

자석영 (紫石英)

학명 Amethyst

자원 자주색의 수정

성분 CaF2 (플루오르화칼슘)

약리 phosphate binder

효능 Inhibition of phosphate-activated glutaminase
➡ glutamate 합성 억제

적응증 Epilepsy

처방예

風引湯: Epilepsy (뇌전증)

REFERENCE

B Antonny and M Chabre. Characterization of the aluminum and beryllium fluoride species which activate transducin. Analysis of the binding and dissociation kinetics. The Journal of Biological Chemistry, April 5, 1992, 267, 6710-6718.

자위 (紫葳)

생약명 Campsitis Flos

자원 꿀풀목 능소화의 줄기 잎

성분 campenoside

약리 추측 Plasmodium falciparum FabI blocker

효능 Inhibition of P. falciparum fatty acid synthesis

적응증 Plasmodium falciparum malaria

처방예

鱉甲煎丸: Plasmodium falciparum malaria (열대열원충 말라리아)

자충 (蟅虫)

학명 EUPOLYPHAGA SINENSIS WALKER (ESW), 별렴과에 속하는 흙바퀴의 암컷 충체

성분 ESW extraction

약리 추측 Erythrocyte C3b receptor (+) modulator

효능 hematoma 제거

적응증 Kaposis sarcoma / Placenta accreta

처방예

大黃蟅虫丸: Kaposis sarcoma (카포시 육종)
下瘀血湯: Placenta accreta (태반유착)

REFERENCE

Yang YF, Wang SQ, Feng MJ, Ning AH, Huang CH. Effects of Eupolyphaga Sinensis Walker on erythrocyte's CR1 activity and anti-cardiolipin antibody level in rats with stagnation of blood. Xi Bao Yu Fen Zi Mian Yi Xue Za Zhi. 2005 Jan;21(1):53-6.

작약 (芍藥)

생약명 PAEONIAE RADIX ALBA

자원 미나리아재비과에 속한 다년생 초본인 작약의 뿌리

성분 paeoniflorin

약리 superoxide scavenger

효능 Inhibition of superoxide-mediated cytotoxicity / Inhibition of ischemia-reperfusion cytotoxicity

적응증 Common cold / Uterine myoma / Colon cancer / 처방예 참고

적응증예

Common cold

➡ skeleton muscle cell
➡ 지속적인 ATP생산
➡ mitochondrial respiration 반복: superoxide 축적
➡ superoxide dismutase2 고갈
➡ superoxide: Fe^{3+}(ferric ions) ▶ Fe^{2+}(ferrous ion) 환원
➡ mitochondria: ferrous ion-induced lipid peroxidation
➡ mitochondria membrane potential damage
➡ ATP 생산 감소

Ischemia-reperfusion cytotoxicity

➡ xanthine oxidase: superoxide 축적
➡ superoxide dismutase1 고갈
➡ superoxide: Fe^{3+}(ferric ions) ▶ Fe^{2+}(ferrous ion) 환원
➡ lipid membrane: ferrous ion-induced peroxidation
➡ Na^+/ K^+ pump activity 감소
➡ 세포부종 & 세포손상

처방예

桂枝湯: Common cold
桂枝茯苓丸: Uterine myoma (자궁근종)
麻子仁丸: Colon cancer (대장암)
當歸芍藥散: Pregnancy hypertention (임신고혈압)
當歸散: Pregnancy essential supplements (임신 필수보충제)
當歸建中湯: Postpartum hypotension (산후저혈압)
當歸四逆湯: Autoimmune hemolytic anemia (자가면역 용혈성빈혈)
當歸四逆加吳茱萸生薑湯: Autoimmune hemolytic anemia-mediated pancreatitis (자가면역 용혈성빈혈-매개 췌장염)
芍藥甘草附子湯: Human T-Lymphotropic Virus (HTLV) infection
芍藥甘草湯: Inclusion body myositis (봉입체근염)
黄芩湯: Cholera

黃芩加半夏生薑湯: Salmonella typhi

REFERENCE

Hsieh CL, Cheng CY, Tsai TH, Lin IH, Liu CH, Chiang SY, Lin JG, Lao CJ, Tang NY. Paeonol reduced cerebral infarction involving the superoxide anion and microglia activation in ischemia-reperfusion injured rats. J Ethnopharmacol. 2006 Jun 30;106(2):208-15. Epub 2006 Feb 3.

재백피 (梓白皮)

학명 Catalpa ovata G. Don

자원 개오동 나무의 근피 또는 수피

성분 β-lapachone

약리 AMPK phosphorylation activator

약리 해설 AMPK phosphorylation

➡ AKT/mTOR pathway inhibition

➡ B-cell: malignant proliferation 억제

적응증 Warm autoantibody-mediated hemolytic anemia

➡ bone marrow B-cell: Epstein-Barr virus infection

➡ Myeloid DCs: IL-12 분비

➡ natural killer cell 유도

➡ natural killer cell: IFN-γ 분비

➡ B-cell proliferation

➡ NKc-generated hydroxyl radical 유출

➡ B-cell: mutation

➡ B-cell: malignant proliferation

➡ B-cell CD20: antigen binding

➡ warm & cold autoantibody 분비

처방예

麻黃連翹赤小豆湯: Warm autoantibody-mediated hemolytic anemia
(온난자가항체-매개 용혈성빈혈)

REFERENCE

Bae JH, Kim JW, Kweon GR, Park MG, Jeong KH, Kim JJ, Moon DG. Corpus Cavernosal Smooth Muscle Relaxation Effect of a Novel AMPK Activator, Beta-Lapachone. J Sex Med. 2010 May 11.

저령 (猪苓)

생약명 POLYPORUS

자원 구멍쟁이버섯과에 속한 진균인 저령의 균핵

성분 ergosterol

약리 Mesangial cell proliferation inhibitor

적응증 Immune complex-mediated glomerulonephritis / Free bile acids-mediated glomerulonephritis / Anti-GBM glomerulonephritis / IgA nephropathy

적응증예

Immune complex-mediated glomerulonephritis

➡ glomerulus: Immune complex 침착
➡ mesangial cell: phagocytosis
➡ mesangial cell: IL-1 분비
➡ glomerulus endothelial cell: VCAM-1 발현
➡ monocyte 유도

➡ 사구체 내피세포 손상
➡ 수출소동맥 저산소증
➡ 수출소동맥 수축
➡ 사구체 손상
➡ monocyte: mesangial cell growth factor 분비
➡ mesangial cell proliferation

처방예

五苓散: Immune complex-mediated glomerulonephritis (면역복합체-매개 사구체신염)
茵蔯五苓散: Free bile acids-mediated glomerulonephritis(자유담즙산-매개 사구체신염)
豬苓湯: Anti-GBM glomerulonephritis (항-기저막 사구체신염)
豬苓散: IgA nephropathy (IgA 신병증)

REFERENCE

Ching-Yuang Lin, Fu-Mei Ku, Yuh-Chi Kuo, Chieh-Fu Chen, Wei-Perng Chen, AnnChen, Ming-Shi Shiao. Inhibition of activated human mesangial cell proliferation by the natural product of Cordyceps sinensis (H1-A): An implication for treatment of IgA mesangial nephropathy. Journal of Laboratory and Clinical Medicine, Volume 13 3, Issue 1, Pages 55-63.

적석지 (赤石脂)

학명 Halloysite

자원 풍화가 진행되어 K이온이 제거된 후 양이온 교환 능력이 커진 갈색 점토 광물

성분 Al_2O_3, $2SiO_2 \cdot 4H_2O$

약리 Cation absorbent

적응증 Cytomegalovirus inclusion colitis / Epilepsy

적응증예

Cytomegalovirus inclusion colitis

➡ colon mucosa: capillary endothelial cells
➡ cytomegalovirus (CMV) replication
➡ inclusion body 형성
➡ capillary endothelial cells: giant cell
➡ 모세혈관 내강 좁아져서 점막상피에 혈류량 감소됨
➡ mucosa cell: necrosis
➡ dead mucosa cell: protein-rich fluid
➡ pus 생성
➡ 수분 흡수 불량

처방예

赤石脂禹餘粮湯: Cytomegalovirus inclusion colitis (사이토메가로바이러스 봉입체대장염)
風引湯: Epilepsy (뇌전증)

REFERENCE

O. Abollino[1], A. Giacomino[1], M. Malandrino[1] and E. Mentasti[1]. The Efficiency of Vermiculite as Natural Sorbent for Heavy Metals. Application to a Contaminated Soil . Water, Air, & Soil Pollution, Volume 181, Numbers 1-4 / 2007:5, page 149-160.

적소두 (赤小豆)

생약명 PHASEOLI SEMEN

자원 콩과에 속하는 덩굴팥, 팥의 성숙한 종자

성분 albumin

약리 추측 immunoglobulin Fc region binder

효능 Inhibition of IgG Fc region & erythrocyte FcR binding / Inhibition of IgG Fc region & complement

적응증 Warm autoantibody-mediated hemolytic anemia / Polyclonal IgM cold agglutinins-mediated hemolytic anemia

적응증예

Polyclonal IgM cold agglutinins-mediated hemolytic anemia

➡ bone marrow B-cell: Epstein-Barr virus infection
➡ Myeloid DCs: IL-12 분비
➡ natural killer cell 유도
➡ natural killer cell: IFN-γ 분비
➡ B-cell proliferation
➡ NKc-generated hydroxyl radical 유출
➡ B-cell: malignant proliferation
➡ bone marrow: acidity ▶ bone marrow injury
➡ B-cell CD20: antigen binding
➡ warm & cold autoantibody 분비
➡ erythrocyte FcR: warm autoantibody (IgG) 부착
➡ IgG coated erythrocyte: macrophage phagocytosis
➡ hemolysis

처방예

麻黃蓮軺赤小豆湯: Warm autoantibody-mediated hemolytic anemia
(온난자가항체-매개 용혈성빈혈)
赤豆當歸散: Polyclonal IgM cold agglutinins-mediated hemolytic anemia
(다클론IgM 한냉응집소-매개 용혈성빈혈)

REFERENCE

Mark S. Dennis†§, Min Zhang†, Y. Gloria Meng¶, Miryam Kadkhodayan‖, Daniel Kirchhofer**, Dan Combs† and Lisa A. Damico†. Albumin Binding as a General Strategy for Improving the Pharmacokinetics of Proteins*. Journal of Biological Chemistry, 2002, September 20, 277, 35035-35043.

정력자 (葶藶子)

생약명 LEPIDII SEMEN

자원 배추과에 속하는 한해살이풀인 꽃다지와 다닥냉이의 여문씨를 말린 것

성분 helveticoside

약리 cardiac glycoside

약리 해설 cardiac glycoside
- ➡ myocardiocyte Na+/ K+ pumps: Na+ out ↓
- ➡ cytoplasm Ca2+ ↑
- ➡ myocardiocyte contraction ↑
- ➡ refractory period of the AV node ↑
- ➡ 심장 수축 짧고 강해짐
- ➡ 확장기 길어짐
- ➡ 대정맥을 통해 유입되는 혈액량이 증가
- ➡ 말초정맥 울혈 해소

적응증 Mesenteric lymphoma / Lung abscess

적응증예

Mesenteric lymphoma

- ➡ chronic infection
- ➡ mesenteric lymph nodes: persistent antigenic stimulation
- ➡ B cell: genetic alteration
- ➡ B cell: neoplastic transformation
- ➡ mesenteric lymphoma
- ➡ mesenteric lymphadenopathy
- ➡ 장정맥 조직액: 장간막 림프절 유입 실패
- ➡ 장정맥 울혈
- ➡ 장폐쇄

처방예

己椒藶黃丸: Mesenteric lymphoma (장간막 림프종)

葶藶大棗瀉肺湯: Lung abscess (폐농양)

REFERENCE

BABULOVA A, BURAN L, SELECKY FV. The cardiotoxic activity of helveticoside, a cardiac glycoside from Erysimum canescens Roth. Arzneimittelforschung. 1963 May; 13:412-4.

제조 (蠐螬, 굼벵이)

학명 Larva Holotrichiae

자원 딱정벌레목 풍뎅이의 유충을 말린 것

성분 fibrinolytic serine protease

약리 fibrinolysis

적응증 Kaposis`s sarcoma

➡ HHV8 infected endothelium: IL-6

➡ fibroblast: NF-κB 활성화 ▶ estrogen receptor 발현 ↑

▶ proliferation ↑

▶ fibrosarcoma cell 전환

➡ fibrosarcoma cell: fibroblast growth factor 분비

➡ spindle cell: tyrosine kinase domain 활성화

➡ spindle cell: proliferation & migration

➡ Kaposi's sarcoma 형성

➡ 이동 조직: skin / mouth / respiratory tract / gastrointestinal tract

➡ Kaposi's sarcoma: lysis

➡ hemorrhagic patches

➡ 합병증: obstruction / organ perforation / sepsis

처방예

大黃蟅虫丸: Kaposis`s sarcoma (카포시 육종)

REFERENCE

1. Kwon TH, Kim MS, Choi HW, Joo CH, Cho MY, Lee BL. A masquerade-like serine proteinase homologue is necessary for phenoloxidase activity in the coleo pteran insect, Holotrichia diomphalia larvae. Eur J Biochem. 2000 Oct;267(20):61 88-96.

2. MOON SUK KIM ; MIN JI BAEK ; MI HEE LEE ; JI WON PARK ; SO YOUNG LEE ; SÖDERHÄLL Kenneth ; BOK LUEL LEE ; A New Easter-type Serine Protease Cleaves a Masquerade-like Protein during Prophenoloxidase Activation in Holotrichia diomphalia Larvae*. THE JOURNAL OF BIOLOGICAL CHEMISTRY Vol. 277, No. 42, Issue of October 18, pp. 39999--40004, 2002.

조협 (皁莢)

생약명 GLEDITSIAE SPINA

자원 콩과에 속하는 낙엽교목인 조각자나무의 가시를 말린 것

성분 triacanthin

약리 추측 Phosphodiesterase (PDE) blocker

약리 해설 기관지 확장증

➡ 가래 축적

➡ Phosphodiesterase blocker

➡ cAMP ↑

➡ 기관지 평활근 이완

➡ 기도 확장

적응증 Bronchiectasis

처방예

皁莢丸: Bronchiectasis (기관지 확장증)

죽여 (竹茹)

생약명 BAMBUSAE CAULIS IN TAENIAM

자원 대과에 속하는 사철푸른 키나무인 참대 곧 왕대의 속껍질을 말린 것

성분 Tyrosine

약리 Dopamine / Norepinephrine / Epinephrine biosynthesis

적응증 Multiple sclerosis

➡ virus linked multiple sclerosis
: hunan herpes virus / varicella zoster virus / Epstein Barr virus / endogenous retrovirus / etc

➡ myelin oligodendrocyte glycoprotein & virus protein

➡ molecular mimicry response

➡ myelin oligodendrocyte glycoprotein: IgG & complement 부착

➡ oligodendrocyte: membrane attack complex 형성

➡ oligodendrocyte H2O2 ↑

➡ oligodendrocyte loss

➡ axon nerve: demyelination

➡ myelin plaque 생성

➡ multiple sclerosis

➡ nerve conduction disorders

➡ 주로 침범되는 부위: 시신경 / 뇌간 / 소뇌 / 척수

처방예

橘皮竹茹湯: Multiple sclerosis (다발성경화증)

REFERENCE

Totsune H, Nakano M, Inaba H. Chemiluminescence from bamboo shoot cut. Biochem Biophys Res Commun. 1993 Aug 16;194(3):1025-9.

죽엽 (竹葉)

생약명 PHYLLOSTACHYS FOLIUM

자원 벼과에 속하는 다년생 상록교목인 솜대의 잎

성분 arundoin

약리 추측 β-amyloid gene expression (-) modulator

효능 Inhibition of amyloidosis

적응증 Secondary tuberculosis / Postpartum EBV activation-mediated mononucleosis

적응증예

Secondary tuberculosis

➡ pulmonary: cavitation
➡ M. tuberculosis: reactivation
➡ systemic spread
➡ pulmonary upper lobe / peripheral lymph node / brain / heart / pancreas / kidney / thyroid / skeletal muscle / bone
➡ M. tuberculosis infected cell: MHC class II 발현
➡ cytotoxic T cell 유도
➡ perforin & granulysin 분비
➡ M. tuberculosis infected cell: Na+/ K+ pump 손상
➡ M. tuberculosis infected cell: necrosis
➡ tissue destruction

➡ amyloidosis
➡ amyloid fibrosis

처방예

竹葉石膏湯: Secondary tuberculosis (이차성 결핵)
竹葉湯: Postpartum EBV activation-mediated mononucleosis
(산후 EBV 활성화-매개 단핵구증)

지모 (知母)

생약명 ANEMARRHENAE RHIZOMA

자원 지모과에 속한 지모의 건조한 근경

성분 timosaponin

약리 추측 nestin (+) modulator

약리 해설 nestin
➡ multi-differentiation 세포에서 발현되는 단백질
➡ progenitor cell: 조직특수성 분화 유도함
➡ 분화예: β-cell / synoviocyte & chondrocyte & cartilage muscle / thyrocyte / locus coeruleus & raphe nucleus

적응증 Type 1 diabetes / Rheumatoid arthritis / Viral thyroiditis / basilar artery hemorrhage-mediated Insomnia

적응증예

Rheumatoid arthritis

➡ synovial tissue: auto-antigen 출현
➡ synovial dendritic cell: phagocytosis
➡ B cell 활성화: auto-antigen specific IgE 생산 ↑
➡ synovial mast cell FcR γ: high affinity IgE Rc

➡ mast cell: Fyn/Gab2/RhoA-signaling pathway 활성화
➡ mast cell: IL-1 & TNF-α 분비
➡ vascular endithelium: VCAM-1 발현
➡ eosinophil 유도: vasoactive amines degranulation ↑
➡ synoviocyte inflammation: IL-8 분비
➡ neutrophil 유도
➡ neutrophil elastase: hyaluronate destruction ▶ synovitis
➡ neutrophil: IL-1 분비
➡ synovial fibroblast 활성화: prostaglandin E2 분비
➡ chodrocyte: copper-zinc superoxide dismutase 소진
▶ superoxide ↑ ▶ chondrocytis & cartilage muscle: 대사 항진
▶ lactate ↑ ▶ cartilage muscle inflammation

처방예

白虎湯: IL-1 mediated Type 1 diabetes
白虎加人蔘湯: Coxsackie B4 virus-mediated Type 1 diabetes
白虎加桂枝湯: Viral thyroiditis (바이러스성 갑상선염)
酸棗仁湯: basilar artery hemorrhage-mediated Insomnia(뇌저동맥 출혈에 의한 불면증)
桂枝芍藥知母湯: Rheumatoid arthritis (류마티스 관절염)

REFERENCE

1. H.Rasmussen[1]. Pattern formation and cell interactions in epidermal development of Anemarrhena asphodeloides (Liliaceae). Nordic Journal of Botany, Volume 6 Issue4, Pages 467 - 477.

2. Rohan K. Humphrey, Nathan Bucay, Gillian M. Beattie, Ana Lopez, Conrad A.Messam, Vincenzo Cirulli, and Alberto Hayek. Characterization and Isolation of Promoter-Defined Nestin-Positive Cells from the Human Fetal Pancreas. Diabetes October 2003 52:2519-2525.

3. Michael Maleski, Susan Hockfield. Glial cells assemble hyaluronan-based pericellular matrices in vitro. Glia Volume 20 Issue 3, Pages 193 - 202.

지실 (枳實)

생약명 AURANTII IMMATURUS FRUCTUS

자원 운향과 상록교목인 산등과 탱자나무의 어린 과실

성분 auraptene

약리 matrix metalloproteinases (MMPs) blocker

효능 Inhibition of extracellular matrix degradation

적응증 Retained placenta / Hepatocellular carcinoma / Alcoholic cirrhosis / Macrophage foam cell formation / Unstable angina / Colon cancer / 처방예 참고

적응증예

Hepatocellular carcinoma

➡ chronic hepatitis B virus & hepatitis C virus infection
➡ virus replicon RNAs
➡ HBV & HCV gene: 간세포 DNA에 삽입
➡ HBV & HCV: NOS2 gene expression ↑
➡ 삽입된 HBV & HCV gene: mutation
➡ 돌연변이된 HBV & HCV gene: mutant protein 생산
➡ mutant protein: p53 binding
➡ p53 inactivation
➡ hepatocyte apoptosis & cell-growth control: 실패
➡ oncogenic hepatocyte: 출현
➡ oncogenic hepatocyte: PDGF 분비
➡ hepatic stellate cell (HSC): 활성화
➡ HSC: matrix metalloproteinases (MMP) 분비
➡ HSC: integrin 분해
➡ HSC: 기저막에서 분리
➡ HSC: oncogenic hepatocyte 쪽으로 이동
➡ HSC: hepatocyte growth factor 분비
➡ oncogenic hepatocyte: tyrosine kinase 활성화

➡ oncogenic hepatocyte: proliferation
➡ hepatocellular carcinoma

처방예

枳實芍藥散: Retained placenta (감입태반)
大柴胡湯: Hepatocellular carcinoma (간암)
梔子大黃湯: Alcoholic cirrhosis (알코올성 간경변)
枳實梔子豉湯: Macrophage foam cell formation (동맥경화증 단계 중 거품세포 생성)
梔子厚朴湯: Atheroma formation (죽종 형성)
枳實梔子大黃豉湯: Fibrous cap formation (섬유덮개 형성)
枳實薤白桂枝湯: Unstable angina (불안정형 협심증)
小承氣湯: Diffuse large B cell lymphoma of gastric MALT
(위장 점막림프조직의 미만성 B세포 림프종)
大承氣湯: Diffuse large B cell lymphoma of small intestine MALT
(소장 점막림프조직의 미만성 B세포 림프종)
厚朴七物湯: Gastrointestinal leiomyosarcoma (위장관 평활근육종)
厚朴三物湯: Adenomatous polyp (선종성 용종)
麻子仁丸: Colon cancer (대장암)

REFERENCE

1. Kawabata K, Murakami A, Ohigashi H. Auraptene decreases the activity of matrix metalloproteinases in dextran sulfate sodium-induced ulcerative colitis in ICR mice. Biosci Biotechnol Biochem, 2006 Dec;70(12):3062-5, Epub 2006 Dec 7.

2. Takuji Tanaka[2], Hiroyuki Kohno, Manabu Murakami, Seiko Kagami and Karam El-Bayoumy. Suppressing Effects of Dietary Supplementation of the Organoselenium 1,4-Phenylenebis(methylene)selenocyanate and the Citrus Antioxidant Aurapteene on Lung Metastasis of Melanoma Cells in Mice[1]. Cancer Research 60, 3713-3716, July 15, 2000.

3. Arai, Soichi; Yasuoka, Akihito; Abe, Keiko. Functional food science and food for specified health use policy in Japan: state of the art. Current Opinion in Lipidology, February 2008, Volume 19, Issue 1, p 69-73.

진피 (秦皮)

생약명 FRAXINI CORTEX

자원 물푸레나무과에 속한 물푸레나무의 가지껍질과 체간부의 껍질

성분 aesculetin

약리 NOD2 gene mutation inhibitor (in small intestinal epithelial cell)

적응증 Crohn's disease

➡ small intestine epithelial cel: Mycobacterium, other pathogenic bacteria 융합
➡ Mycobacterium, other pathogenic bacteria: unusual peptidoglycan 생성
➡ 상피세포 NOD2 gene mutation (NOD2: nucleotide-binding oligomerization domain 2)
➡ Mycobacterium, other pathogenic bacteria: 면역반응 시작됨
➡ 상피세포 NF-kB pathway
➡ macrophage 침착
➡ macrophage granuloma 형성: TNF-α
➡ 소장상피세포 / 술잔세포 / 근육층 / Mycobacterium, other pathogenic bacteria : apoptosis
➡ granulomatous colitis

처방예

白頭翁湯: Crohn's disease (크론병)

REFERENCE

1. Ewa Kupidlowska. The Effects of Two Disubstituted Coumarins on Mitosis and Respiration in Meristematic Cells. Pharmaceutical Biology 2001, Vol. 39, No. 4, Pages 273-283.

2. Wei-Jun Ding, Yun Deng, Hao Feng, Wei-Wei Liu, Rong Hu, Xiang Li, Zhe-Ming Gu, Xiao-Ping Dong. Biotransformation of aesculin by human gut bacteria and identification of its metabolites in rat urine. World J Gastroenterol 2009 March 28; 15(12): 1518-1523.

창포 (菖蒲)

생약명 ACORI GRAMINEI RHIZOMA

자원 천남성과에 속한 여러해살이풀

성분 asarone

약리 HMG-CoA reductase blocker

약리 해설 신우신염을 일으키는 병원성 세균
➡ E. coli / Enterococcus faecalis / Streptococcus
➡ HMG-CoA reductase을 이용해 증식함

효능 Antibacterial activity of E. coli / Enterococcus faecalis / Streptococcus

적응증 Pyelonephritis
➡ kidney pyelum: E. coli / Enterococcus faecalis / streptococcus infection
➡ E. coli / Enterococcus faecalis / streptococcus: HMG-CoA reductase gene 활성화
➡ isopentenyl pyrophosphate (IPP) & dimethylallyl pyrophosphate (DMAPP) 생성
➡ cholesterol biosynthesis
➡ cell growth
➡ pyelonephritis
➡ 혈장단백 유출

처방예

蒲灰散: Pyelonephritis (신우신염)

REFERENCE

1. Author:Rodriguez-Paez, L.; Juarez-Sanchez, M.; Antunez-Solis, J.; Baeza, I.; Wong, C. [alpha]-Asarone inhibits HMG-CoA reductase, lowers serum LDL-cholesterol levels and reduces biliary CSI in hypercholesterolemic rats.(cholesterol saturation index). International Journal of Phytotherapy & Phytopharmacology Article date:June 1, 2003.

2. M. Kooa, S.H. Kima, N. Leea, M.Y. Yoo, S.Y. Ryu, D.Y. Kwon and Y.S. Kim. 3-Hydroxy-3-methylglutaryl-CoA (HMG-CoA) reductase inhibitory effect of Vitisvinifera. Fitoterapia, Volume 79, Issue 3, April 2008, Pages 204-206.

3. Autumn Sutherlin,[1] Matija Hedl,1 Barbara Sanchez-Neri,[1] John W. Burgner II,[2] Cynthia V. Stauffacher,[2] and Victor W.Rodwell[1*]. Enterococcus faecalis 3-Hydroxy -3-Methylgluaryl Coenzyme A Synthase, an Enzyme of Isopentenyl Diphosphate Biosynthesis†. J Bacteriol. 2002 August; 184(15): 4065−4070.

4. MICHIHIRO FUKUSHIMA AND MASUO NAKANO*. Effects of a mixture of oganis ms, Lactobacillus acidophilus or Streptococcus faecalis on cholesterol metabolismin rats fed on a fat- and cholesterol-enriched diet. British Journal of Nutrition (1996), 76, 857467.

천궁 (川芎)

생약명 CNIDII RHIZOMA

자원 산형과 다년생 초목인 천궁의 뿌리를 말린 것

성분 cnidilide

약리 α-adrenergic receptor blocker

약리 해설 혈관평활근 α-adrenergic Rc 자극
➡ 짧고 약한 수축 (경련) 발생
➡ 출혈 & 허혈 부위: α-adrenergic Rc 흥분 지속
➡ 짧고 약한 수축 지속
➡ 허혈 심해짐

적응증 Pregnancy hypertention / Pregnancy essential supplements / Uterine Bleeding / Cerebral infarct / Basilar artery hemorrhage-mediated Insomnia

적응증예

Cerebral infarct

➡ 허혈부위 혈관내피세포: oxidative stress ▶ VCAM-1 발현 ▶ monocyte 부착
▶ 모세혈관 폐쇄 ▶ erythrocyte 정체
▶ 적혈구 골격단백질 불안정화
▶ deformity erythrocyte 생성
▶ met-hemoglobin 생성: nitric oxide 소진
▶ 혈관평활근: oxidative stress
▶ α-adrenergic Rc Ca channel 자극
▶ 혈관평활근 경련
▶ 허혈 ↑

처방예

當歸芍藥散: Pregnancy hypertention (임신고혈압)
當歸散: Pregnancy essential supplements (임신 필수보충제)
膠艾湯: Uterine Bleeding (자궁출혈)
候氏黑散: Cerebral infarction (뇌경색)
酸棗仁湯: Basilar artery hemorrhage-mediated Insomnia(뇌저동맥 출혈에 의한 불면증)

REFERENCE

1. Duan X, Zhou L, Wu T, Liu G, Qiao J, Wei J, Ni J, Zheng J, Chen X, Wang Q. Chinese herbal medicine suxiao jiuxin wan for angina pectoris. Cochrane Database of Systematic Reviews 2008, Issue 1. Art. No.: CD004473. DOI: 10.1002/14651858.

2. Shafi Mussaa, Tash Priorc, Nicholas Alp, Kathryn Wood, Keith M. Channon and David P. Taggart. Duration of action of antispasmodic agents: novel use of amouse model as an in vivo pharmacological assay. European Journal of Cardio-Thoracic Surgery, Volume 26, Issue 5, November 2004, Pages 988-994.

초목 (椒目)

생약명 Zanthoxyli Semen

자원 초피나무 종자

성분 xanthoxin

약리 경련독

효능 Improvement of bowel obstruction

적응증 Mesenteric lymphoma / Ascariasis

적응증예

Mesenteric lymphoma

➡ chronic infection
➡ mesenteric lymph nodes: persistent antigenic stimulation
➡ B cell: genetic alteration
➡ B cell: neoplastic transformation
➡ mesenteric lymphoma
➡ mesenteric lymphadenopathy
➡ 장정맥 조직액: 장간막 림프절 유입 실패
➡ 장정맥 울혈
➡ 장폐쇄

처방예

己椒藶黃丸: Mesenteric lymphoma (장간막 림프종)
烏梅丸: Ascariasis (회충증)

촉초 (蜀椒)

학명 Zanthoxylum piperitum

자원 초피나무의 열매 껍질 = 山椒, 川椒

성분 sanshool

약리 Potassium leak channel blocker

효능 Inhibition of K+ efflux

효능 해설 신경세포 K+ leak channel ▶ K+ efflux ▶ 활동전위 발생 ▶ 근수축, K+ leak channel 차단 ▶ 근수축 억제

적응증 Intussusception / Toxoplasmosis

처방예

大健中湯: Intussusception (장 중첩)
升麻鱉甲湯: Toxoplasmosis (톡소플라즈마증)

REFERENCE

1. Elizabeth M. Adler. How Sanshool Produces One Singular Sensation. Sci. Signal., 1 July 2008, Vol. 1, Issue 26, p. ec237.

2. Diana M Bautista, Yaron M Sigal, Aaron D Milstein, Jennifer L Garrison, Julie A Zorn, Pamela R Tsuruda, Roger A Nicoll & David Julius. Pungent agents from Szechuan peppers excite sensory neurons by inhibiting two-pore potassium channels. Nature Neuroscience 11, 772–779 (1 July 2008) | doi:10.1038/nn.2143.

촉칠 (蜀漆)

기원 조팝나무 (Spiraea prunifolia Sieb. et. Zucc. var simpliciflora Nakai) 줄기

성분 dichroine / halofuginone

약리 Vasodilation / Collagen synthesis inhibitor

적응증 Hyperthemia / Malaria

처방예

桂枝去芍藥加蜀漆牡蠣救逆湯: Rapid hypernatremia (급속 고나트륨혈증)
蜀漆散: Plasmodium malariae & vivas & ovale malaria
(사일열원충 & 삼일열원충 & 난형열원충)
牡蠣澤瀉湯: Lymphedema (림프부종)

REFERENCE

Hson-Mou Chang,Paul Pui-Hay,Sih-Cheng Yao. Pharmacology and Applications of Chinese Material Medical. VOL II.

총백 (葱白)

생약명 ALLII RADIX

자원 백합과에 속하는 여러해살이 풀인 파의 인경

성분 allicin

약리 factor VII, IX, X absorbent

효능 Inhibition of intravenous thrombin formation

적응증 Henoch−Schönlein purpura / Henoch−Schönlein purpura-associated colitis & paralytic ileus / Portal vein thrombosis

적응증예

Henoch-Schönlein purpura

➡ GI tract (주로: 공장 & 회장): small arterioles & venules
➡ circulating IgA deposition
➡ antibody-dependent cell-mediated cytotoxicity (ADCC)
➡ macrophage 유도
➡ IL-8 분비
➡ neutrophil 유도
➡ neutrophil degranulation
➡ small arterioles & venules: endothelium 손상
➡ extrinsic pathway: prothrombin 활성화 via factor VII, IX, X
➡ thrombin 생성
➡ 장허혈

처방예

白通湯: Henoch−Schönlein purpura (헤노호-쉐라인 자반증)
白通四逆加猪膽汁湯: Henoch−Schönlein purpura-associated colitis & paralytic ileus (헤노호-쉐라인 자반증에 연관된 대장염 & 장마비)
旋覆花湯: Portal vein thrombosis (간문맥 혈전증)

REFERENCE

J. KLEIJNEN, P. KNIPSCHILD & G. TER RIET. Garlic, onions and cardiovascular risk factors. A review of the evidence from human experiments with emphasis on commercially available preparations. Br. J. clin. Pharmac. (1989), 28, 535-544.

치자 (梔子)

생약명 GARDENIAE FRUCTUS

자원 꼭두서니과에 속하는 상록활엽관목인 치자나무나 동속식물의 성숙한 과실

성분 crocin

약리 Low-Density Lipoprotein (LDL) antioxidant & conjugated-bilirubin oxidizer

효능 Inhibition of LDL oxidation & Inhibition of conjugated-bilirubin oxidation

적응증 Coronary arteris spasm / Atherosclerosis / Intrahepatic cholangiocarcinoma / Klatskin tumor

적응증예

Atherosclerosis

➡ blood stream: LDL ▶ Monocyte ROS burst & other free radical 접촉
➡ free radical: LDL 공격
➡ LDL 자체 항산화 인자(carotenoid/ α-tocopherol/ cryptoxanthin/ ubiquinol-10) 고갈
➡ LDL: FUFAs lipid peroxidation
➡ ox-LDL 생성
➡ 혈관내피 ox-LDL Rc: ox-LDL 부착 & 내피 밑으로 이동
 # paraoxonase1 ▶ ox-LDL 환원 ▶ 혈류로 방출
 # 대식세포 탐식 ▶ paraoxonase2 ▶ ox-LDL 환원 ▶ 혈류로 방출
➡ paraoxonase1 & paraoxonase2 고갈
➡ ox-LDL 탐식한 대식세포
➡ Mp foam cell 형성
➡ cholesterol crystal 축적
➡ Mp foam cell: MMP 분비
➡ 혈관내피 matrix 분해
➡ 평활근 이동
➡ 이동된 평활근세포: cholesterol crystal & 대식세포 분해소체 ▶ endocytosis
➡ cholesterol crystal을 free cholesterol로 전환시켜 자체 활용
➡ cholesterol crystal & 대식세포의 분해소체가 현저히 많아지면 평활근세포 증식함

➡ Atheroma 내부: 신생혈관 생성
➡ Atheroma formation
➡ 신생혈관 출혈
➡ lipid core: tissue factor ↑
➡ 평활근 종양화
➡ collagen 분비
➡ Fibrous cap formation

처방예

梔子豉湯: Coronary arteris spasm (관상동맥 경련)
梔子甘草豉湯: Coronary arteris spasm & Myocardial ischemia (심근허혈)
梔子生薑豉湯: Coronary arteris spasm & Myocardial referfusion (심근재관류)
枳實梔子豉湯: Macrophage foam cell formation (동맥경화증 단계 중 거품세포 생성)
梔子厚朴湯: Atheroma formation (죽종 형성)
枳實梔子大黃豉湯: Fibrous cap formation (섬유덮개 형성)
茵蔯蒿湯: Intrahepatic cholangiocarcinoma (간내담도암)
大黃硝石湯: Klatskin tumor (간문부 담관암)

REFERENCE

He SY, Qian ZY, Tang FT, Wen N, Xu GL, Sheng L. Effect of crocin on experimental atherosclerosis in quails and its mechanisms. Life Sci, 2005 Jul 8; 77(8):907-21. Epub 2005 Mar 28.

택사 (澤瀉)

생약명 ALISMATIS RHIZOMA

자원 택사과에 속하는 다년생 소택식물인 질경이택사나 택사의 괴경

성분 alisol

약리 angiotensin II receptor blocker

효능 Inhibition of vasoconstriction

적응증 Hypertension / Pregnancy hypertention / Immune complex-mediated glomerulonephritis / Endothelin-1 mediated Renal failure / 처방예 참고

적응증예

Hypertension

➡ stress
➡ corticosteroids ↑
➡ angiotensinogen levels ↑
➡ angiotensin II persistence in blood
➡ vascular smooth muscle: type 1 ANG II receptor 자극
➡ vascular smooth muscle: contraction
➡ vascular smooth muscle: NADH / NADPH oxidase ↑
➡ redox-sensitive transcription 활성화
➡ vascular smooth muscle: VCAM-1 발현
➡ leukocyte & monocyte adhesion
➡ inflammation
➡ 혈관 내강 좁아짐

처방예

澤瀉湯: Hypertension
當歸芍藥散: Pregnancy hypertention (임신고혈압)
五苓散: Immune complex-mediated glomerulonephritis (면역복합체-매개 사구체신염)
豬苓湯: Anti-GBM glomerulonephritis (항-기저막 사구체신염)
茵蔯五苓散: Free bile acids-mediated glomerulonephritis (유담즙산-매개 사구체신염)
八味腎氣丸: Endothelin-1 mediated Renal failure
茯苓澤瀉湯: Decompensated heart failure (보상기전 실패 심부전)

REFERENCE

C. Hsu, J. Yang, L. Yang. Effect of "Dang-Qui-Shao-Yao-San" a Chinese medicinal prescription for dysmenorrhea on uterus contractility in vitro. Phytomedicine, Volume 13, Issue 1, Pages 94-100.

택칠 (澤漆)

생약명 EUPHORBIAE HELIOSCOPIAE HERBA

자원 대극과에 속한 일년생 또는 이년생 초본인 등대풀

성분 quercetin

약리 추측 β-defensin (+) modulator

약리 해설 β-defensin ➡ 점막세포에서 분비하는 항균, 항바이러스 펩타이드
➡ respiratory syncytial virus envelope 분해
➡ RSV: bronchiol epithelium 침입 억제

적응증 RSV (respiratory syncytial virus) bronchiolitis

처방예

澤漆湯: RSV bronchiolitis (호흡기 세포융합 바이러스 세기관지염)

파두 (巴豆)

생약명 CROTONIS FRUCTUS

자원 대극과 식물인 파두의 종자

성분 phorbol ester

약리 Squamous cell PKC activator

약리 해설 편평상피세포암
➡ Protein kinase C 소실
➡ p53 down-regulation
➡ cell growth 주기 계속됨

➡ phorbol ester: Protein kinase C 활성화
➡ p53 발현 증가
➡ 편평상피세포암: apoptosis

적응증 Head and neck cancer / Esophageal squamous cell carcinoma / Squamous cell lung carcinoma / Anal cancer / Esophageal adenocarcinoma / Small cell lung carcinoma / Gastrointestinal stromal tumor / Epiglottitis

처방예

走馬湯: Squamous cell carcinoma (편평세포암)
(head and neck cancer / esophageal squamous cell carcinoma / squamous cell lung carcinoma / anal cancer)
三物備急丸: Esophageal adenocarcinoma & Small cell lung carcinoma
& Gastrointestinal stromal tumor (식도암 / 소세포폐암 / 위장관간질 종양)
三物小白散: Epiglottitis (후두개염)

REFERENCE

1. Vipin Yadav*, Nicole C. Yanez, Sarah E. Fenton, and Mitchell F. Denning*. Loss of Protein Kinase C Gene Expression in Human Squamous Cell Carcinomas. A Laser Capture Microdissection Study. American Journal of Pathology, doi:10.2253/aipath.2010.090816.

2. Zhang G, Kazanietz MG, Blumberg PM, Hurley JH. Crystal structure of the cys2 activator-binding domain of protein kinase C delta in complex with phorbol ester. Cell. 1995 Jun 16;81(6):917-24.

3. U Kikkawa, Y Takai, Y Tanaka, R Miyake and Y Nishizuka. Protein kinase C as apossible receptor protein of tumor-promoting phorbol esters. The Journal of Biological Chemistry, 1983 October 10, 258, 11442-11445.

패모 (貝母)

생약명 FRITILLARIAE CIRRHOSAE BULBUS

자원 나리과에 속하는 여러해살이 풀인 조선패모와 부전패모, 기타 패모속 식물의 비늘줄기를 말린 것

성분 verticine

약리 추측 Calcium ATPase blocker

약리 해설 Haemophilus influenzae & Trichomonas vaginalis
➡ Calcium ATPase 차단
➡ 세포내 대사 정지
➡ 균독성 약화됨

적응증 Epiglottitis / Trichomoniasis in pregnancy

적응증예

Trichomoniasis in pregnancy

➡ pregnancy
➡ 혈액량 & 적혈구 증가
➡ Iron deficiency & vitB 12 deficiency
➡ 적혈구 골격단백질 결합
➡ deformity erythrocyte 생성
➡ 산소포화도 감소
➡ 무증상 trichomonas vaginalis: 영양불량
➡ gene transformation: tyrosinase 활성화
➡ 이동에 필요한 actin cytoskeleton 형성
➡ 편모 운동성 증가
➡ <u>병원성 전환</u>
➡ trichomonasis: 방광염 / 미숙한 태막의 파열 / 임신초기의 조산 / 자궁내부 성장지연

처방예

三物小白散: Epiglottitis (후두개염)
當歸貝母苦蔘丸: Trichomoniasis in pregnancy (임신부 트리코모나스증)

패장 (敗醬)

생약명 PATRINAE RADIX

자원 두해살이 풀, 마타리과의 다년생 초본식물

성분 oleanolic acid

약리 PPAR (peroxisome proliferator-activated receptors) activator

효능 p53 inhibition

적응증 Appendicitis (충수염)

➡ bacterial infection
➡ Yersinia spp / Campylobacter spp / Salmonella spp / etc
➡ bacteria antibody 출현
➡ appendix endothelium: HLA-B27 (MHC class I allele) 발현
➡ molecular mimic response
➡ HLA-B27: bacteria antibody 부착
➡ antibody-dependent cellular cytotoxicity
➡ macrophage 유도: phagocytosis
➡ TNF-α 분비
➡ appendix endothelium: TNF Rc 부착
➡ 세포막 대사 증가 & 미토콘드리아 대사 증가
➡ reactive oxygen species ↑
➡ NF-κB ↑
➡ p53 활성화
➡ appendix endothelium: apoptosis

처방예

薏苡附子敗醬散: Appendicitis (충수염)

REFERENCE

Sudhakar Chintharlapalli1, Sabitha Papineni2, Indira Jutooru2, Alan McAlees3 and Stephen Safe12. Structure-dependent activity of glycyrrhetinic acid derivatives as peroxisome proliferator−activated receptor γ agonists in colon cancer cells. Mol Cancer Ther May 2007 6; 1588.

포부자 (炮附子)

생약명 ACONITI IATERALIS PREPARATA RADIX

자원 미나리아재비과에 속하는 다년생 초본인 부자의 건조한 자근을 구운 것

성분 aconitine

약리 추측 neutrophil` Voltage-gated proton channels blocker

약리 해설 Voltage-gated proton channels

➡ 식균작용에 의해 증가된 세포내 H+을 세포외로 방출시키는 채널

➡ Voltage-gated proton channels 차단

➡ H+ 방출 억제

➡ 세포내 pH ↓

➡ 세포대사 정지됨

효능 Inhibition of neutrophil metabolism

적응증 c-ANCA associated vasculitis / Endothelin-1 mediated renal failure / Small intestine stenosis in Behcet's Disease / 처방에 참고

적응증예

c-ANCA associated vasculitis

➡ virus & bacteria infection: IL-1 ↑

➡ neutrophil 활성화: 세포막에 proteinase 3 발현
➡ medium-size vessel: c-ANCA bind proteinase3 expressed neutrophil
➡ p-ANCA * neutrophil complex
➡ complement 유도
➡ vessel endothelial cell: H_2O_2-mediated VCAM-1 발현
➡ neutrophil adhesion
➡ neutrophil phagocytosis
➡ medium-size vessel vasculitis

처방예

眞武湯: c-ANCA associated vasculitis (항호중구 세포질항체-매개 혈관염)
附子湯: p-ANCA associated vasculitis (핵주위-항호중구 세포질항체-매개 혈관염)
八味腎氣丸: Endothelin-1 mediated renal failure
桂枝加附子湯: Acute EBV infection
附子硬米湯: Small intestine stenosis in Behcet's Disease (베체트 소장협착증)
桂枝附子湯: Influenza myositis (인플루엔자 근염)
甘草附子湯:Coxsackie virus-mediated polymyositis & polyarthritis (다발성근염&관절염)
麻黃附子甘草湯: Early autoimmune response in tissue
麻黃附子細辛湯: Early autoimmune response in erythrocyte
白朮附子湯: Myoglobin-mediated renal failure
大黃附子湯: Distal extrahepatic cholangiocarcinoma (원위부 간외담관암)
附子瀉心湯: Cholecystitis (담낭염)
桂枝去芍藥加麻黃細辛附子湯: Autoimmune response-mediated Methemoglobinemia
桂枝去芍藥加附子湯: IL-1 mediated Cardiac toxicity

해백 (薤白)

생약명 ALLII MACROSTEMI BULBUS

자원 백합과에 속한 다년생 초본인 산달래와 염부추, 산부추의 뿌리줄기

성분 vitamin B1

약리 Pyruvate dehydrogenase & Oxoglutarate dehydrogenase의 coenzymes

효능 Activation of TCA cycle

적응증 Unstable angina / Myocardial infarction

적응증예

Myocardial infarction

➡ coronary artery: atherosclerotic plaque
➡ atherosclerotic plaque: macrophage ↑
➡ plaque rupture
➡ plaque 내부의 tissue factor 노출
➡ platelet independent thrombus formation
➡ plaque 위로 thrombus 축적
➡ platelet thrombin Rc: thrombus 부착
➡ plaque 위로 platelet-thrombin complex 형성
➡ platelet-thrombin complex 분리
➡ micro-emboli 작용
➡ coronary artery branch: 폐쇄
➡ coronary artery: 내강 좁아짐 (완전경색)
➡ myocardiocyte ischemia
➡ TCA cycle ↓
➡ myocardial infarction
➡ 허혈부위 심근세포: 섬유아세포로 분화됨

처방예

枳實薤白桂枝湯: Unstable angina (불안정형 협심증)
栝蔞薤白白酒湯: Myocardial infarction (심근경색)
栝蔞薤白半夏湯: Myocardial infarction & micro-emboli (심근경색 & 미세혈전)

REFERENCE

Yoon Sojung. Scientists disclose 54 Korean foods that fight cancer. Science / Tech, June 23, 2007.

행인 (杏仁)

생약명 ARMENIACAE AMARUM SEMEN

자원 벚나무과에 속하는 살구나무와 산살구나무의 건조한 종자

성분 benzoic acid

약리 Hydroxyl radical scavenger

효능 Inhibition of hydroxyl radical-mediated cytotoxicity

적응증 Colon cancer / Emphysema / Asthma / Reactive arthritis / 처방예 참고

적응증예

Asthma

➡ bronchial endothelium: allergen attack
➡ dendritic cell: antigen 제시
➡ immature T cell: antigen 전달 받음
➡ immature T cell: T-helper type 2 (Th2) cells 분화
➡ Th2 cells: chemokine 분비 ▶ eosinophil 유도
➡ eosinophil granule 활성화: degranulation & eosinophil peroxidase (EPO) 활성화
➡ EPO generated hydroxyl radical 생성
➡ extracellular matrix: hydroxyl radical 유출
➡ bronchial endothelium: Na+/ K+ pumps 손상
➡ bronchitis

처방예

桂麻各半湯: *IFN-a* resistant viral infection
桂枝二麻黃一湯: *heat shock protein*-resistant viral infection
麻黃湯: *heat shock protein & IFN-a* resistant viral infection
大靑龍湯: *IFN-γ* resistant viral infection
麻子仁丸: Colon cancer (대장암)
厚朴麻黃湯: Emphysema (폐기종)
麻黃蓮軺赤小豆湯: Warm autoantibody-mediated hemolytic anemia

(온난자가항체-매개 용혈성빈혈)
麻黃杏仁甘草石膏湯: Asthma (천식)
麻黃杏仁薏苡甘草湯: Reactive arthritis (반응성 관절염)

REFERENCE

Akihisa Sakumot[1], Gen-ichi Tsuchihashi[1]. Radiation-induced Reaction in an Aqueous Benzoic Acid Solution. II. Determination of Products by Isotope Dilution Method. Bulletin of the Chemical Society of Japan, Vol.34, No.5(1961)pp.663-667.

향시 (香豉)

생약명 SANTALI ALBAE LIGNUM

자원 콩과에 속한 일년생 초본인 콩의 성숙한 종자를 발효 가공하여 건조한 것

성분 L-arginine

효능 Synthesis of nitric oxide

적응증 Coronary arteris spasm / Atherosclerosis

적응증예

Coronary arteris spasm

➡ blood stream: LDL ▶ Monocyte ROS burst & other free radical 접촉
➡ free radical: LDL 공격
➡ LDL 자체 항산화 인자(carotenoid/ α-tocopherol/ cryptoxanthin/ ubiquinol-10) 고갈
➡ LDL: FUFAs lipid peroxidation
➡ ox-LDL 생성
➡ ox-LDL: 관상동맥 혈관내피 ox-LDL Rc 부착
➡ 대식세포 탐식: fever

➡ 관상동맥 혈관내피: nitric oxide 분사
➡ ox-LDL을 떨어뜨림
➡ nitric oxide 고갈
➡ 관상동맥 혈관 확장력 ↓
➡ vasospasm: agony
➡ 협심증

처방예

梔子豉湯: Coronary arteris spasm (관상동맥 경련)
梔子甘草豉湯: Coronary arteris spasm & Myocardial ischemia (심근허혈)
梔子生薑豉湯: Coronary arteris spasm & Myocardial referfusion (심근재관류)
枳實梔子豉湯: Macrophage foam cell formation (동맥경화증 단계 중 거품세포 생성)
枳實梔子大黃豉湯: Fibrous cap formation (섬유덮개 형성)
梔子厚朴湯: Atheroma formation (죽종 형성)

활석 (滑石)

학명 Talc

자원 층상 규산염 광물로 경도가 가장 약한 광물

성분 $Mg_3(Si_4O10)(OH)_2$

약리 Nitrogen group & Nucleic acid absorbent

약리 해설 Talc는 Nitrogen group과 염을 잘 형성하기 때문에 사구체신염으로 인한 단백질 손실을 막아주며 혈액속의 바이러스 핵산을 제거해 줌

적응증 Anti-GBM glomerulonephritis / Bornavirus late infection

적응증예

anti-GBM glomerulonephritis

➡ glomerular basement membrane: IgG autoantibodies

➡ complement 유도
➡ GBM injury
➡ mesangial cell: GBM에서 이탈
➡ mesangial cell proliferation
➡ mesangial cell: proteinase 분비
➡ elastic laminin 손상
➡ crescent formation
➡ 사구체 모세혈관 손상: thrombus formation
➡ Bowman's capsule: 단백질 & 당 유출 ▶ thirst
➡ 수출소동맥 저산소증
➡ 수출소동맥 수축
➡ 사구체내 압력 ↑
➡ 사구체 손상 ↑

처방예

豬苓湯: Anti-GBM glomerulonephritis (항-기저막 사구체신염)
百合滑石散: Bornavirus late infection

REFERENCE

1. Ashton et al. Multi-purpose body powder composition. United States Patent 4913896, November, 1984 - 4485092.

2. Sattar SA, Westwood JC. Comparison of talc-Celite and polyelectrolyte 60 invirus recovery from sewage: development of technique and experiments with poliovirus (type 1, Sabin)-contaminated multilitre samples. Can J Microbiol. 1976 Nov;22(11):1620-7.

황금 (黃芩)

생약명 SCUTELLARIAE RADIX

자원 꿀풀과의 여러해살이 풀인 황금의 뿌리

성분 baicalin

약리 Peroxynitrite ($ONOO^-$) scavenger

효능 Inhibition of peroxynitrite-mediated cytotoxicity

적응증 Cholera / Gastric ulcer / Duodenal ulcer / Viral hepatitis (type A, B) / Type C hepatitis / Viral fulminant hepatitis / Cirrhosis / Hepatocellular carcinoma / Pregnancy essential supplements / 처방예 참고

적응증예

Hepatocellular carcinoma

➡ chronic hepatitis B virus & hepatitis C virus infection
➡ virus replicon RNAs
➡ HBV & HCV gene: 간세포 DNA에 삽입
➡ HBV & HCV: NOS2 gene expression ↑
➡ nitric oxide + superoxide
➡ peroxynitrite ($ONOO^-$) ↑
➡ 삽입된 HBV & HCV gene: mutation
➡ 돌연변이된 HBV & HCV gene: mutant protein 생산
➡ mutant protein: p53 binding
➡ p53 inactivation
➡ hepatocyte apoptosis & cell-growth control: 실패
➡ oncogenic hepatocyte: 출현

처방예

黃芩湯: Cholera
黃芩加半夏生薑湯: Salmonella typhi
六物黃芩湯: Pathogenic E. coli infection
黃連湯: Group A streptococcus (GAS) infection (그룹 A 연쇄상구균감염증)

乾薑黃連黃芩人參湯: Staphylococcal food poisoning (포도구균 식 중독)
葛根黃連黃芩湯: Botulism (보튤리누스 독소증)
半夏瀉心湯: Gastric ulcer (위궤양)
生薑瀉心湯: Duodenal ulcer (십이지장궤양)
甘草瀉心湯: Peptic ulcer-complicated perforation (소화성궤양에 합병된 천공)
瀉心湯: H.pylori-mediated stomach bleeding
附子瀉心湯: Cholecystitis (담낭염)
小柴胡湯: Viral hepatitis (type A, B) (바이러스성 간염)
柴胡桂枝湯: Type B hepatitis-mediated immune complex disease
柴胡加芒硝湯: Type C hepatitis (C형 간염)
柴胡加龍骨牡蠣湯: Viral fulminant hepatitis (바이러스성 전격성간염)
柴胡桂枝乾薑湯: Liver cirrhosis (간경변)
大柴胡湯: Hepatocellular carcinoma (간암)
大黃蟅虫丸: Kaposis sarcoma (카포시 육종)
當歸散: Pregnancy essential supplements (임신 필수보충제)
侯氏黑散: Cerebral infraction (뇌경색)
黃土湯: Immune thrombocytopenic purpura (면역성 혈소판감소 자반증)
王不留行散: Tetany (파상풍)

REFERENCE

1. DAE HYUN KIM, KI HO CHO, SANG KWAN MOON, YOUNG SUK KIM, DONG HYUN KIM, JAE SUE CHOI, HAE YOUNG CHUNG. Cytoprotective mechanism of baicalin against endothelial cell damage by peroxynitrite. Journal of pharmacy and pharmacology, 2005, vol. 57, no12, pp. 1581-1590.

2. Rui Hai Liu, James R. Jacob 1, Joseph H. Hotchkiss 3, Paul J. Cote 2, John L. Gerin 2 and Bud C. Tennant 1. Woodchuck hepatitis virus surface antigen induces nitric oxide synthesis in hepatocytes: possible role in hepatocarcinogenes is. Oxford Journals Life Sciences & Medicine Carcinogenesis Volume 15, Number 12 Pp. 2875-2877.

3. Keigo Machida,1 Kevin T.-H. Cheng,1 Vicky M.-H. Sung,1 Ki Jeong Lee,1 Alexandra M. Levine,2 and Michael M. C. Lai1*. Hepatitis C Virus Infection Activates the Immunologic (Type II) Isoform of Nitric Oxide Synthase and Thereby Enhances DNA Damage and Mutations of Cellular Genes. Journal of Virology, August 2004, p. 8835-8843, Vol. 78, No. 16.

황기 (黃芪)

생약명 ASTRAGALI RADIX

자원 콩과에 속하는 다년생 초본인 단너삼의 건조한 뿌리

성분 astragaloside

약리 Tissue plasminogen activator (+) modulator

효능 Fibrinolysis of capillaritis-mediated fibrin

적응증 Chromohidrosis / Axon terminal capillaritis / Skeletal smooth muscle capillaritis-mediated disseminated intravascular coagulation / Chronic right heart failure-mediated systemic congestion / 처방예 참고

적응증예

Axon terminal capillaritis

➡ axon terminal: capillary congestion
➡ capillaritis
➡ fibrin formation
➡ neuron ischemia
➡ neuritis
➡ axon terminal: acetylcholine 분비 ↓
➡ skeletal muscle fiber: 자극 감소
➡ skeletal muscle fiber: total enzyme 감소
➡ lactate dehydrogenase ↓ / superoxide dismutase ↓ / glutathione ↓ / c-AMP ↓
➡ lactate ↑ / superoxide ↑ / hydrogen peroxide ↑ / glucolysis ↓
➡ ATP ↓
➡ skeletal muscle fiber: 수축 실패
➡ paralysis

처방예

黃耆芍藥桂枝苦酒湯: Chromohidrosis (색깔 땀 분비증)
黃耆桂枝五物湯: Axon terminal capillaritis (축삭종말 모세혈관염)

黃耆建中湯: Skeletal smooth muscle capillaritis-mediated disseminated intravascular coagulation (골격평활근 모세혈관염-매개 파종성 혈관내응고증)
桂枝加黃耆湯: Eccrine sweat gland capillaritis (에크린분비선 모세혈관염)
防己茯苓湯: Chronic right heart failure-mediated systemic congestion (전신울혈)
防己黃耆湯: Right heart failure-mediated venous congestion (정맥울혈)

REFERENCE

Zhang WJ, Woita J, Binder BR. Regulation of the fibrinolytic potential of cultured human umbilical vein endothelial cells: astragaloside IV downregulates plasminogen activator inhibitor-1 and upregulates tissue-type plasminogen activator expression. J Vasc Res,1997 Jul-Aug;34(4):273-80.

황련 (黃連)

생약명 COPTIDIS RHIZOMA

자원 미나리아재비과의 다년생 초본인 깽깽이 풀의 뿌리줄기

성분 berberine

약리 sortase inhibitor

효능 Inhibition of bacterial peptidoglycan synthesis

효능 해설 sortase

➡ 세균 세포벽 성분인 peptidoglycan을 만드는 효소
➡ 그람양성 세균 세포벽 80~90%: peptidoglycan
➡ peptidoglycan 합성 억제
➡ 삼투압에 취약해져 용균됨

적응증 Group A streptococcus (GAS) infection / Staphylococcal food poisoning /

Botulism / Gastric ulcer / Duodenal ulcer / Gastric MALT lympoma / Gastric adenocarcinoma / Cholecystitis / Bacterial endocarditis / Crohn's disease / 처방예 참고

적응증예

Gastric adenocarcinoma

➡ Stomach body & antrum: Helicobacter pylori 감염
➡ Helicobacter pylori: 병원성 균으로 형질전환
➡ H. pylori peptidoglycan: type IV secretion system 형성
➡ gastric ulcer 반복
➡ gastric mucosal cells: metaplasia (intestine epithelium)
➡ chronic atrophic gastritis
➡ gastric mucosal cells: syndecan 소실
➡ gastric mucosal cells: phenotypic transition
➡ fibroblast-like cell 전환
➡ fibroblast-like cell: collagenase 분비
➡ invasion & metastasis

처방예

黄連湯: Group A streptococcus (GAS) infection (그룹 A 연쇄상구균감염증)
乾薑黄連黄芩人參湯: Staphylococcal food poisoning (포도구균 식 중독)
葛根黄連黄芩湯: Botulism (보툴리누스 독소증)
半夏瀉心湯: Gastric ulcer (위궤양)
生薑瀉心湯: Duodenal ulcer (십이지장궤양)
甘草瀉心湯: Peptic ulcer-complicated perforation (소화성궤양에 합병된 천공)
瀉心湯: H.pylori-mediated stomach bleeding
大黄黄連瀉心湯: Gastric MALT lympoma (위장 점막림프종)
小陷胸湯: Gastric adenocarcinoma (위암)
附子瀉心湯: Cholecystitis (담낭염)
黄連阿膠湯: Bacterial endocarditis (세균성 심내막염)
白頭翁湯: Crohn's disease (크론병)
白頭翁加甘草阿膠湯: Postpartum Crohn's disease (산후 크론병)

REFERENCE

Luciano A. Marraffini,1 Andrea C. DeDent,2 and Olaf Schneewind2*. Sortases and the Art of Anchoring Proteins to the Envelopes of Gram-Positive Bacteria. MICRO BIOLOGY AND MOLECULAR BIOLOGY REVIEWS, Mar. 2006, p. 192--221.

황백 (黃栢)

생약명 PHELLODENDRI CORTEX

자원 운향과식물인 황벽나무의 나무껍질

성분 phellodendrine

약리 추측 Monocyte / Macrophage / Neutrophil CD14 blocker

약리 해설 혈액 Monocyte / Macrophage / Neutrophil CD14
➡ LPS & bacterial antigen 전달
➡ Monocyte / Macrophage / Neutrophil: cytokine
➡ T cell 분화
➡ TNF-α 분비
➡ sepsis
➡ multiple organ dysfuction

효능 Sepsis

적응증 Crohn's disease / Postpartum Crohn's disease / Klatskin tumor

적응증예

Klatskin tumor

➡ hilar bile duct cholangiocyte: Gut bacterial translocation
➡ chronic cholangitis

➡ cholangiocyte: adenomatous hyperplasia
➡ adenomatous cholangiocyte : EGF autocrine
➡ tyrosine kinase domain 활성화 ▶ 세포 증식
➡ hilar bile duct: cholangiocarcinoma
➡ hilar bile duct: 압력 상승
➡ diconjugated bilirubin: 혈 중 역류
▶ 혈 중 unconjugated bilirubin ↑ & translocated bacteria: 혈류 이동
▶ sepsis

처방예

白頭翁湯: Crohn's disease (크론병)
白頭翁加甘草阿膠湯: Postpartum Crohn's disease (산후 크론병)
大黃硝石湯: Klatskin tumor (간문부 담관암)

후박 (厚朴)

생약명 MAGNOLIAE CORTEX

자원 목련과에 속하는 낙엽교목인 나무의 줄기 또는 뿌리껍질을 말린 것

성분 honokiol

약리 VEGF receptor blocker

효능 Inhibition of angiogenesis & extracellular remodelling

적응증 Adenomatous polyp / Pancreatic ductal adenocarcinoma / Emphsema / Lung adenocarcinoma & Large cell lung carcinoma / Atheroma formation / Colon cancer / Unstable angina / Diffuse large B cell lymphoma of gastric MALT / Diffuse large B cell lymphoma of small intestine MALT / Plasmodium palciparum malaria

적응증예

Pancreatic ductal adenocarcinoma

➡ duct cell: proliferation
➡ NF-kB pathway: anti-apoptosis gene ↑
➡ KRAS mutation
➡ INK4A gene loss: p53 protein 생산 안됨
➡ duct cell: neogenesis
➡ heparanase 분비
➡ duct cell: heparan sulfate 분해
➡ TGF-β 분리됨: TGF-β mediated cell apoptosis 실패
➡ pancreatic ductal adenocarcinoma 지속
➡ 세포질내: hydrogen peroxide ↑
➡ VEGF expression ↑ : angiogenesis
➡ pancreatic ductal adenocarcinoma 성장

처방예

厚朴三物湯: Adenomatous polyp (선종성 용종)
厚朴七物湯: Gastrointestinal leiomyosarcoma (위장관 평활근육종)
厚朴生薑半夏甘草人蔘湯: Pancreatic ductal adenocarcinoma (췌장암)
厚朴麻黃湯: Emphsema (폐기종)
厚朴大黃湯: Lung adenocarcinoma & Large cell lung carcinoma(폐선암 & 대세포폐암)
梔子厚朴湯: Atheroma formation (죽종 형성)
麻子仁丸: Colon cancer (대장암)
枳實薤白桂枝湯: Unstable angina (불안정형 협심증)
小承氣湯: Diffuse large B cell lymphoma of gastric MALT (위장 점막림프조직의 미만성 B세포 림프종)
大承氣湯: Diffuse large B cell lymphoma of small intestine MALT (소장 점막림프조직의 미만성 B세포 림프종)
鱉甲煎丸: Plasmodium palciparum malaria (열대열원충 말라리아)

REFERENCE

LIU, Y.; CHEN, L.; HE, X.; FAN, L.; YANG, G.; CHEN, X.; LIN, X.; DU, L.; LI, Z.; YE, H.; MAO, Y.; ZHAO, X.; WEI, Y. Enhancement of therapeutic effectiveness by combining liposomal honokiol with cisplatin in ovarian carcinoma. International Journal of Gynecological Cancer, July/August 2008, Volume 18, Issue 4, p652-659.

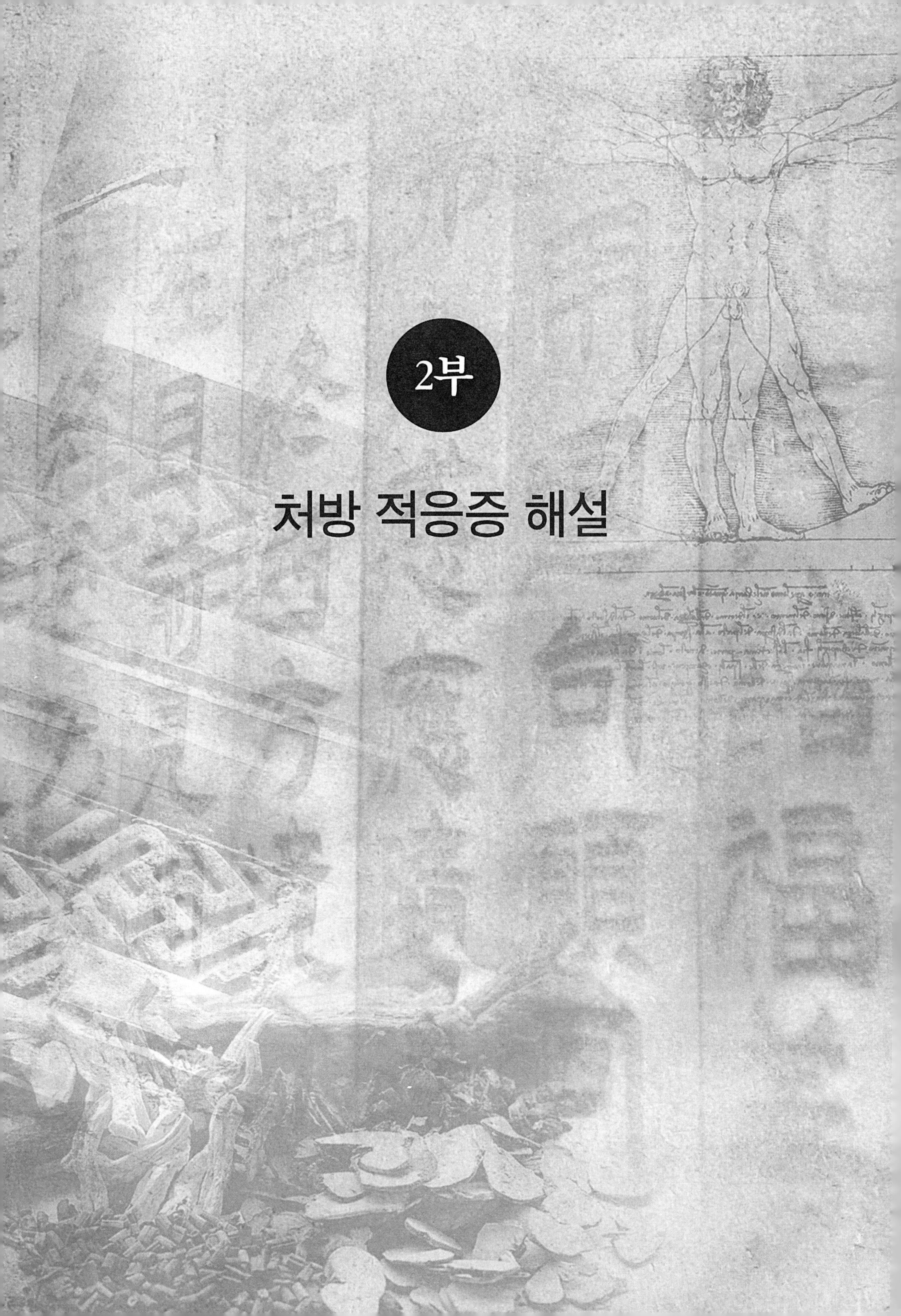

2부

처방 적응증 해설

갈근가반하탕 (葛根加半夏湯)

원문 太陽 與 陽明 合病, 不下利, 但 嘔 者, 葛根加半夏湯 主之。

원문 해설 림프절 감염과 점막림프조직 감염이 동반되어 설사는 없고 구역만 있는 경우에는 갈근가반하탕을 쓴다.

적응증 Enterovirus-mediated Meningoencephalitis (장바이러스-매개 뇌수막염)

병태 & 증상

Enterovirus

➡ respiratory MALT infection: enterovirus replication
➡ respiratory MALT destruction: MALT 상피세포 상환 ▶ free sulfate : neusea
➡ lymph node infection: enterovirus replication
➡ neurotropism target
➡ astrocyte 감염
➡ IgG mediated cellular response
➡ microglia 유도: TNF-α 분비: no sweating / coldness
➡ Astrocyte apoptosis
➡ microglia: nitric oxide 분비
➡ BBB breakdown
➡ 뇌실질의 대사산물이 뇌척수액으로 유출
➡ 뇌수막 압력 ↑ : neck-back stiffness
➡ meningitis
➡ astrocyte apoptosis ↑↑
➡ synapse에서 glutamate 축적
➡ postsynaptic neuron NMDA Rc: glutamate 자극
➡ postsynaptic neuron: glutamate excitotoxicity
➡ 피질 손상
➡ encephalitis

처방 목표 heat shock protein 활성화: 림프절 바이러스 증식 억제 / microglia secretion 억제 / NMDA Rc 차단 / MALT 상피세포 상환 촉진: enterovirus 림프절감염 억제

처방 구성 葛根 四兩 / 麻黃 三兩 / 炙甘草 二兩 / 芍藥 二兩 / 桂枝 二兩 / 生薑 二兩 / 半夏 半升 / 大棗 十二枚

처방 약리

계지 / 작약 / 생강 / 대조 / 구감초

heat production ➡ heat shock protein 활성화 (계지탕 참고)

마황 ephedrine ➡ Epinephrine receptors agonist
➡ adenylate cyclase 활성화
➡ cAMP ↑
➡ microglia secretion 억제

갈근 daidzein ➡ NMDA receptor blocker

반하 triterpenoid ($C_{30}H_{48}O_7S$)
➡ Rho GTPase family transcription promotor
➡ focal adhesion 생성
➡ 상피세포 이동 촉진

갈근탕 (葛根湯)

원문 太陽病, 項背強几几, 無汗 惡風, 葛根湯 主之。太陽 與 陽明 合病 者, 必 自下利, 葛根湯 主之。

원문 해설 림프절 감염병으로 목과 등이 뻣뻣해지고 땀없이 추위를 타는 경우에는 갈근탕을 쓴다. 림프절 감염과 점막림프조직 감염이 같이 된 경우에는 반드시 설사를 하게 되며 갈근탕을 쓴다.

적응증 Mosquito-borne encephalitis virus
& Enterovirus-mediated Meningoencephalitis
(모기-매개 뇌염바이러스 & 장바이러스-매개 뇌수막염)

병태 & 증상

Mosquito-borne encephalitis virus & Enterovirus
: lymph node & MALT infection

➡ lymph node & MALT: replication
➡ neurotropism target
➡ Astrocyte 감염
➡ IgG mediated cellular response
➡ Microglia 유도: TNF-α 분비: no sweating / coldness
➡ Astrocyte apoptosis
➡ Microglia: nitric oxide 분비
➡ BBB breakdown
➡ 뇌실질의 대사산물이 뇌척수액으로 유출
➡ 뇌수막 압력 : neck-back stiffness
➡ meningitis
➡ Astrocyte apoptosis ↑↑
➡ synapse: glutamate 축적
➡ postsynaptic neuron NMDA Rc: glutamate 부착
➡ postsynaptic neuron: glutamate excitotoxicity
➡ 피질 손상
➡ encephalitis

처방 목표 heat shock protein 활성화: 바이러스 증식 억제 / microglia secretion 억제 / NMDA Rc 차단

처방 구성 葛根 四兩 / 麻黃 三兩 / 桂枝 二兩 / 生薑 三兩 / 炙甘草 二兩 / 芍藥 二兩 / 大棗 十二枚

처방 약리

계지 / 작약 / 생강 / 대조 / 구감초 heat production ➡ heat shock protein 활성화

마황 ephedrine ➡ Epinephrine receptors agonist
➡ adenylate cyclase 활성화
➡ cAMP ↑
➡ microglia secretion 억제

갈근 daidzein ➡ NMDA receptor blocker

갈근황금황련탕 (葛根黃芩黃連湯)

원문 太陽病, 桂枝證 , 醫 反 下之 , 利遂 不止 , 脈 促 者, 表未解 也 , 喘 而 汗出 者 , 葛根黃芩黃連湯 主之 。

원문 해설 림프절 감염병으로 계지증(근육증상)이 있으면서 설사가 그치지 않고 맥이 급하고 체표증상이 낫지 않으면서 호흡곤란이 있는 경우에는 갈근황금황련탕을 쓴다.

적응증 Botulism (보툴리누스 독소증)

병태 & 증상

Botulism

➡ Clostridium botulinum (G+): food poisoning ➡ diarrhea
➡ botulinum toxin
➡ heavy chain: 운동신경 말단의 NMDA Rc에 부착 후 endocytosis 됨
➡ light chain: acetylcholine의 방출에 관여하는 synaptosome associated protein 절단
➡ 운동신경 말단: acetylcholine degranulation 실패
➡ neuromuscular junction: acetylcholine ↓
➡ 근육 자극 감소
➡ 근육세포 ATP
➡ 근육세포: Na+/ K+ pump 손상
➡ 근육세포 부종
➡ Severe botulism
➡ respiration muscles paralysis: dyspnea
➡ macrophage: Clostridium botulinum 식균
➡ extracellular peroxynitrite ($ONOO^-$) ↑
➡ tissue damage

처방 목표 Clostridium botulinum 살균 / NMDA Rc 차단 ➡ botulinum toxin 운동신경 유입 억제시킴 / 근육세포: Na+/ K+ pump 활성화 / extracellular peroxynitrite ($ONOO^-$) 제거

처방 구성 葛根 半斤 / 炙甘草 二兩 / 黃芩 三兩 / 黃連 三兩

처방 약리

황련 berberine ➡ sortase inhibitor
➡ Clostridium botulinum: peptidoglycan 합성 억제
➡ 삼투압성 용균 유도

갈근 daidzein ➡ ionotropic glutamate receptor blocker
➡ botulinum toxin의 운동신경 유입 억제

구감초 18β-24-Hydroxyglycyrrhetinic acid ➡ HSD11B2 inhibitor
➡ cortisol 분해 억제
➡ mineralocorticoid receptors 자극 지속
➡ 근육세포 Na+/ K+ pumps 전사 활성화

황금 baicalin ➡ peroxynitrite ($ONOO^-$) scavenger
➡ macrophage 식균 후 조직 손상 억제

감강령출탕 (甘薑苓朮湯)

원문 腎著 之 病, 其人 身體重, 腰中冷, 如 坐水中, 形 如 水 狀, 反 不渴, 小便 自利, 飮食 如故, 病屬 下焦, 身勞 汗出, 衣裡 冷濕, 久久 得之, 腰以下 冷痛, 腹 重 如 帶 五千錢, 甘薑苓朮湯 主之。

원문 해설 신장 사구체혈관에 혈전이 쌓여서 병이 생기면 몸이 무거워지고 허리부위가 냉해지며 물속에 들어가 앉아 있는 것 같고 갈증은 없으며 소변이 저절로 나오면서 음식이 여전하면 병이 하초에 있는 것이다. 일을 하면 땀이 나면서 옷이 냉한 땀으로 젖고 병이 만성이 된다. 허리 이하가 냉하며 아프고 무거운 전대를 배에 두른 듯 보이는 경우에는감강령출탕을 쓴다.

적응증 p-ANCA mediated crescentic glomerulonephritis
(핵주위 항호중구 세포질 항체-매개 반월상 사구체신염)

병태 & 증상

p-ANCA mediated crescentic glomerulonephritis

➡ p-ANCA (perinuclear neutrophil cytoplasmic antibody)
➡ target: neutrophil myeloperoxidase (MPO)
➡ viral infection: IL-1 & TNF-α ↑
➡ neutrophil 활성화 & B cell 활성화
➡ myeloperoxidase 생성 ↑ & p-ANCA 생성 ↑
➡ neutrophil & p-ANCA: complex 형성
➡ 사구체 혈관내피에 침착
➡ 사구체 혈관내피: VCAM-1 발현
➡ 사구체 혈관내피: neutrophil 부착
➡ neutrophil phagocytosis
➡ HClO 분비 via H2O2
➡ 사구체 혈관내피 손상
➡ vasculitis
➡ thrombus formation

처방 목표 p-ANCA 생성 억제 / VCAM-1 차단 / HClO 분비 억제 / thrombus 제거

처방 구성 甘草 二兩 / 白朮 二兩 / 乾薑 四兩 / 茯苓 四兩

처방 약리

감초 glycyrrhetinic acid

➡ 11-beta-hydroxysteroid dehydrogenase1 (HSD11B1) inhibitor
➡ glucocorticoid 작용
➡ B cell: IκBα 생성
➡ NF-κB 억제
➡ 항체 생성 억제

백출 atractylon ➡ vascular cell adhesion molecule-1 (VCAM-1) blocker

건강 shogaol ➡ neutrophil H2O2 scavenger
➡ HClO 분비 억제

복령 pachymic acid ➡ glycoprotein IIb/IIIa (gpIIb/IIIa) (-) modulator
➡ thrombus formation 억제

감맥대조탕 (甘麥大棗湯)

원문 婦人 臟躁, 喜 悲 傷 欲 哭, 象 如 神 靈 所 作, 數 欠 伸, 甘麥大棗湯 主之。

원문 해설 부인이 행동과 말이 조급하고 시끄러우며, 슬퍼하기를 잘하여 소리 높여 우는데, 그 모습이 신령굿 하는 것 같으며, 자주 하품하며 기지개를 켜는 경우에는 감맥대조탕을 쓴다.

적응증 Bipolar affective disorder (양극성 정동장애)

병태 & 증상

Bipolar affective disorder

➡ Vitamin B6 부족
➡ Pyridoxal phosphate
➡ γ-aminobutyric acid (GABA) & dopamine 생성
➡ GABA 부족 ▶ 신경 흥분, 근육 경직: excitement, yawn, stretching
& dopamine 부족 ▶ 슬픔: sorrow

처방 목표 Vitamin B6 보충 / GABA & dopamine 생성 촉진 / GABA & dopamine 전도 촉진

처방 구성 甘草 三兩 / 小麥 一升 / 大棗 十枚

처방 약리

소맥 Vitamin B6 source

감초 glycyrrhetinic acid
➡ 11-beta-hydroxysteroid dehydrogenase1 (HSD11B1) inhibitor
➡ glucocorticoid 작용
➡ GABA & dopamine synthesis 촉진

대조 cAMP ➡ electrical impulses 생성 활성화

감초건강탕 (甘草乾薑湯)

원문 傷寒 脈浮 , 自汗出 , 小便 數 , 心煩 , 微 惡寒 , 脚 攣急 , 反 與 桂枝, 欲 攻其表 , 此 誤也 。得之 便厥 , 咽中乾 , 煩躁 吐逆 者, 作 甘草乾薑湯 與之 。

원문 해설 세포병변성 감염증으로 맥이 뜨고 땀나고 소변이 잦으며 마음이 괴롭고 약 간 오한이 들며 다리가 땅기어 오므라드는 경우에 계지를 병용하지 않는다. 계지로 체열을 올리면 병이 악화된다. 병의 초기에 곧바로 수족냉증이 나타나고 목구멍이 건조하며 괴롭고 구토하는 경우에는 감초건강탕을 병용하여 쓴다.

적응증 Sjogren's syndrome (쇼그렌 증후군)

병태 & 증상

➡ exocrine glands cell: endogenous retrovirus 활성화
➡ Anti-SSA/Ro & anti-SSB/La antibodies 출현
➡ neutrophil 유도
➡ neutrophil phagocytosis
➡ HClO 분비 via H2O2
➡ exocrine glands: 세포막 손상
➡ Na+/ K+ pump 손상
➡ 세포부종
➡ exocrine glands inflammation: throat dryness, vommiting
➡ blood H2O2: hypotension ▶ hand & feet coldness

처방 목표 HClO 분비 억제 / Na+/ K+ pump 활성화

처방 구성 炙甘草 四兩 / 乾薑 二兩

처방 약리

구감초 18β-24-Hydroxyglycyrrhetinic acid
➡ HSD11B2 inhibitor
➡ cortisol 분해 억제
➡ mineralocorticoid receptors 자극 지속
➡ Na+/ K+ pumps 전사 촉진

건강 shogaol ➡ neutrophil H2O2 scavenger
➡ HClO 분비 억제

감초마황탕 (甘草麻黃湯)

원문 裡水, 越婢加朮湯 主之, 甘草麻黃湯 亦 主之。

원문 해설 피하 부종이 있을 때는 월비가출탕이나 감초마황탕을 쓴다.

적응증 Type I hypersensitive reaction: first sensitization

병태 & 증상

Type I hypersensitive reaction: first sensitization

➡ allergen 침입
➡ B cell IgE Rc: allergen binding
➡ B cell: allergen specific IgE 생산
➡ mast cell FcR γ: IgE binding
➡ mast cell FcR γ: IgE ▶ allergen: single binding
➡ mast cell: calcium channel
➡ calcium influx
➡ membrane-bound adenylate cyclase 활성화
➡ cAMP ↑
➡ cAMP-dependent protein kinase 활성화
➡ cAMP ↓
➡ granule-membrane protein: phospholylation
➡ granule swelling
➡ plasma membrane: granule fusion
➡ histamine degranulation
➡ vasodilation
➡ body fluid influx: body swelling

처방 목표 allergen specific IgE 생산 억제 / histamine granulation 억제

처방 구성 甘草 二兩 / 麻黃 四兩

처방 약리

감초 glycyrrhetinic acid
➡ 11-beta-hydroxysteroid dehydrogenase1 (HSD11B1) inhibitor

➡ glucocorticoid 작용
➡ B cell: IκBα 생성
➡ NF-κB 억제
➡ 항체 생성 억제

마황 ephedrine ➡ Epinephrine receptors agonist
➡ adenylate cyclase 활성화
➡ cAMP ↑
➡ histamine degranulation 억제

감초부자탕 (甘草附子湯)

원문 風濕 相搏，骨節 疼煩，掣 痛 不得 屈伸，近 之 則 痛 劇，汗出 短氣，小便 不利，惡風 不欲 去衣，或 身 微 腫 者，甘草附子湯 主之。

원문 해설 백혈구 공격으로 세포내부종이 있고 관절이 쑤시는데, 너무 아파서 구부렸다 폈다를 할 수 없고 근처를 만지기만 해도 통증이 심하고, 땀나고 호흡이 짧아지며 소변이 개운치 않고 추워서 옷 벗기가 싫으며 혹 몸이 약간 붓는 경우에는 감초부자탕을 쓴다.

적응증 Coxsackie virus-mediated polymyositis & polyarthritis
(다발성근염 & 다발성관절염)

병태 & 증상

Coxsackie virus polymyositis & polyarthritis

➡ skeletal muscle cell & joint: Coxsackie virus infection
➡ IgG antibodies 출현
➡ neutrophil 유도
➡ neutrophil: monocyte chemoattractant protein-1 (MCP-1) 분비
➡ endothelial cell: VCAM-1 발현
➡ monocyte 유도
➡ Coxsackie virus infected cell: phagocytosis ▶ IL-1 : sweating, coldness
➡ ROS burst

➡ myositis & arthritis
➡ polymyositis: myoglobinuria & hyperlactemia
  : sychnuria & shortness of breath, edema

처방 목표 neutrophil MCP-1 분비 억제 / VCAM-1 발현 억제 / hyperlactemia 교정

처방 구성 炮附子 二枚 / 白朮 二兩 / 桂枝 四兩 / 炙甘草 二兩

처방 약리

포부자 aconitine

➡ 약리추측: neutrophil` Voltage-gated proton channels blocker
  (식균작용에 의해 증가된 세포내 proton을 세포외로 방출시키는 채널)
➡ Voltage-gated proton channels 차단
➡ 호중구내 수소이온 축적
➡ neutrophil 대사 억제
➡ monocyte chemoattractant protein-1 (MCP-1) 분비 억제

백출 atractylon ➡ vascular cell adhesion molecule-1 (VCAM-1) blocker

계지 cinnamic acid ➡ lactate oxidizer
  ➡ Cori cycle: pyruvate 전환 촉진

구감초 18β-24-Hydroxyglycyrrhetinic acid
  ➡ HSD11B2 inhibitor
  ➡ cortisol 분해 억제
  ➡ mineralocorticoid receptors 자극 지속
  ➡ H+ 배출

감초사심탕 (甘草瀉心湯)

원문 傷寒 / 中風 / 醫 反 下 之, 其 人 下利 日 數 十 行, 穀 不化, 腹中 雷鳴, 心 下 痞硬 而 滿, 乾嘔, 心煩 不 得 安。醫 見 心下痞, 謂 病 不 盡, 復 下 之, 其 痞 益 甚, 此 非 結 熱, 但 以 胃中虛, 客氣 上逆, 故 使 硬 也, 甘草瀉心湯 主之。

원문 해설 세포병변성 감염증으로 Hypothalamic set point가 상승되어 있는데 잘못하여 위장관 점막림프구를 배출시키면 설사를 하루에 수십 번 하게 되고, 소화가 안 되고 뱃속에서 꼬르륵 소리가 진동하며 속 쓰림이 있으면서 명치 밑이 단단해지고 팽만감과 구역이 있고 괴롭고 편하지 않다. 속 쓰림이 있고 병이 낫지 않았는데 다시 사하제를 쓰면 속 쓰림이 더 심해지며 단지 속이 빈 것 같으면 복막염이 되지 않은 것으로 천공이 아직 윗부분에 있는 것이며 복부가 단단해진다. 감초사심탕을 쓴다.

적응증 Peptic ulcer-complicated perforation (소화성궤양에 합병된 천공)

병태 & 증상

Peptic ulcer complicated perforation

➡ 위장, 십이지장: Helicobacter pylori 정착
➡ Helicobacter pylori: 병원성 균으로 형질전환
➡ Helicobacter pylori: Cag pathogenicity island (Cag PAI) 유전자 활동
➡ H. pylori peptidoglycan: type IV secretion system 형성
➡ peptidoglycan: macrophage 유도
➡ extracellular peroxynitrite ($ONOO^-$)
➡ 상피세포 & 점막세포 손상
➡ mucin 분비 ↓ : heartburn
➡ Helicobacter pylori: CagE gene
➡ epithelial cell: IL-8 분비
➡ neutrophil 유도 ▶ neutrophil phagocytosis
➡ HClO 분비 via H2O2
➡ ulcer 진행: 근육층 손상
➡ 위산 공격
➡ 천공: collapse felling & stiffness

처방 목표 H. pylori peptidoglycan 합성 억제 / extracellular $ONOO^-$ 제거 / 상피 &점막세포 상환 촉진 / HClO 분비 억제 / 위산 분비 억제 / 점막근층 ~ 근육층 재생 촉진

처방 구성 炙甘草 四兩 / 黃芩 三兩 / 半夏 半升 / 大棗 十二枚 / 黃連 一兩 / 乾薑 三兩

처방 약리

황련 berberine ➡ sortase inhibitor
➡ H. pylori: peptidoglycan 합성 억제
➡ 병독성 감소됨

황금 baicalin ➡ peroxynitrite ($ONOO^-$) scavenger

반하 triterpenoid ($C_{30}H_{48}O_7S$)
➡ Rho GTPase family transcription promotor
➡ focal adhesion 생성
➡ 상피세포 이동 촉진

건강 shogaol ➡ neutrophil H_2O_2 scavenger
➡ HClO 분비 억제

구감초 18β-24-Hydroxyglycyrrhetinic acid ➡ HSD11B2 inhibitor
➡ cortisol 분해 억제
➡ mineralocorticoid receptors 자극 지속
➡ H+ 배출
➡ 위산 분비 감소

대조 c-AMP ➡ Protein kinase A avtivator
➡ ATP 합성 촉진
➡ cell cycle ↑

감초탕 (甘草湯)

원문 少陰病 , 二 三 日 , 咽痛 者, 甘草湯 主之 。

원문 해설 항체매개 세포독성이 시작되고 2~3일후 인후통이 있는 경우에는 감초탕을 쓴다.

적응증 Viral pharyngitis (바이러스성 인두염)

병태 & 증상

Viral pharyngitis

➡ numerous viruses
➡ pharynx: lymph glands infection
➡ B cell: IgM 생성
➡ 보체 유도
➡ 보체의존성 세포용해
➡ virus infected lymph glands: necrosis
➡ swollen lymph glands: sore throat

처방 목표 IgM 생성을 억제시킴

처방 구성 甘草 二兩

처방 약리

감초 glycyrrhetinic acid

➡ 11-beta-hydroxysteroid dehydrogenase1 (HSD11B1) inhibitor
➡ glucocorticoid 작용
➡ IκBα 생성
➡ NF-κB 억제
➡ B cell 대사 억제
➡ 항체 생성 억제

건강부자탕 (乾薑附子湯)

원문 下之後，復發汗，晝日 煩躁 不得眠，夜 而 安靜，不嘔 不渴，無 表證，脈 沉微，身 無 大熱 者, 乾薑附子湯 主之。

원문 해설 치료 후 다시 땀이 나고 낮에는 괴로워 잠들지 못하고, 밤이 되면 편해진다. 구역과 갈증이 없고 체표증상도 없이 맥이 가라앉고 약하면서 고열이 없는 경우에는 건강부자탕을 쓴다.

적응증 Adenovirus infection

병태 & 증상

lymph node macrophage: adenovirus infection

➡ macrophage: adenovirus vector 삽입
➡ macrophage 활성화
➡ macrophage: inflammatory protein-2 & CKC chemkine 분비
➡ neutrophil 유도
➡ neutrophil phagocytosis
➡ HClO 분비 via H2O2: 낮시간에 증가
➡ tissue injury: agony

처방 목표 macrophage: inflannatory protein-2 & CKC chemkine 분비 억제 / HClO 분비 억제

처방 구성 乾薑 一兩 / 附子 一枚

처방 약리

부자 hypaconitine
➡ 약리 추측 : macrophage` Voltage-gated proton channels blocker
(식균작용에 의해 증가된 세포내 proton을 세포외로 방출시키는 채널)
➡ proton 방출 억제
➡ 세포내 pH ↓ 감소
➡ macrophage 대사 억제
➡ inflannatory protein-2 & CKC chemkine 분비 억제

건강 shogaol ➡ neutrophil H2O2 scavenger
➡ HClO 분비 억제

건강인삼반하환 (乾薑人參半夏丸)

원문 妊娠 嘔吐 不止 , 乾薑人參半夏丸 主之 。

원문 해설 임신 중에 구토가 멈추지 않는 경우에는 건강인삼반하탕을 쓴다.

적응증 Cytomegalovirus-mediated placental villitis (태반 융모세포염)

병태 & 증상

Cytomegalovirus-mediated placental villitis

➡ placental villi: CMV infection
➡ specific CMV antibody 출현
➡ neutrophil 유도
➡ neutrophil phagocytosis
➡ HClO 분비 via H2O2
➡ villitis: gonadotropin ↑: vomit
➡ 영양막 세포: 섬유소 분비
➡ villous calcification
➡ villous tissues: TGF-β ↑
➡ villous calcification 억제

처방 목표 HClO 분비 억제 / villitis 복구 / villous tissues TGF-β 발현 증가

처방 구성 乾薑 一兩 / 人參 一兩 / 半夏 二兩

처방 약리

건강 shogaol ➡ neutrophil H2O2 scavenger
➡ HClO 분비 억제

반하 triterpenoid (C30H48O7S)
➡ Rho GTPase family transcription promotor
➡ focal adhesion 생성
➡ 영양막 세포 상환 촉진

인삼 panax ginsenoside
➡ Transforming growth factor β (TGF-β) (+) modulator
➡ villous calcification 억제

건강황금황련인삼탕 (乾薑黃芩黃連人參湯)

원문 傷寒 本 自寒下, 醫 復 吐 下 之, 寒格, 更 逆 吐 下, 若 食 入 口 即 吐, 乾薑黃芩黃連人參湯 主之。

원문 해설 세포병변성 감염증에서 물설사를 하는데, 최토제를 쓰거나 사하제를 쓰면 물설사도 그치지 않고 음식을 먹는 즉시 구토하는 경우에는 건강황금황련인삼탕을 쓴다.

적응증 Staphylococcal food poisoning (포도구균 식 중독)

병태 & 증상

Staphylococcal food poisoning

➡ intestinal epithelium: staphylococcus aureus infection
➡ staphylococcal enterotoxins
➡ macrophage 유도
➡ staphylococcus aureus 식균: nitric oxide 생성
➡ 세포간질: peroxynitrite ($ONOO^-$) 유출
➡ 상피손상
➡ macrophage inflammatory protein-1α 분비
➡ neutrophil 유도
➡ staphylococcus aureus 식균
➡ neutrophil phagocytosis
➡ HClO 분비 via H2O2
➡ staphylococcus aureus: survival & mutant
➡ 점막 손상: diarrhea
➡ staphylococcal mutant: enterotoxins 분비
➡ T cell 활성화
➡ T cell: cytokine 분비 ▶ vomiting

처방 목표 staphylococcus aureus 항균 / $ONOO^-$ 제거 / HClO 분비 억제 / 손상된 점막 재생

처방 구성 乾薑 / 黃芩 / 黃連 / 人參 各 三兩

처방 약리

황련 berberine ➡ sortase inhibitor
➡ staphylococcus aureus peptidoglycan 합성 억제
➡ 삼투압성 용균

황금 baicalin ➡ peroxynitrite ($ONOO^-$) scavenger

건강 shogaol ➡ neutrophil H2O2 scavenger
➡ HClO 분비 억제

인삼 panax ginsenoside

➡ Transforming growth factor β (TGF-β) (+) modulator
➡ cell proliferation 촉진

계령오미감초거계가강신하탕 (桂苓五味甘草去桂加薑辛夏湯)

원문 咳滿即止，而更復渴，衝氣復發者，以細辛、乾薑為熱藥也，服之當遂渴，而渴反止者，為支飲也。支飲者法當冒，冒者必嘔，嘔者復內半夏以去其水。

원문 해설 기침과 심장부위의 팽만감이 가라앉고서, 다시 갈증이 시작되면서 심장독성이 재발하는 경우에도 세신과 건강으로 갈증이 없어져야 하며 반대로 갈증이 그치지 않을 때에는 수분정체가 있는 것이며, 환자는 머리가 무거울 것이고, 구역이 생길 것이므로 반하를 추가한다.

적응증 Chronic left heart failure-mediated alveolar-capillary barrier damage
(만성좌심부전-매개 폐포-모세혈관 장벽 손상)

병태 & 증상

Pneumonia complications-mediated alveolar-capillary barrier damage

➡ pneumonia
➡ alveolar macrophage: IL-8
➡ 폐포 간질: neutrophil 유도
➡ neutrophil phagocytosis
➡ HClO 분비 via H2O2
➡ alveolar-capillary barrier: damage
➡ 폐포 간질: erythrocyte 유입
➡ Met hemoglobin 형성 ▶ 혈관 수축
➡ alveolitis
(폐포 간질: fibroblast 이동 ▶ collagen 분비: thirsty, neusea)
➡ 폐포환기량 저하

➡ pulmonary artery pressure ↑
➡ 좌심실: out flow ↓
➡ 좌심실 심첨부: thrombus formation

처방 목표 alveolar macrophage 대사 억제 / HClO 분비 억제 / Met hemoglobin 환원 / 폐포 세포 상환 촉진 / 폐포환기량 증가 / 좌심실 심첨부: thrombus 억제
처방 구성 茯苓 四兩 / 甘草 二兩 / 細辛 二兩 / 乾薑 二兩 / 五味子 半升 / 半夏 半升

처방 약리

감초 glycyrrhetinic acid

➡ 11-beta-hydroxysteroid dehydrogenase1 (HSD11B1) inhibitor
➡ glucocorticoid 작용
➡ IκBα 생성
➡ NF-κB 억제
➡ alveolar macrophage 대사 억제

건강 shogaol ➡ neutrophil H2O2 scavenger
➡ HClO 분비 억제

세신 eugenol ➡ Met-Hb reducer
➡ Rho GTPase family transcription promotor
➡ focal adhesion 생성
➡ 폐포 세포 상환 촉진

오미자 schizandrin ➡ acetylcholinesterase inhibitor
➡ 횡격막근 수축 강화

복령 pachymic acid ➡ glycoprotein IIb/IIIa (gpIIb/IIIa) (-) modulator
➡ thrombus formation 억제

계령오미감초탕 (桂苓五味甘草湯)

원문 青龍湯 下 已, 多唾 口燥, 寸脈 沉, 尺脈 微, 手足 厥逆, 氣 從 小腹 上衝 胸咽, 手足 痹, 其 面 翕熱 如 醉狀, 因 復 下 流 陰股, 小便 難, 時 復 冒 者, 與 茯苓桂枝五味甘草湯, 治 其 氣 衝。

원문 해설 청룡탕으로 치료한 뒤에, 침이 많아지고 입이 마르며, 촌맥은 가라앉고 척맥은 약하며, 손발이 심하게 차가워지고, 아랫배에서 심장부위로 치밀어 오르는 듯한 기운이 있으며, 손발이 저리고, 얼굴은 술 취한 듯이 열감이 있고, 이런 열감이 넓적다리 부위로 다시 내려가며, 소변이 힘들고 때때로 머리가 무거운 경우에는 복령계지오미감초탕을 써서 심장 독성을 치료한다.

적응증 Pneumonia complications-mediated hypoxemia (폐렴합병증-매개 저산소혈증)

병태 & 증상

Pneumonia complications-mediated hypoxemia

➡ pneumonia
➡ 폐포 손상
➡ 폐포환기량 저하
➡ pulmonary artery pressure ↑
➡ 좌심실: out flow ↓
➡ 좌심실 심첨부: thrombus formation

➡ 혈 중산소 농도 감소
➡ hypoxemia
➡ artery pressure 지속 : cold hands and feet, face hot flashes
, urine retension, head heavy
➡ peripheral tissue: ischemic damage
➡ lactatemia: cardiac toxicity

처방 목표 폐포환기량 증가 / 좌심실 심첨부: thrombus 억제 / lactatemia 교정

처방 구성 茯苓 四兩 / 桂枝 四兩 / 炙甘草 三兩 / 五味子 半升

처방 약리

오미자 schizandrin ➡ acetylcholinesterase inhibitor
➡ 횡격막근 수축 강화

복령 pachymic acid ➡ glycoprotein IIb/IIIa (gpIIb/IIIa) (-) modulator
➡ thrombus formation 억제

계지 cinnamic acid ➡ lactate oxidizer
➡ pyruvate 전환
➡ Cori cycle 활성화
➡ lactatemia 교정

구감초 18β-24-Hydroxyglycyrrhetinic acid
➡ 11-beta-hydroxysteroid dehydrogenase2 (HSD11B2) inhibitor
➡ aldosterone 생리작용과 동일
➡ H+ secretion

계지가갈근탕 (桂枝加葛根湯)

원문 太陽病 , 項背 強几几 , 反 汗出 惡風 者, 桂枝加葛根湯 主之 。

원문 해설 림프절 감염병으로 목과 등이 뻣뻣해지고 땀이 나며 추위를 타는 경우에는 계지가갈근탕을 쓴다.

적응증 IFN-a mediated Meningoencephalitis (뇌수막염)

병태 & 증상

Measles virus / Mumps virus / Rubella virus

➡ meningeal infection
➡ meningeal macrophage phagocytosis
➡ macrophage: IL-1 분비: sweating / coldness
➡ fever: heat shock protein activation
➡ macrophage내 복제된 바이러스 단백질 분해 & 세포밖에서 바이러스 입자 포획
➡ Astrocyte infection

➡ Astrocyte: IFN-a 분비
➡ microglia 유도: nitric oxide 분비
➡ BBB breakdown
➡ 뇌실질의 대사산물이 뇌척수액으로 유출
➡ 뇌수막 압력 ↑: neck-back stiffness
➡ meningitis
➡ nitric oxide: Astrocyte EAAT expression ↓
➡ synapse에서 glutamate 축적
➡ postsynaptic neuron ionotropic glutamate Rc: glutamate 자극
➡ postsynaptic neuron: glutamate excitotoxicity ↑
➡ encephalitis

처방 목표 heat shock protein 활성화 : 바이러스 증식 억제 / microglia secretion 억제 / ionotropic glutamate Rc 차단

처방 구성 葛根 四兩 / 桂枝 三兩 / 芍藥 三兩 / 生薑 三兩 / 炙甘草 二兩 / 大棗 十二枚 / 麻黃 三兩

처방 약리

계지 / 작약 / 생강 / 대조 / 구감초 heat production
➡ heat shock protein 활성화 (계지탕 참고)

마황 ephedrine ➡ epinephrine receptors agonist
➡ microglia secretion 억제

갈근 ionotropic glutamate receptor blocker

계지가계탕 (桂枝加桂湯)

원문 燒針 令 其 汗 / 針處 被 寒 / 核 起 而 赤 者 / 必 發 奔豚 , 氣從 少腹 上衝 心 者 / 灸 其 核 上 各 一 壯 / 與 桂枝加桂湯 。

원문 해설 온침을 놓아 발한시킴: 땀이 없는 발열 지속되어 온침으로 땀구멍 열어줌 / 침자리가 냉해짐: 온침으로 땀구멍 연 곳만 땀나고 냉해짐 / 침자리가 빨갛게 돋아남: 체표가 차가워진 후 지방세포가 분해되는 것 / 분돈증 생김 (새끼 돼지가 이리저리 달리는 모습을 표현 한 것) / 분돈증은 아랫배에서 심장 쪽으로 치밀어 오르는 듯한

고통이 생긴다. / 빨갛게 돋은 침 자리에 뜸을 한 장씩 뜸 (뜨겁게 해주면 지방세포 분해 멈춤) / 계지가계탕을 같이 쓴다.

적응증 Lipacidemia-mediated Cardiac toxicity (지방산혈증-매개 심장독성)

병태 & 증상

TNF-α mediated viral infection

➡ TNF-α: hypotension 유도됨 ▶ 땀구멍 닫힘 ▶ 발열 지속 됨
➡ TNF-α: Insulin resistance
➡ 복강 지방세포 / 큰말초 지방세포 / 골격근 세포 / 간세포 : Lipolysis ↑
➡ 혈 중 유리 지방산 ↑
➡ 심근: 유리 지방산 산화 ↓, 포도당 산화 ↓
➡ 심근: lactate & H+축적
➡ 심근 수축력 ↓
➡ Lipacidemia mediated Cardiac toxicity

처방 목표 Lipolysis 억제 / 심근의 lactate을 pyruvate로 전환

처방 구성 桂枝 五兩 / 芍藥 三兩 / 生薑 三兩 / 炙甘草 二兩 / 大棗 十二枚

처방 약리

뜸 lipolysis 억제

계지 / 작약 / 생강 / 대조 / 구감초 heat production ➡ lipolysis 억제

계지 cinnamic acid ➡ lactate oxidizer
➡ pyruvate 전환 촉진

계지가대황탕 (桂枝加大黃湯)

원문 本 太陽病，醫 反 下 之，因 爾 腹滿 時 痛 者，屬 太陰 也，桂枝加芍藥湯 主 之；大 實 痛 者，桂枝加大黃湯 主之。

원문 해설 본래 림프절 감염병인데 의사가 반대로 위장관 점막림프절을 배출시킨 후, 복부팽만감과 복통이 반복되면 태음병(자가항체독성병)이 된 것으로 계지가작약탕을 쓰고, 변비가 있으면서 복통이 있는 경우에는 계지가대황탕을 쓴다.

적응증 Autoimmune enteropathy & colon cancer (자가면역성 장병증 & 대장암)

병태 & 증상

Autoimmune enteropathy & colon cancer

➡ small bowel : intra-epithelial lymphocyte
➡ enterocyte : MHC class II molecule 발현
➡ autoantigen 발현 (tumor suppressor gene)
➡ T cell 활성화
➡ : p56kk activation : H2O2 mediation
  ➡ Phospholipase C activation
  ➡ diacylglycerol & Inositol trisphosphate 생성
  ➡ diacylglycerol ▶ Ras GTPase ↑ : superoxide mediation
  ➡ Inositol trisphosphate ▶ endoplasmic reticulum: calcium 분비
  ➡ T cell transcription ↑
➡ B cell 활성화
➡ anti-enterocyte antibody 생성됨
➡ enterocyte : autoantibody 부착
➡ enterocyte : 세포내 대사 ↓
➡ enterocyte : SOD ↓
➡ superoxide ↑
➡ superoxide로 인해 Fe3+(ferric ions)가 Fe2+(ferrous ion)로 환원됨
➡ Ferrous ion-induced lipid peroxidation in mitochondria
➡ mitochondria membrane potential damage
➡ enterocyte : lactate ↑ ▶ ATP ↓
➡ Na+/ K+ pump 손상
➡ enterocyte 손상
➡ persistent diarrhea & tumor suppressor gene 손상
➡ colon cancer

처방 목표 T cell 대사 억제 / superoxide 제거 / enterocyte lactate 교정 / colon cancer 성장 억제

처방 구성 桂枝 三兩 / 大黃 二兩 / 芍藥 六兩 / 生薑 三兩 / 炙甘草 二兩 / 大棗 十二枚

처방 약리

생강 gingerol ➡ T cell H_2O_2 scavenger : p56kk 억제됨

작약 paeoniflorin ➡ superoxide scavenger
➡ T cell Ras GTPase 감소됨 & enterocyte superoxide 제거

대조 c-AMP ➡ inhibition of granular organelles phosphorylation
➡ T cell endoplasmic reticulum: calcium 분비 억제

구감초 18β-24-Hydroxyglycyrrhetinic acid
➡ HSD11B2 inhibitor
➡ cortisol 분해 억제
➡ mineralocorticoid receptors 자극 지속됨
➡ enterocyte Na+/ K+ pumps 활성화

계지 cinnamic acid ➡ lactate oxidizer
➡ pyruvate 전환 촉진

대황 emodin ➡ tyrosine kinase blocker
➡ colon cancer 성장 억제

REFERENCE

Susumu Ishikawaa, Ichiro Kobayashib, Jun-Ichi Hamadaa, Mitsuhiro Tadaa, Atsuko Hiraia, Keiji Furuuchia, Yoko Takahashia, Yi Baa and Tetsuya Moriuchia . Interaction of MCC2, a novel homologue of MCC tumor suppressor, with PDZ-domain Protein AIE-75. Gene, Volume 267, Issue 1, 4 April 2001, Pages 101-110.

계지가부자탕 (桂枝加附子湯)

원문 太陽病 , 發汗 , 遂漏 不止 , 其人 惡風 , 小便 難 , 四肢 微急 , 難 以 屈伸 者, 桂枝加附子湯 主之 。

원문 해설 림프절 감염병에서 땀이 줄줄 흐르고 추위를 타며 소변이 안 나오고 팔다리가 땅겨서 굽혔다 폈다하기가 힘든 경우에는 계지가부자탕을 쓴다.

적응증 Acute EBV infection

병태 & 증상

Acute EBV infection

➡ pharynx: EBV infection (Epstein-Barr virus)
➡ pharynx: 1차증식
➡ 전신 lymphoreticular system: B cell ➡ 2차증식
➡ EBV infected B cell: IL-1 autocrine & paracrine: sweating, coldness
➡ EBV replication
➡ EBV antibody 출현
➡ neutrophil 유도
➡ neutrophil: cathepsin 분비
➡ lymphoreticular ststem tissue 손상: limbs ache
➡ Kidney의 세뇨관 간질: EBV infection
➡ acute interstitial nephritis
➡ acute oliguric renal failure

처방 목표 heat shock protein 활성화: EBV replication 억제 / neutrophil: cathepsin 분비 억제

처방 구성 桂枝 三兩 / 芍藥 三兩 / 炙甘草 三兩 / 生薑 三兩 / 大棗 十二枚 / 炮附子 一枚

처방 약리

계지 cinnamic acid ➡ 골격근세포 lactate을 pyruvate로 환원

작약 paeoniflorin ➡ 골격근세포 superoxide scavenger

생강 gingerol ➡ 골격근세포 hydrogen peroxide scavenger

대조 cAMP ➡ 골격근세포 glycogenolysis 촉진

구감초 18β-24-Hydroxyglycyrrhetinic acid -〉 골격근세포 Na-K pumps 활성화

계지/ 작약/ 생강/ 대조/ 구감초 ➡ 골격근 ATP 생산 증가

➡ heat shock protein 활성화
➡ EBV replication 억제

포부자 aconitine

➡ 약리추측 : neutrophil` Voltage-gated proton channels blocker
(식균작용에 의해 증가된 세포내 proton을 세포외로 방출시키는 채널)
➡ Voltage-gated proton channels 차단
➡ 호중구내 수소이온 축적
➡ neutrophil 대사 억제
➡ cathepsin 분비 억제

계지가용골모려탕 (桂枝加龍骨牡蠣湯)

원문 夫失精家少腹弦急，陰頭寒，目眩，髮落，脈極虛芤遲，為清穀亡血，失精。脈得諸芤動微緊，男子失精，女子夢交，桂枝加龍骨牡蠣湯主之。

원문 해설 성인이 체액을 손실하면 아랫배가 당기고 생식기 부위가 차가우며, 어지럽고 탈모가 생긴다. 맥이 거의 잡히지 않고 느리고 비어 있는 것은 구토, 설사, 출혈 등으로 체액을 손실했기 때문이다. 맥이 비어 있고 누르면 약간 급한 경우에는 남녀의 잠자리가 원인이고 계지가용골모려탕을 쓴다.

적응증 Hypernatremia-mediated hypotension (고나트륨혈증-매개 저혈압)

병태 & 증상

Hypernatremia-mediated hypotension

➡ 체액 손실: 위장관 / 피부 / 기관지 / 요로 / 생식기 / 출혈
➡ hypovolemic hypernatremia
➡ hypotension
➡ tissue ischemia: myalgia, cold hands and feet, dizziness, hair loss
➡ ischemia cell: lactate ↑ & superoxide ↑ & hydrogen peroxide & cAMP
➡ NF-κB 활성화
➡ ischemia cell: inflammation

➡ lactatemia
➡ acidosis

처방 목표 lactate 교정 / superoxide 제거 / hydrogen peroxide 제거 / c-AMP 보충 / NF-κB 억제 / acidosis 교정 / Hypernatremia 교정

처방 구성 桂枝 三兩 / 芍藥 三兩 / 生薑 三兩 / 甘草 二兩 / 大棗 十二枚 / 龍骨 三兩 / 牡蠣 三兩

처방 약리

계지 cinnamic acid ➡ lactate oxidizer
➡ pyruvate 전환 촉진

작약 paeoniflorin ➡ superoxide scavenger

생강 gingerol ➡ hydrogen peroxide scavenger
대조 c-AMP ➡ protein kinase A avtivator
➡ activation of glycogenolysis

감초 glycyrrhetinic acid
➡ 11-beta-hydroxysteroid dehydrogenase1 (HSD11B1) inhibitor
➡ glucocorticoid 작용
➡ IκBα 생성
➡ NF-κB 억제

용골 CaCO3 ➡ NaHCO3 공급원 ➡ 산증 교정

모려 NaCl ➡ hyponatremia & hypernatremia 교정

계지가작약탕 (桂枝加芍藥湯)

원문 本太陽病，醫反下之，因爾腹滿時痛者，屬太陰也，桂枝加芍藥湯主之。

원문 해설 본래 림프절 감염병인데 의사가 반대로 위장관 점막림프세포를 배출시킨 후,그로 인해 복부팽만감과 복통이 반복되면 태음병(자가항체독성병)이 된 것이며 계지가작약탕을 쓴다.

적응증 Autoimmune enteropathy (자가면역성 장병증)

병태 & 증상

Autoimmune enteropathy

➡ small bowel: intra-epithelial lymphocyte ↓
➡ enterocyte: MHC class II molecule 발현 ↑
➡ T cell 활성화
: p56kk activation : H2O2 mediation
　➡ Phospholipase C activation
　➡ diacylglycerol & Inositol trisphosphate 생성
　➡ diacylglycerol ➡ Ras GTPase ↑ : superoxide mediation
　➡ Inositol trisphosphate ➡ endoplasmic reticulum: calcium 분비
　➡ T cell transcription ↑
➡ B cell 활성화
➡ anti-enterocyte antibody 생성됨
➡ enterocyte : autoantibody 부착
➡ enterocyte : 세포내 대사 ↓
➡ enterocyte : SOD ↓
➡ superoxide ↑
➡ superoxide로 인해 Fe^{3+}(ferric ions)가 Fe^{2+}(ferrous ion)로 환원됨
➡ Ferrous ion-induced lipid peroxidation in mitochondria
➡ mitochondria membrane potential damage
➡ enterocyte: lactate ↑
➡ ATP ↓
➡ Na^+/ K^+ pump 손상
➡ enterocyte 손상
➡ persistent diarrhea

처방 목표 T cell 대사 억제 / superoxide 제거 / enterocyte lactate 교정

처방 구성 桂枝 三兩 / 芍藥 六兩 / 炙甘草 二兩 / 大棗 十二枚 / 生薑 三兩

처방 약리

생강 gingerol ➡ T cell H2O2 scavenger: p56kk 억제됨

작약 paeoniflorin ➡ superoxide scavenger
➡ T cell Ras GTPase 감소됨 & enterocyte superoxide 제거

대조 cAMP ➡ inhibition of granular organelles phosphorylation
➡ T cell endoplasmic reticulum: calcium 분비 억제

구감초 18β-24-Hydroxyglycyrrhetinic acid
➡ HSD11B2 inhibitor
➡ cortisol 분해 억제
➡ mineralocorticoid receptors 자극 지속
➡ enterocyte Na+/ K+ pumps 활성화

계지 cinnamic acid ➡ lactate oxidizer
➡ pyruvate 전환 촉진

계지가황기탕 (桂枝加黃耆湯)

원문 黃汗之病, 兩脛自冷 ; 假令發熱, 此屬歷節。食已汗出, 又身常暮臥盜汗出者, 此勞氣也。若汗出已反發熱者, 久久其身必甲錯 ; 發熱不止者, 必生惡瘡。若身重, 汗出已輒輕者, 久久必身目瞤, 目瞤即胸中痛, 又從腰以上必汗出, 下無汗, 腰髖弛痛, 如有物在皮中狀, 劇者不能食, 身疼重, 煩躁, 小便不利, 此為黃汗, 桂枝加黃耆湯主之。

원문 해설 누런 땀이 있고 양쪽 종아리가 차가우면서 열이 나는 것은 노화가 원인이며밥 먹을 때 땀을 흘리며 저녁에 자려할 때도 땀이 나는 것은 과로가 원인이다. 만약 땀을 흘

린 이후에 발열을 계속 하면 피부에 반드시 부스러기가 생기고 열이 그치지 않으면 반드시 악창이 생긴다. 만약 몸이 무거운데 땀이 난 뒤에는 가벼워지고 병이 오래되면 반드시 몸에서 쥐가 나고 눈꺼풀이 떨리게 된다, 눈꺼풀이 떨리면 이어서 흉통이 생기며, 허리 윗부분은 반드시 땀을 흘리고 아랫부분은 땀이 없으며, 허리와 엉덩이 부위가 땅기고 아프고, 피부 밑에 물체가 있는 듯이 보이고, 심하면 먹지 못하고 몸이 아리면서 무거우며, 마음이 괴롭고 불편하며, 소변이 불편하다. 이상의 증상은 황한병으로 생긴 것으로 계지가황기탕을 쓴다.

적응증 Eccrine sweat gland capillaritis (에크린분비선 모세혈관염)

병태 & 증상

ATP & fever 생산 ↑

➡ 땀선 모세혈관 수축: 증발열 억제
➡ capillary constriction ↑↑
➡ eccrine sweat gland: myoepithelium ischemia
➡ myoepithelium: 수축력 감소
➡ 땀분비 감소
➡ 식사 & 수면: acethylcholine ↑
➡ eccrine sweat gland 자극
➡ myoepithelium: 수축 ▶ 허혈 손상
➡ eccrine sweat gland: 땀분비 정지
➡ 진피 & 표피 모세혈관 / 수분 이동 & apocrine sweat gland: sweating,
하체에는 apocrine sweat gland 없음: 下無汗
➡ capillary congestion
➡ lymphocyte 유도
➡ capillaritis
➡ fibrin formation
➡ fibrin embolism
➡ multiple infarcts : muscle / heart / iliolumbar artery / gastrointestinal brain / kidney

처방 목표 myoepithelium ischemia 개선 / lymphocyte 이동 억제 / fibrin 용해

처방 구성 桂枝 三兩 / 芍藥 三兩 / 生薑 三兩 / 大棗 十二枚 / 甘草 二兩 / 黃耆 二兩

처방 약리

계지 / 작약 / 생강 / 대조 ➡ myoepithelium ischemia 개선

감초 glycyrrhetinic acid

➡ HSD11B1 inhibitor

➡ cortisol 분해 억제

➡ glucocorticoid receptors 자극 지속됨

➡ IκBα 생성

➡ NF-κB 억제

➡ leukocyte 이동 억제됨

황기 astragaloside ➡ Tissue plasminogen activator (+) modulator

➡ fibrinolysis

계지가행자탕 (桂枝加厚朴杏子湯)

원문 太陽病，下之 微 喘者，表未解 故也，桂枝加厚朴杏子湯 主之.

원문 해설 림프절 감염병을 치료한 후 천식 증상을 보일 때는 아직 바이러스 증식이 있는 것이므로 계지가행자탕을 쓴다.

적응증 Airway remodeling-mediated Asthma (기도 개형-매개 천식)

병태 & 증상

Airway remodeling-mediated Asthma

➡ airway endothelial cell: Rhinovirus infection

➡ airway endothelial cell: rhinovirus replication

➡ IgA: Rhinovirus coated airway endothelial cell 결합

➡ complement 유도

➡ airway endothelial cell: MAC (membrane attack complement) 형성

➡ airway endothelial cell: mitochondria 대사 항진

➡ hydroxyl radical ↑ : airway endothelial cell apoptosis

➡ 천식 환자의 경우

➡ airway endothelial cell: VEGF 분비

➡ airway smooth muscle cell: VEGF Rc 부착

➡ Rho kinase 활성화

➡ smooth muscle cell: proliferation
➡ 기관지 평활근 두꺼워짐
➡ Airway remodeling

처방 목표 heat shock protein 활성화: rhinovirus replication 억제시킴 / hydroxyl radical 제거 / VEGF Rc 차단

처방 구성 桂枝 三兩 / 炙甘草 二兩 / 生薑 三兩 / 芍藥 三兩 / 大棗 十二枚 / 厚朴(炙) 二兩 / 杏仁 五十枚

처방 약리

계지 / 작약 / 생강 / 대조 / 구감초 : heat shock protein 생성 촉진
행인 : benzoic acid ➡ hydroxyl radical scavenger

후박 : honokiol ➡ VEGF receptor blocker

계지감초용골모려탕 (桂枝甘草龍骨牡蠣湯)

원문 火 逆 下 之，因 燒 針 煩躁 者, 桂枝甘草龍骨牡蠣湯 主之。

원문 해설 발열 중에 뜸을 뜨거나 온침을 놓으면 땀구멍이 열려 땀이 나게 되는데 이런 치료는 잘못된 것이고 화역이라 하며 계지감초용골모려탕을 쓴다.

적응증 Rapid hyponatremia (급속 저나트륨혈증)

병태 & 증상

Rapid hyponatremia

➡ IL-1 mediated fever
➡ 땀: water loss
➡ 물 섭취 않으면: 고장성 탈수 / 물 섭취하면: 등장성 탈수
➡ hyponatremia
➡ 세포외액이 세포내부로 이동됨

➡ 뇌세포의 경우 세포내의 유기성 삼투질(organic osmolytes)을 감소시켜 뇌세포부종을 교정함
➡ Rapid hyponatremia 경우
➡ 유기성 삼투질을 통한 뇌세포부종의 교정단계를 거치지 못하고 뇌세포 부종이 진행됨
➡ neuron: Na+ & water accumulation
➡ Na+/ K+ pump: dysfunction
➡ 뇌세포 부종
➡ 두개내압 ↑
➡ 신경학적 증상 발생
➡ & 소변량 감소: H+ 분비 ↓
➡ acidosis

처방 목표 rapid hyponatremia 교정

➡ CNS 증상 있을 때는 hypertonic saline (3~5%) 투여 / acidosis 교정/ Na+/ K+ pump 활성화 / lactate 대사 촉진 ➡ 뇌신경 대사 촉진

처방 구성 桂枝 一兩 / 炙甘草 二兩 / 牡蠣 二兩 / 龍骨 二兩

처방 약리

모려 NaCl ➡ hyponatremia & hypernatremia 교정

용골 $CaCO_3$ -> $NaHCO_3$ 공급원 -> 산증 교정

구감초 18β-24-Hydroxyglycyrrhetinic acid

➡ HSD11B2 inhibitor
➡ cortisol 분해 억제
➡ mineralocorticoid receptors 자극 지속
➡ Na+/ K+ pumps 전사 활성화

계지 cinnamic acid ➡ lactate oxidizer

➡ pyruvate 전환 촉진
➡ 뇌신경세포 대사기능 촉진

계지감초탕 (桂枝甘草湯)

원문 發汗 過多, 其人 叉 手 自 冒 心, 心下悸, 欲 得 按 者, 桂枝甘草湯 主之。

원문 해설 땀을 많이 흘린 후 두 손을 깍지 껴서 가슴을 덮게 되고, 심장이 두근거려서계속 누르게 되는 경우에는 계지감초탕을 쓴다.

적응증 Lactacidemia-mediated cardiomyopathy (지방산혈증-매개 심근병증)

병태 & 증상

IL-1을 증가시키는 virus infection

➡ Hypothalamic set point ↑
➡ smooth muscle heat production: ATP 합성
➡ cortisol
➡ sweat glands 자극
➡ sweating
➡ muscle: lactate ↑
➡ liver & kidney: Cori cycle에서 lactate 처리
➡ Cori cycle 포화
➡ blood: hyperlactation
➡ lactacidemia
➡ myocardiocyte: ATP생산에 lactate의 참여가 증가됨
➡ myocardiocyte: lactate ↑
➡ low pH
➡ ATP
➡ Na+/ K+ pump 손상
➡ 심근세포 부종
➡ 심장 박동 불규칙해짐: palpitation
➡ lactacidemia mediated cardiomyopathy

처방 목표 심근 lactate 교정 / 심근 Na+/ K+ pump 활성화

처방 구성 桂枝 四兩 / 炙甘草 二兩

처방 약리

계지 cinnamic acid ➡ lactate oxidizer
➡ pyruvate 전환 촉진

구감초 18β-24-Hydroxyglycyrrhetinic acid
➡ HSD11B2 inhibitor
➡ cortisol 분해 억제
➡ mineralocorticoid receptors 자극 지속
➡ Na+/ K+ pumps 전사 촉진

계지거계가복령백출탕 (桂枝去桂加茯苓白朮湯)

원문 服 桂枝湯，或 下 之，仍 頭項 強痛，翕翕 發熱，無汗, 心下 滿 微痛 ，小便 不利 者, 桂枝去桂加茯苓白朮湯 主之 。

원문 해설 계지탕을 복용한 후나 혹은 위장관 점막림프절을 배출한 후에 머리와 목이 대단히 아프고, 찌는 듯이 발열하고, 땀은 없이 심장 밑이 부풀듯이 약간 아프고 소변이 잘 나오지 않는 경우에는 계지거계가복령백출탕을 쓴다.

적응증 Kawasaki disease

병태 & 증상

Kawasaki disease

➡ Staphylococcus aureus / Streptococcus pyogenes / retrovirus: superantigen
➡ T cell Rc 부착
➡ p56kk activation: H2O2 mediation
➡ Phospholipase C activation
➡ diacylglycerol & Inositol trisphosphate 생성
➡ diacylglycerol ➡ Ras GTPase ↑ : superoxide mediation
➡ Inositol trisphosphate ➡ endoplasmic reticulum: calcium 분비
➡ T cell transcription ↑
➡ TNF-α 분비: fever / no sweating

➡ 혈관내피세포: VCAM-1 발현
➡ monocyte 부착후 내피하 침윤: 주로 관상동맥 & 콩팥 동맥 & 신경계 혈관
: coronary arteritis & kidney arteritis & neuritis
➡ monocyte: ROS 분비
➡ 혈관내피세포: Na+/ K+ pump 손상
➡ 혈관내피세포 부종
➡ 혈관내피 손상
➡ 혈소판 응집
➡ thrombus formation

처방 목표 T cell 대사 억제 / 혈관내피세포 VCAM-1 차단 / 혈관내피세포 Na+/ K+ pump 활성화 / thrombus 제거

처방 구성 芍藥 三兩 / 炙甘草 二兩 / 生薑 三兩 / 茯苓 三兩 / 白朮 三兩 / 大棗 十二枚

처방 약리

생강 gingerol ➡ H2O2 scavenger: T cell p56kk 억제됨

작약 paeoniflorin ➡ superoxide scavenger: T cell Ras GTPase 감소됨

대조 cAMP ➡ inhibition of granular organelles phosphorylation
➡ T cell endoplasmic reticulum: calcium 분비 억제

구감초 18β-24-Hydroxyglycyrrhetinic acid
➡ HSD11B2 inhibitor
➡ cortisol 분해 억제
➡ mineralocorticoid receptors 자극 지속
➡ 혈관내피세포: Na+/ K+ pumps 전사 촉진

백출 atractylon ➡ vascular cell adhesion molecule-1 (VCAM-1) blocker

복령 pachymic acid ➡ glycoprotein IIb/IIIa (gpIIb/IIIa) (-) modulator
➡ thrombus formation 억제

계지거작약가마황세신부자탕 (桂枝去芍藥加麻黃細辛附子湯)

원문 氣分, 心下堅, 大如盤, 邊 如 旋杯, 水飲 所作, 桂枝去芍藥加麻黃細辛附子湯 主之 。

원문 해설 호흡이 편하지 않으면서 심장 밑이 큰 쟁반처럼 단단하고 가장자리가 국 담는 대접처럼 오목해져 있는 것은 흉막강에 삼출액이 고인 것으로 계지거작약가마황세신부자탕을 쓴다.

적응증 Autoimmune response-mediated Methemoglobinemia

병태 & 증상

Autoimmune response-mediated Methemoglobinemia

➡ Early autoimmune response for erythrocyte
➡ erythrocyte C3b Rc: C3b coated immune complex 부착
➡ natural killer cell FcR III: erythrocyte 부착
➡ natural killer cell: IFN-γ 분비
➡ neutrophil 유도
➡ neutrophil: IL-12 분비
➡ natural killer cell: degranulation
➡ natural killer cell: IFN-γ 분비 촉진
➡ erythrocyte 손상
➡ erythrocyte hemoglobin: methemoglobin 전환
➡ Methemoglobinemia
➡ shortness of breath
➡ 횡격막근 수축 빈도 ↑: hydrogen peroxide ↑, lactate ↑
➡ 횡격막근 피로
➡ 횡격막근 수축력 ↓
➡ 복강을 아래로 밀어내리는 힘이 약해지고 흉곽이 확장되지 못하고 수축됨
➡ 흉골 함몰

처방 목표 항체 생성 억제 / neutrophil: IL-12 분비 억제 / natural killer cell: degranulation 억제 / methemoglobin 환원 / 횡격막근 피로 개선

처방 구성 桂枝 三兩 / 生薑 三兩 / 甘草 二兩 / 大棗 十二枚 / 麻黃 二兩 / 細辛 二兩 / 炮附子 一枚

처방 약리

감초 glycyrrhetinic acid

➡ 11-beta-hydroxysteroid dehydrogenase1 (HSD11B1) inhibitor

➡ glucocorticoid 작용

➡ IκBα 생성

➡ NF-κB 억제

➡ B cell 항체 형성 감소

포부자 aconitine

➡ 약리추측: neutrophil` Voltage-gated proton channels blocker
(식균작용에 의해 증가된 세포내 proton을 세포외로 방출시키는 채널)

➡ Voltage-gated proton channels 차단

➡ 호중구내 수소이온 축적

➡ neutrophil 대사 억제

➡ IL-12 분비 억제

마황 ephedrine ➡ Epinephrine receptors agonist

➡ adenylate cyclase 활성화

➡ cAMP ↑

➡ Natural killer cell: degranulation 억제

세신 eugenol ➡ methemoglobin reducer

계지 cinnamic acid ➡ lactate oxidizer

➡ pyruvate 전환 촉진

➡ 횡격막근 lactate 교정

생강 gingerol ➡ hydrogen peroxide scavenger

➡ 횡격막근 수축력 증가

대조 c-AMP ➡ protein kinase A avtivator

➡ 횡격막근 glycogenolysis 촉진

계지거작약가부자탕 (桂枝去芍藥加附子湯)

원문 太陽病，下之後，脈促，胸滿, 若 微寒 者, 桂枝去芍藥加附子湯 主之。

원문 해설 림프절 감염병이 나은 후 맥박이 빨라지고 가슴부위가 뻐근해지고 약간 오한이 나는 경우에는 계지거작약가부자탕을 쓴다.

적응증 IL-1 mediated Cardiac toxicity

병태 & 증상

lymph node: virus infection

➡ lymph node macrophage: IL-1 ↑
➡ cortisol ↑
➡ epinephrine 작용시간 ↑
➡ myocardiocyte: 수축빈도 ↑
➡ mitochondrial respiration 반복되면서 superoxide 발생
➡ superoxide dismutase에 의해 hydrogen peroxide 생성
➡ Catalase, GSH-Px 작용으로 H2O와 O2로 전환
➡ Catalase, GSH-Px 고갈
➡ hydrogen peroxide 축적
➡ 저농도 hydrogen peroxide: PKC을 자극하여 PKC mediated signal 활성화
, 고농도 hydrogen peroxide: PKC가 억제되어 PKC mediated 근수축 감소
➡ intracellular lactate ↑
➡ ATP ↓
➡ Na+/ K+ pumps 손상
➡ myocardiocyte apoptosis: IL-6 분비 -> chills
➡ neutrophil 유도
➡ neutrophil ; cathepsin 분비
➡ 심근 손상

처방 목표 hydrogen peroxide 제거 / intracellular lactate 교정 / Na+/ K+ pump 활성화 / 심근 수축력 회복 / neutrophil ; cathepsin 분비 억제

처방 구성 桂枝 三兩 / 炙甘草 二兩 / 生薑 三兩 / 大棗 十二枚 / 炮附子 一枚

처방 약리

생강 gingerol ➡ hydrogen peroxide scavenger

계지 cinnamic acid ➡ lactate oxidizer
➡ pyruvate 전환 촉진

구감초 18β-24-Hydroxyglycyrrhetinic acid
➡ HSD11B2 inhibitor
➡ cortisol 분해 억제
➡ mineralocorticoid receptors 자극 지속
➡ Na+/ K+ pumps 활성화

대조 c-AMP ➡ Ca-dependent contraction 회복

포부자 aconitine
➡ 약리추측: neutrophil` Voltage-gated proton channels blocker
(식균작용에 의해 증가된 세포내 proton을 세포외로 방출시키는 채널)
➡ Voltage-gated proton channels 차단
➡ 호중구내 수소이온 축적
➡ neutrophil 대사 억제

계지거작약가촉칠모려용골구역탕 (桂枝去芍藥加蜀漆牡蠣龍骨救逆湯)

원문 傷寒 脈浮，醫 以 火迫劫 之，亡陽，必 驚狂，臥起 不安 者，桂枝去芍藥加蜀漆牡蠣龍骨救逆湯 主之。

원문 해설 세포병변성 감염증에서 맥이 뜨는데 온침이나 부황으로 치료한 경우, 뇌세포 내액이 고갈되어 반드시 미친 사람처럼 되고 극도로 불안해지는 경우에는 계지거작약가촉칠모려용골구역탕을 쓴다.

적응증 Rapid hypernatremia (급속 고나트륨혈증)

병태 & 증상

Rapid hypernatremia

➡ TNF-α mediated fever
➡ 땀 없는 발열
➡ 과호흡: water loss
➡ Na 소실은 없으면서 물만 소실된 경우
➡ hypernatremia
➡ 세포내액이 세포밖으로 배출됨
➡ 천천히 발생된 고나트륨혈증: 뇌세포는 inositol, glutamine과 같은 유기성 삼투질을 생산하여 세포내 삼투압을 높여서 세포내액을 보존함
➡ rapid hypernatremia
➡ 뇌세포에서 유기성 삼투질을 만들기 전에 뇌세포액이 세포 밖으로 배출됨
➡ 뇌세포 위축: agitation, confusion, seizure, coma
➡ 과호흡: PaCO2 ↑ , PaO2 ↓
➡ hypoxemia
➡ brain: H2O2 ↑ & c-AMP ↓
➡ brain: Na+/ K+ pump 손상
➡ tissue ischemia: lactate ↑
➡ lactacidemia
➡ acidosis

처방 목표 체열 발산 / rapid hypernatremia 교정 / brain H2O2 감소시킴 / brain c-AMP 공급 / Na+/ K+ pump 활성화 / lactacidemia 교정 / acidosis 교정

처방 구성 桂枝 三兩 / 炙甘草 二兩 / 生薑 三兩 / 大棗 十二枚 / 牡蠣 五兩 / 蜀漆 三兩 / 龍骨 四兩

처방 약리

촉칠 dichronine ➡ Vasodilation: 체열 떨어뜨림

모려 NaCl ➡ hyponatremia & hypernatremia 교정

생강 gingerol ➡ hydrogen peroxide scavenger

대조 c-AMP ➡ Protein kinase A acvtivator
➡ neuron: ATP 생산 촉진

구감초 18β-24-Hydroxyglycyrrhetinic acid

➡ HSD11B2 inhibitor

➡ cortisol 분해 억제

➡ mineralocorticoid receptors 자극 지속

➡ Na+/ K+ pumps 전사 촉진

계지 cinnamic acid ➡ lactate oxidizer

➡ Cori cycle: pyruvate 전환 촉진

용골 $CaCO_3$ ➡ $NaHCO_3$ 공급원 ➡ 산증 교정

REFERENCE

J I Sznajder, A Fraiman, J B Hall, W Sandera, G Schmidt, G Crawford, A Nahum, P Factor, and L D Wood. Increased hydrogen peroxide in the expired breath of patients with acute hypoxemic respiratory failure. CHEST September 1989 vol. 96 no. 3 606-612.

계지거작약탕 (桂枝去芍藥湯)

원문 太陽病 , 下之後 , 脈促, 胸滿 者, 桂枝去芍藥湯 主之 。

원문 해설 림프절 감염병이 나은 후 맥박이 빨라지고 가슴부위가 뻐근해지는 경우에는계지거작약탕을 쓴다.

적응증 IL-1 mediated Cardiac toxicity

병태 & 증상

lymph node: virus infection

➡ lymph node macrophage: IL-1 ↑

➡ cortisol ↑

➡ epinephrine 작용시간 ↑

➡ myocardiocyte: 수축빈도 ↑

➡ mitochondrial respiration 반복되면서 superoxide 발생

➡ superoxide dismutase에 의해 hydrogen peroxide 생성

➡ Catalase, GSH-Px 작용으로 H2O와 O2로 전환
➡ Catalase, GSH-Px 고갈
➡ hydrogen peroxide 축적
➡ 저농도 hydrogen peroxide: PKC 자극 ▶ PKC mediated signal 활성화
➡ 고농도 hydrogen peroxide: PKC 억제 ▶ 근수축 감소
➡ intracellular lactate ↑
➡ ATP ↓
➡ Na+/K+ pumps 손상
➡ 심근 수축력 감소

처방 목표 hydrogen peroxide 제거 / intracellular lactate 교정 / Na+/K+ pump 활성화 / 심근 수축력 회복

처방 구성 桂枝 三兩 / 炙甘草 二兩 / 生薑 三兩 / 大棗 十二枚

처방 약리

생강 gingerol ➡ hydrogen peroxide scavenger

계지 cinnamic acid ➡ lactate oxidizer
➡ pyruvate 전환 촉진

구감초 18β-24-Hydroxyglycyrrhetinic acid
➡ HSD11B2 inhibitor
➡ cortisol 분해 억제
➡ mineralocorticoid receptors 자극 지속
➡ Na+/ K+ pumps 전사 촉진

대조 c-AMP ➡ Ca-dependent contraction 회복

계지마황각반탕 (桂枝麻黃各半湯)

원문 太陽病，得 之 八 九 日，如 瘧 狀，發熱 惡寒，熱多 寒少，其 人 不 嘔, 清 便 欲 自 可，一 日 二 三 度 發。脈 微 緩 者，為 欲 愈 也 ; 脈 微 而 惡寒 者，此 陰 陽 俱 虛，不 可 更 發汗 更 下 更 吐 也 ; 面色 反 有 熱 色 者， 未 欲 解 也, 以 其 不能 得 小 汗出，身 必 癢，宜 桂枝麻黃各半湯。

원문 해설 림프절 감염증이 8~9일이 경과한 뒤, 학질 같이 발열과 오한이 있는데, 열이 많고 오한은 적다. 구역이 없고 대소변도 정상인데, 하루에 2~3회씩 발열과 오한이 반복된다. 맥이 약하고 느린 경우에는 나으려고 하는 것이며, 맥이 약하고 오한이 있는 경우에는 체열상승도 약하고, 면역세포의 활동력도 약한 것이므로, 발한법 (계지탕)과 사하법 (망초), 최토법 (과체산)을 계속 쓰지 않는다. 얼굴색이 열이 있는 것처럼 보이면 아직 낫지 않은 것이며, 땀이 조금도 나지 않아 몸이 가려워 지는데 계지마황각반탕을 쓴다.

적응증 *IFN*-a resistant viral infection

병태 & 증상

Virus infection

➡ lymph node immune cell: virus infection ➡ IL-1 분비: 발열 유도
➡ lymph node immune cell: heat shock protein 활성화 ▶ virus replication 억제
➡ 만약, 초기 heat shock protein: 바이러스 억제 실패
➡ virus infected immune cell: virus replication 지속
➡ 만약, IFN-a: 회피 바이러스인 경우
➡ Natural killer cell 유도: 실패
➡ IL-1 지속
➡ fever
➡ B cell proliferation
➡ 중화 항체 출현
➡ virus infected cell: antibody 부착
➡ immature Natural killer cell 유도
➡ immature Natural killer cell: TRAIL-dependent secretion
: fever / coldness / no sweating
➡ antibody coated virus infected cell: TRAIL 작동
▶ 당대사 급격한 증가

▶ lactate ↑

▶ mitochondria ROS ↑

▶ mitochondria dysfunction

▶ apoptosis

➡ NKc-generated hydroxyl radical 유출

➡ tissue damage

처방 목표 발열 유도를 통해 B cell proliferation 촉진 / immature Natural killer cell: TRAIL-dependent secretion 억제 / hydroxyl radical 제거

처방 구성 桂枝 一兩 十六銖 / 芍藥 / 生薑 / 炙甘草 / 麻黃 各 一兩 / 大棗 四枚 / 杏仁 二十四枚

처방 약리

계지 / 작약 / 생강 / 대조 / 구감초: heat production ➡ B cell proliferation 촉진

➡ 항체 생성 촉진

마황 ephedrine ➡ Epinephrine receptors agonist

➡ adenylate cyclase 활성화

➡ cAMP ↑

➡ NKc secretion 억제

행인 benzoic acid ➡ hydroxyl radical scavenger

계지복령환 (桂枝茯苓丸)

원문 婦人 宿 有 癥病, 經斷 未及 三月, 而 得 漏下 不止, 胎動 在 臍上 者, 為 癥 痼 害。妊娠 六月 動 者, 前 三月 經水 利 時, 胎 也。下 血 者, 後 斷 三月 衃 也。所 以 血 不 止 者, 其 癥 不 去 故 也, 當 下 其 癥, 桂枝茯苓丸 主之。

원문 해설 오랫동안 근종이 있는 부인이 생리가 3개월째 없는데(임신12주) 대하가 생겨 그치지 않는 것은 태아가 위치를 바로잡지 못해 계속 움직이기 때문에 생기는 것으로 근종 때문이다. 임신 6개월에 태동이 있으며 3개월 전부터 출혈이 있는 것은 태아가 편

한 위치를 잡기 위해 움직이기 때문이다. 근종이 있어 생리양이 많던 부인이 생리가 3개월째 없는 경우는(임신12주) 근종이 커질 것이다. 따라서 임신 중에 하혈이 그치지 않으면 근종을 제거해야 되며 계지복령환을 쓴다.

적응증 Uterine myoma (자궁근종)

병태 & 증상

Uterine myoma

➡ normal myocyte
➡ tumor initiator: genetic factor (?)
➡ somatic mutation
➡ mutated myocyte
➡ estrogen & progesterone
➡ mitogenesis
➡ clonal expansion
➡ myoma
➡ myoma: estrogen receptor mediated rapidly growth
➡ myoma tissue: ischemic-reperfusion
➡ lactate 축적 / superoxide 증가
➡ manganese superoxide dismutase & glutathione peroxidase 고갈
➡ myoma tissue: oxidant stress
➡ necrosis
➡ huge myoma: deep vein thrombosis
& 임신 1~2분기에 자궁출혈을 일으키고 자연유산율이 증가됨
& 임신 3분기에 조산율이 증가됨

처방 목표 myoma estrogen receptor 차단 / lactate 제거 / superoxide 제거 / myoma: ROS scanenger enzyme 생산 증가시킴 / thrombosis 억제

처방 구성 桂枝 / 茯苓 / 牡丹 / 芍藥 / 桃仁 各 等分

처방 약리

도인 amygdalin,
➡ 체내 활성 성분: thiocyanate (amygdalin metabolite)
➡ 4S estrogen receptor (ER): 5S estrogen receptor 전환 억제
(5S dimer: estrogen 고친화성)

계지 cinnamic acid ➡ lactate oxidizer
➡ pyruvate 전환 촉진

작약 paeoniflorin ➡ superoxide scavenger

목단피 β-Sitosterol
➡ manganese superoxide dismutase & glutathione peroxidase (+) modulator

복령 pachymic acid ➡ glycoprotein IIb/IIIa (gpIIb/IIIa) (-) modulator
➡ thrombus formation 억제

계지부자탕 (桂枝附子湯)

원문 傷寒 八 九 日 , 風濕 相搏 , 身體 疼煩 , 不能 自轉側, 不嘔 不渴, 脈 浮虛 而 澀 者 , 桂枝附子湯 主 之 。若 其人 大便硬 , 小便 自利 者 , 去桂加白朮湯 主 之 。

원문 해설 세포병변성 감염증이 8~9째 백혈구 공격으로 세포내부종이 발생하여 몸이 쑤시고 아프며 움직일 수 없게 된 경우, 구역과 갈증이 없으며 맥이 뜨면서 부족하고 막히는 맥상이면 계지부자탕으로 치료한다. 만약 대변이 굳고 소변이 저절로 나오면 거계가백출탕을 쓴다.

적응증 Influenza myositis (인플루엔자 근염)

병태 & 증상

Influenza myositis

➡ skeletal muscle cell: Influenza virus infection
➡ macrophage: Influenza virus 탐식
➡ macrophage: IL-8 분비
➡ neutrophil 유도: cathepsin 분비
➡ Influenza virus infected skeletal muscle cell: 기저막에서 분리됨
➡ skeletal muscle cell: mitochondria dysfunction
➡ intracellular lactate ↑ : lactatemia

➡ ATP ↓
➡ xanthine oxidase mediated superoxide 축적
➡ superoxide dismutase에 의해 hydrogen peroxide 생성
➡ Na+/ K+ pumps 손상
➡ 골격근세포 부종
➡ myositis: myalgias, severe pain

처방 목표 neutrophil: cathepsin 분비 억제 / intracellular lactate 교정 / Cori cycle을 통한 lactatemia 교정 / hydrogen peroxide 제거 / Na+/ K+ pumps 활성화 / ATP 생산 촉진

처방 구성 桂枝 四兩 / 炮附子 三枚 / 生薑 三兩 / 大棗 十二枚 / 炙甘草 二兩, 去桂加白朮湯: 炮附子 三枚 / 白朮 四兩 / 生薑 三兩 / 炙甘草 二兩 / 大棗 十二枚

처방 약리

포부자 aconitine
➡ 약리추측: neutrophil` Voltage-gated proton channels blocker
(식균작용에 의해 증가된 세포내 proton을 세포외로 방출시키는 채널)
➡ Voltage-gated proton channels 차단
➡ 호중구내 수소이온 축적
➡ neutrophil 대사 억제

계지 cinnamic acid ➡ lactate oxidizer
➡ pyruvate 전환 촉진

생강 gingerol ➡ hydrogen peroxide scavenger

구감초 18β-24-Hydroxyglycyrrhetinic acid
➡ HSD11B2 inhibitor
➡ cortisol 분해 억제
➡ mineralocorticoid receptors 자극 지속
➡ Na+/ K+ pumps 전사 촉진

대조 c-AMP ➡ Protein kinase A avtivator
➡ activation of glycogenolysis

계지이마황일탕 (桂枝二麻黃一湯)

원문 服 桂枝湯，大汗出，脈 洪大者，與 桂枝湯，如 前法。
若 形 似 瘧，一日 再發者，汗出 必解，宜 桂枝二麻黃一湯。

원문 해설 계지탕 복용 후 땀을 많이 흘렸는데 맥이 넓고 크면 다시 계지탕을 쓴다. 만약 증상이 학질 같이 하루 두 번씩 발열 한다면 땀을 나게 해서 풀어주어야 하며 계지이마황일탕을 쓴다.

적응증 heat shock protein-resistant viral infection

병태 & 증상

Virus infection

➡ lymph node immune cell: virus infection ▶ IL-1 분비: 발열 유도
➡ lymph node immune cell: heat shock protein 활성화 ▶ virus replication 억제

➡ 만약, heat shock protein: 회피 바이러스인 경우
➡ virus infected immune cell: virus replication 지속
➡ IFN-a 분비: fever
➡ NKc activation
➡ Natural killer cell: degranulation
➡ IFN-γ
➡ virus infected cell: IFN-γ Rc binding
➡ virus infected immune cell 세포막: FAS 작동
➡ virus infected immune cell : TRAIL 작동
▶ 당대사 급격한 증가
▶ mitochondria ROS ↑
▶ mitochondria dysfunction
▶ apoptosis
➡ extracellular hydroxyl radical 유출
➡ tissue damage

처방 목표 발열 유도를 통해 B cell proliferation 촉진 / NKc degranulation 억제 / extracellular hydroxyl radical 제거

처방 구성 桂枝 一兩 十七銖 / 芍藥 一兩 六銖 / 麻黃 十六銖 / 生薑 一兩 六銖 / 杏仁 十六個 / 炙甘草 一兩 二銖 / 大棗 四枚

처방 약리

계지 / 작약 / 생강 / 대조 / 구감초: heat production ➡ B cell proliferation 촉진
➡ 항체 생성 촉진

마황 ephedrine ➡ Epinephrine receptors agonist
➡ adenylate cyclase 활성화
➡ cAMP ↑
➡ NKc degranulation 억제

행인 benzoic acid ➡ hydroxyl radical scavenger

계지이월비일탕 (桂枝二越婢一湯)

원문 太陽病, 發熱 惡寒, 熱多 寒少, 脈微弱者, 此 無陽也, 不可 發汗, 宜 桂枝二越婢一湯 。

원문 해설 림프절 감염병으로 발열하고 오한이 있는데, 발열은 많고 오한이 적으며 맥이 아주 약할 때에는 면역력이 약해 IL-1이 적어서 생기는 증상이므로이런 경우에는 발열만 동원해서는 안 되므로 계지이월비일탕을 쓴다.

적응증 IL-1 deficiency-mediated viral infection

병태 & 증상

Virus infection

➡ immature dendritic cell (iDC): virus phagocytosis
➡ iDC: virus replication
➡ iDC: IL-1 ↑ ▶ fever ▶ heat shock protein 활성화: 바이러스 증식 억제

➡ 만약 IL-1 생산 ↓: 無陽
➡ virus replication 지속
➡ iDC: IFN-α
➡ NKc 유도
➡ NKc: TNF-α 분비: fever ↑
➡ iDC: mature DC 전환

➡ mature DC: MHC class II molecule에 바이러스 항원 발현
➡ Th2 cell: 항원 전달됨
➡ macrophage 활성화
➡ virus 전파 ↑

처방 목표 iDC: virus replication 억제 / NKc secretion 억제 / Th2 cell apoptosis 유도

처방 구성 桂枝 / 芍藥 / 麻黃 / 炙甘草 各 十八銖 / 大棗 四枚 / 生薑 一兩 二銖 / 石膏 二十四銖

처방 약리

계지 / 작약 / 생강 / 대조 / 구감초: heat production
➡ iDC: virus replication 억제

마황 ephedrine ➡ Epinephrine receptors agonist
➡ adenylate cyclase 활성화
➡ cAMP ↑
➡ NKc secretion 억제

석고 $CaSO_4$ ➡ calcium mediated T-cell apoptosis 유도

계지인삼탕 (桂枝人參湯)

원문 太陽病, 外證 未除, 而 數 下之, 遂 協熱 而 利, 利下 不止, 心下 痞硬, 表裡 不解 者, 桂枝人參湯 主之.

원문 해설 림프절 감염병에서 체표증상이 있어서 수차례 치료했는데도 열이 가시지 않으면서 설사하는데, 설사가 그치지 않고 명치 밑이 쓰린 경우는 체표와 장부가 낫지 않은 것이므로 계지인삼탕을 쓴다.

적응증 Rotavirus enteritis (로타바이러스 장염)

병태 & 증상

Rotavirus enteritis

➡ 소장 enterocyte: rotavirus infection
➡ enterocyte: integrin 발현
➡ rotavirus fusion & endocytosis
➡ rotavirus replication
➡ enterocyte: IL-8 분비
➡ neutrophil 유도
➡ neutrophil degranulation
➡ enterocyte: 손상
➡ 선와세포 (crypt cell) 증식후 융모끝으로 이동
➡ 미성숙한 선와세포로 소장상피가 대체됨
➡ 미성숙한 선와세포: Na+/ K+ pump activity ↓
➡ glucose coupled Na transport 장애
➡ 수분, 전해질 흡수 ↓ & lactase ↓
➡ 설사 & 젖산혈증

처방 목표 enterocyte integrin 차단 / neutrophil degranulation 억제 / 선와세포 Na+/ K+ pump 활성화 / 선와세포 성숙 촉진 / 젖산혈증 교정

처방 구성 桂枝 四兩 / 炙甘草 四兩 / 白朮 三兩 / 人參 三兩 / 乾薑 三兩

처방 약리

백출 atractylon ➡ integrin blocker

건강 shogaol ➡ neutrophil H2O2 scavenger
➡ neutrophil degranulation 억제

구감초 18β-24-Hydroxyglycyrrhetinic acid
➡ HSD11B2 inhibitor
➡ cortisol 분해 억제
➡ mineralocorticoid receptors 자극 지속
➡ Na+/ K+ pumps 전사 촉진

인삼 panax ginsenoside
➡ Transforming growth factor β (TGF-β) (+) modulator
➡ cell development 촉진

계지 cinnamic acid ➡ lactate oxidizer

➡ Cori cycle: pyruvate 전환 촉진
➡ lactatemia 교정

계지작약지모탕 (桂枝芍藥知母湯)

원문 諸肢節疼痛，身體尫羸，脚腫如脫，頭眩短氣，溫溫欲吐，桂枝芍藥知母湯主之。

원문 해설 모든 관절이 쑤시고 아프며, 혹 같이 불거져서 괴롭고, 다리가 부어서 빠질 듯하며, 머리가 어지럽고 호흡이 짧으며, 토하고 싶은 경우에는 계지작약지모탕을 쓴다.

적응증 Rheumatoid arthritis (류마티스 관절염)

병태 & 증상

Rheumatoid arthritis

➡ synoviocyte: auto-antigen 발현
➡ synovial dendritic cell: phagocytosis
➡ B cell 활성화
➡ B cell: auto-antigen specific IgE 생산 ↑
➡ synovial mast cell FcR γ: high affinity IgE Rc
▶ auto-antigen: mutiple binding
➡ mast cell: Fyn/Gab2/RhoA-signaling pathway 활성화
➡ microtubule polymerization via hydrogen peroxide
➡ 세포질 granule: translocation
➡ plasma membrane: granule fusion
➡ vasoactive amines degranulation
: histamine / serine proteases / serotonin / heparin
➡ vasodilation: body fluid influx
➡ synovial tissue: swelling
➡ mast cell: IL-1 & TNF-α 분비
➡ vascular endothelium: VCAM-1 발현
➡ eosinophil 유도
➡ eosinophil: vasoactive amines degranulation ↑

➡ synoviocyte inflammation: IL-8 분비
➡ neutrophil 유도
➡ neutrophil elastase: hyaluronate destruction ▶ synovitis
➡ neutrophil: IL-1 분비 ▶ dizziness, shortness of breath, vomitting
➡ synovial fibroblast 활성화
➡ synovial fibroblast: prostaglandin E2 분비
➡ chodrocyte: copper-zinc superoxide dismutase 소진
▶ superoxide ↑ ▶ chondrocytis
& cartilage muscle: 대사 항진 ▶ lactate ↑ ▶ cartilage muscle inflammation

처방 목표 auto-antigen specific IgE 생산 억제 / mast cell: hydrogen peroxide 제거 / mast cell & eosinophil: degranulation 억제 / VCAM-1 차단 / neutrophil: elastase 분비 억제 / synovial fibroblast: prostaglandin E2 생성 억제 / chodrocyte: superoxide 제거 / cartilage muscle: lactate 교정 / synoviocyte & chondrocyte & cartilage muscle: 다분화 촉진

처방 구성 桂枝 四兩 / 芍藥 三兩 / 甘草 二兩 / 麻黃 二兩 / 生薑 五兩 / 白朮 五兩 / 知母 四兩 / 防風 四兩 / 炮附子 二枚

처방 약리

감초 glycyrrhetinic acid
➡ 11-beta-hydroxysteroid dehydrogenase1 (HSD11B1) inhibitor
➡ glucocorticoid 작용
➡ B cell: IκBα 생성
➡ NF-κB 억제
➡ 항체 생성 억제

생강 gingerol ➡ hydrogen peroxide scavenger

마황 ephedrine ➡ Epinephrine receptors agonist
➡ adenylate cyclase 활성화
➡ cAMP ↑
➡ degranulation 억제

백출 atractylon ➡ vascular cell adhesion molecule-1 (VCAM-1) blocker

포부자 aconitine

➡ 약리추측: neutrophil` Voltage-gated proton channels blocker
(식균작용에 의해 증가된 세포내 proton을 세포외로 방출시키는 채널)
➡ Voltage-gated proton channels 차단
➡ 호중구내 수소이온 축적
➡ 호중구내 대사 억제
➡ elastase 분비 억제

방풍 deltoin ➡ cyclooxygenase-2 blocker

작약 paeoniflorin ➡ superoxide scavenger

계지 cinnamic acid ➡ lactate oxidizer
➡ pyruvate 전환

지모 timosaponin
➡ nestin (+) modulator
➡ multi-differentiation 세포에서 발현되는 단백질
➡ synovium progenitor cell: nestin 발현
➡ synoviocyte & chondrocyte & cartilage muscle: 다분화 촉진

상한잡병론이 저술된 후한(後漢)시대의 도량 단위

부피: 1승 (升) = 약 198 ml
1두 (斗) = 10승 = 1980 ml

무게: 1수 (銖) = 1/6 푼 = 0.65 g
1푼 (分) = 1/4 량 = 3.9 g
1량 (兩) = 약 14.16 g
1근 (斤) = 16 량 = 226.56 g
1균 (鈞) = 30 근 = 480 량 = 6796.8 g
1석 (石) = 4균 =1920 량
1방촌비 (方寸匕) = 가로, 세로, 높이 2.3cm되는 수저에 담는 용량

길이: 1 척 (尺) = 23㎝

계지탕 (桂枝湯)

원문 熱自發, 汗自出, 嗇嗇惡寒, 淅淅惡風, 翕翕發熱, 鼻鳴乾嘔, 桂枝湯 主之 。

원문 해설 발열하고 땀을 흘리는데, 오싹한 오한이 있으면서 춥고, 화끈거리는 발열이 있으면서, 코가 막히고 구역이 있는 경우에는 계지탕을 쓴다.

적응증 Common cold

병태 & 증상

Common cold

➡ lymph node: virus infection
➡ dendritic cell & macrophage: virus phagocytosis
➡ virus replication
➡ dendritic cell & macrophage: interleukin-1 분비: nausea
➡ Hypothalamus 자극
➡ prostaglandins E2 분비: nasal congestion
➡ Hypothalamic set point ↑
➡ smooth muscle heat production: chills
& vasocontriction: coldness
➡ fever
➡ virus infected cell: heat shock protein 발현 ↑
➡ 세포질내 복제된 바이러스 단백질 분해 & 세포밖에서 바이러스 입자 포획
➡ virus 억제
➡ 혈 중 IL-1: 땀샘을 통해 배출: sweating

골근육 생리

➡ 지속적인 ATP생산
➡ mitochondrial respiration 반복되면서 superoxide 축적
➡ superoxide dismutase에 의해 hydrogen peroxide 생성
➡ Catalase, GSH-Px 작용으로 H2O와 O2로 전환
➡ Catalase, GSH-Px 고갈
➡ hydrogen peroxide 축적
➡ 저농도 hydrogen peroxide: PKC 활성화 ▶ PKC mediated signal 활성화,
고농도: PKC 억제 ▶ PKC mediated 근수축발생 감소

➡ superoxide dismutase2 고갈
➡ superoxide로 인해 Fe3+(ferric ions)가 Fe2+(ferrous ion)로 환원됨.
➡ Ferrous ion-induced lipid peroxidation in mitochondria
➡ mitochondria membrane potential damage
➡ 세포질의 pyruvate: mitochondria 유입 실패
➡ lactate로 환원됨
➡ intracellular lactate ↑
➡ 근육내 수소이온 증가로 pH ↓
➡ 해당효소 glucose 6-phosphate와 phosphofructokinase 활성 ↓
➡ glycogenolysis ↓
➡ ATP 생산 ↓
➡ Na-K pumps activity ↓
➡ 근육세포 부종

처방 목표 골근육 ATP 생성 촉진: heat shock protein 활성화 / superoxide 제거/ hydrogen peroxide 제거 / intracellular lactate 교정 / glycogenolysis 촉진 / Na-K pumps 활성화

처방 구성 桂枝 三兩 / 芍藥 三兩 / 炙甘草 二兩 / 生薑 三兩 / 大棗 十二枚

처방 약리

작약 paeoniflorin ➡ superoxide scavenger

생강 gingerol ➡ hydrogen peroxide scavenger

계지 cinnamic acid ➡ lactate oxidizer
➡ pyruvate 전환 촉진

대조 cAMP ➡ glycogenolysis 촉진

구감초 18β-24-Hydroxyglycyrrhetinic acid
➡ HSD11B2 inhibitor
➡ cortisol 분해 억제
➡ mineralocorticoid receptors 자극 지속
➡ Na+/ K+ pumps 전사 촉진

고주탕 (苦酒湯)

원문 少陰病 , 咽中傷 , 生瘡 , 不能 語言 , 聲 不 出 者, 苦酒湯 主之 。

원문 해설 항체매개 독성병으로 목구멍이 상하고 헐어서 말하기가 힘들고, 못 알아듣게 목소리가 나오는 경우에는 고주탕을 쓴다.

적응증 Laryngitis (후두염, 후두: 기도 입구의 연골 & 점막 조직)

병태 & 증상

Laryngitis

➡ virus infection
➡ B cell: IgM 생성
➡ 보체 유도
➡ 보체의존성 세포용해
➡ 후두: 점막세포 & cartilage 손상

처방 목표 손상된 점막부위로 세포상환 촉진시킴 / 손상된 연골 재생

처방 구성 半夏 十四枚 / 雞子 一枚 / 苦酒 (식초)

처방 약리

반하 triterpenoid ($C_{30}H_{48}O_7S$)

➡ Rho GTPase family transcription promotor
➡ focal adhesion 생성
➡ 세포 상환 촉진

계자 (계란흰자): methionine

식초 CH_3COOH

➡ methionine + CH_3COOH: 천연유기유황 dimethyl sulfone 합성
➡ 체내에서 연골성분을 이어주는데 필수적인 sulfur 공급원

과루모려산 (栝蔞牡蠣散)

원문 百合病, 渴不差者, 用後方主之, 栝蔞牡蠣散方。

원문 해설 백합병에서 갈증이 낫지 않을 경우에는 과루모려산을 쓴다.

적응증 Bornavirus interneuron infection

병태 & 증상

Bornavirus interneuron infection

➡ interneuron endosome: acidic environment
➡ interneuron endosome: bornavirus endocytosis
➡ bornavirus infected interneuron: nucleus
➡ DNA polymerase: bornavirus RNA replication --> hydroxyl group 소모: thirst
➡ cytoplasm: subgenomic RNAs
➡ ribosome: post-transcription
➡ bornavirus replication

처방 목표 interneuron endosome: acidic environment 중화 / ribosome: post-transcription 차단

처방 구성 栝蔞根 / 牡蠣 等分

처방 약리

모려 NaCl ➡ endosome pH 중화시킴

과루근 trichosanthin ➡ ribosome inactivating protein
➡ ribosome: post-transcription 억제

과루해백반하탕 (栝蔞薤白半夏湯)

원문 胸痹 不 得 臥, 心痛 徹 背 者, 栝蔞薤白半夏湯 主之。

원문 해설 가슴부위에 마비감이 있고 누울 수가 없으며 심장통증이 등까지 뻗치는 경우에는 과루해백반하탕을 쓴다.

적응증 Myocardial infarction & micro-emboli (심근경색 & 미세혈전)

병태 & 증상

Myocardial infarction & micro-emboli

➡ coronary artery: atherosclerotic plaque
➡ atherosclerotic plaque: macrophage ↑
➡ plaque rupture
➡ plaque 내부의 tissue factor 노출
➡ platelet independent thrombus formation
➡ plaque 위로 thrombus 축적
➡ platelet thrombin Rc: thrombus 부착
➡ plaque 위로 platelet-thrombin complex 형성
➡ platelet-thrombin complex 분리
➡ micro-emboli 작용
➡ coronary artery branch: 폐쇄
➡ coronary artery: 내강 좁아짐 (완전경색)
➡ myocardiocyte ischemia
➡ TCA cycle ↓
➡ myocardial infarction: chest pain, pulmonary edema, pain radiation
➡ 허혈부위 심근세포: 섬유아세포로 분화됨

처방 목표 micro-emboli 용해 / coronary artery 내강 확장 / TCA cycle 촉진 / 심근세포의 섬유아세포로 분화 억제

처방 구성 栝蔞實 一枚 / 薤白 三兩 / 半夏 半升 / 白酒 一斗

처방 약리

반하 triterpenoid ($C_{30}H_{48}O_7S$)

➡ Rho GTPase family transcription promotor

➡ heparan sulfate 생성 촉진
➡ heparin 유사 작용
➡ micro-emboli 용해

백주 alcohol ➡ vasodilator

해백 vitamin B1
➡ Pyruvate dehydrogenase & Oxoglutarate dehydrogenase의 coenzymes
➡ TCA cycle 활성화

과루실 cucurbitacin
➡ endothelium actin-disrupting agent
➡ endothelium ▶ fibroblast 분화 억제
➡ 심근세포의 섬유아세포로 분화 억제

과루해백백주탕 (栝蔞薤白白酒湯)

원문 胸痹 之 病，喘 息 咳 唾，胸 背 痛，短氣，寸口脈 沉 而 遲， 關上 小 數，栝蔞薤白白酒湯 主之。

원문 해설 가슴부위에 마비감을 만드는 병에 걸리면 호흡이 곤란해지고 기침과 가래가생기며 가슴에서 등쪽으로 뻗치는 통증이 오고 호흡이 짧아진다, 촌구맥이 가라앉아 있으면서 느리고, 관상맥이 약간 단단하고 빠르면 과루해백백주탕을 쓴다.

적응증 Myocardial infarction (심근경색)

병태 & 증상

Myocardial infarction

➡ coronary artery: atherosclerotic plaque
➡ atherosclerotic plaque: macrophage
➡ plaque rupture
➡ plaque 내부의 tissue factor 노출
➡ platelet independent thrombus formation

➡ plaque 위로 thrombus 축적
➡ coronary artery: 내강 좁아짐 (완전경색)
➡ myocardiocyte ischemia
➡ TCA cycle ↓
➡ myocardial infarction: chest pain, pulmonary edema, pain radiation
➡ 허혈부위 심근세포: 섬유아세포로 분화됨

처방 목표 coronary artery 내강 확장 / TCA cycle 촉진 / 심근세포의 섬유아세포로 분화 억제

처방 구성 栝蔞實 一枚 / 薤白 半斤 / 白酒 七升

처방 약리

백주 alcohol ➡ vasodilator

해백 vitamin B1
➡ Pyruvate dehydrogenase & Oxoglutarate dehydrogenase의 coenzymes
➡ TCA cycle 활성화

과루실 cucurbitacin
➡ endothelium actin-disrupting agent
➡ endothelium ▶ fibroblast 분화 억제
➡ 심근세포의 섬유아세포로 분화 억제

과체산 (瓜蔕散)

원문 病 如 桂枝證 , 頭不痛 , 項 不 強 , 寸 脈 微浮 , 胸中 痞硬 , 氣上衝 喉咽 不 得 息 者 , 此 為 胸 有寒 也 , 當 吐 之, 瓜蔕散 主之 。

원문 해설 병이 계지탕증처럼 보이는데 두통은 없고 목 부위의 강직도 없으며 맥은 약간 떠있으면서 가슴부위가 쓰리면서 단단하고 인후가 불편하여 호흡이 곤란한 경우에는 가슴부위에 허혈이 있는 것이므로 최토시켜야 하며 과체산을 쓴다.

적응증 Cytomegalovirus infection in 인후상피 & 기관지상피 & 식도상피

병태 & 증상

Cytomegalovirus infection in 인후상피 & 기관지상피 & 식도상피

➡ 인후상피 & 기관지상피 & 식도상피: cytomegalovirus infection
➡ 모세혈관 내피세포: 재감염
➡ 모세혈관 내피세포: 봉입체 세포로 전환
➡ 내피세포 부종
➡ 모세혈관 내강 좁아짐
➡ 적혈구 흐름 늦어짐
➡ cytomegalovirus 항체: 적혈구 응집
➡ 조직 허혈
➡ 인후부종 / 기도부종 / 식도부종

처방 목표 봉입체세포 배출 / 적혈구 응집 억제

처방 구성 瓜蒂 一分 / 赤小豆 一分

처방 약리

과체 elaterin ➡ 최토제

적소두 (팥) albumin, 약리추측 ➡ immunoglobulin Fc region binder
➡ IgG Fc region: erythrocyte FcR 부착 억제
➡ 적혈구 응집 억제

괄루계지탕 (栝蔞桂枝湯)

원문 太陽病, 其 證 備, 身體 強, 几几然, 脈 反 沉 遲, 此 為 痙, 栝蔞桂枝湯 主之。

원문 해설 림프절 감염병의 증상이 전부 구비되어 있고, 팔다리에 강직감이 있으며, 목이 뻣뻣하여 자연스럽게 움직이지 못하고, 맥상은 반대로 느린 경우에는 이완성마비가 오려고 하는 것이므로 괄루계지탕을 쓴다.

적응증 Poliomyelitis (회백수염, 소아마비)

병태 & 증상

Poliomyelitis

➡ small intestinal epithelium: poliovirus infection
➡ mesenteric lymph node: replication
 ▶ IL-1: fever / nausea / headache / stomachache
➡ first viremia
➡ 항체 출현: 대부분 더 진행되지 않고 불현성감염으로 종료
➡ 1%: secondary viremia
➡ spinal cord motor neuron 침범
➡ motor neuron: poliovirus infection
➡ motor neuron: NF-κB ▶ nucleus translocation
➡ motor neuron ribosomes: poliovirus RNA & protein 번역 활성화
➡ poliovirus replication: spastic paralysis
➡ motor neuron lysis: 주로, anterior horn cell ▶ 사지골격근 지배
➡ spinal cord myelitis: neck & back stiffness
➡ axon terminal: acetylcholine 분비 ↓
➡ skeletal muscle fiber: 자극 감소
➡ skeletal muscle fiber: total enzyme 감소
➡ lactate dehydrogenase ↓ / superoxide dismutase ↓ / glutathione ↓ / c-AMP↓
➡ lactate ↑ / superoxide ↑ / hydrogen peroxide ↑ / glucolysis ↓
➡ ATP ↓
➡ skeletal muscle fiber: 수축 실패
➡ flaccid paralysis

처방 목표 NF-κB ▶ nucleus translocation 억제 / motor neuron ribosomes: poliovirus RNA & protein 번역 억제 / lactate 교정 / superoxide 제거 / hydrogen peroxide 제거 / c-AMP 보충

처방 구성 栝蔞根 二兩 / 桂枝 三兩 / 芍藥 三兩 / 甘草 二兩 / 生薑 三兩 / 大棗 十二枚

처방 약리

감초 glycyrrhetinic acid
 ➡ 11-beta-hydroxysteroid dehydrogenase1 (HSD11B1) inhibitor
 ➡ glucocorticoid 작용
 ➡ IκBα 생성

➡ NF-κB 억제

괄루근 trichosanthin ➡ ribosome inactivating protein
➡ poliovirus RNA & protein 번역 억제

계지 cinnamic acid ➡ lactate oxidizer
➡ pyruvate 전환

작약 paeoniflorin ➡ superoxide scavenger

생강 gingerol ➡ hydrogen peroxide scavenger

대조 c-AMP ➡ glycolysis 촉진

괄루구맥환 (栝蔞瞿麥丸)

원문 小便 不利 者, 有 水氣, 其人 若渴, 栝蔞瞿麥丸 主之。

원문 해설 소변이 불편하고 수독이 있으며 갈증이 나는 경우에는 괄루구맥환을 쓴다.

적응증 Glomerulosclerosis (사구체 경화증)

병태 & 증상

Glomerulosclerosis

➡ Immune complex mediated glomerulonephritis & anti-GBM glomerulonephritis
➡ mesangial cell proliferation
➡ mesangial cell: ribosome을 활성화시켜 collagen 합성
➡ mesangium: extracellular matrix ↑
➡ extracellular matrix & capillary endothelial cell 접촉면 ↑
➡ capillary endothelial cell: vWF 발현 ↑
➡ platelet 1차 응집: cytokine
➡ neutrophil 유도
➡ neutrophil: ADP 분비

➡ platelet 2차 응집: thrombus formation
➡ capillary endothelial cell: hypoxia
➡ capillary endothelial cell: plasminogen activator inhibitor-1 (PAI-1) 분비
➡ fibrin 축적
➡ mesnagium & 사구체간질: fibrosis
➡ 세뇨관 허혈
➡ 세뇨관 상피세포 손상

처방 목표 fibroblast의 collagen 합성 억제 / neutrophil: ADP 분비 억제 / thrombus formation 억제 / plasminogen activator inhibitor-1 (PAI-1) 분비 억제 / 세뇨관 상피세포 허혈 개선

처방 구성 栝蔞根 二兩 / 茯苓 三兩 / 薯蕷 三兩 / 炮附子 一枚 / 瞿麥 一兩

처방 약리

괄루근 trichosanthin ➡ ribosome inactivating protein
➡ collagen 합성 억제

포부자 aconitine
➡ 약리추측: neutrophil` Voltage-gated proton channels blocker
(식균작용에 의해 증가된 세포내 proton을 세포외로 방출시키는 채널)
➡ Voltage-gated proton channels 차단
➡ 호중구내 수소이온 축적
➡ neutrophil 대사 억제
➡ ADP 분비 억제

복령 pachymic acid ➡ glycoprotein IIb/IIIa (gpIIb/IIIa) (-) modulator
➡ thrombus formation 억제

구맥 dianoside ➡ plasminogen activator inhibitor-1 (-) modulator
➡ fibrin 억제

산약 diosgenin ➡ GLUT1 (+) modulator
➡ 세뇨관내 glucose 유입 증가
➡ ATP 증가
➡ 세뇨관 상피세포 생존

교애탕 (膠艾湯)

원문 婦人 有 漏下 者，有 半產 後 因 續 下血 都 不絕 者，有 妊娠 下血 者，假令 妊娠 腹中痛，為 胞 阻，膠艾湯 主之。

원문 해설 자궁점막하근종에 의한 출혈이 있거나, 유산 후 탈락막 기저층에서의 심한 출혈이 있거나, 임신 중에 출혈이 있으면서 배가 아픈 경우는 전치태반이나 태반조기박리가 있는 것으로서 모두 교애탕을 쓴다.

적응증 Uterine bleeding (자궁출혈)

병태 & 증상

Uterine Bleeding

➡ 자궁점막하근종 / 유산후 탈락막 기저층 / 전치태반
➡ 자궁벽 근육 압박
➡ uterin wall: smooth muscle ▶ NF-κB 활성화
➡ uterin wall: smooth muscle ▶ inflammation
➡ intra-uterine artery: 손상
➡ hemorrhage
➡ intra-uterine: erythrocyte 유출
➡ 적혈구 골격단백질 손상
➡ complement 부착
➡ complement cascade: membrane attack complement (MAC) 생성
➡ MAC mediated erythrocyte lysis
➡ hematoma 생성
➡ 조직 허혈: superoxide 생성
➡ 혈관평활근: α-adrenergic Rc Ca channel 자극
➡ vasospasm
➡ severe bleeding

처방 목표 uterin wall smooth muscle: NF-κB 억제 / uterin wall: smooth muscle 합성 촉진 / 적혈구 골격단백질 유지 / superoxide 제거 / α-adrenergic Rc 차단 / 혈관수축 / 조혈

처방 구성 芎藭 二兩 / 阿膠 二兩 / 甘草 二兩 / 艾葉 三兩 / 當歸 三兩
芍藥 四兩 / 乾地黃 四兩

처방 약리

감초 glycyrrhetinic acid

➡ 11-beta-hydroxysteroid dehydrogenase1 (HSD11B1) inhibitor
➡ glucocorticoid 작용
➡ IκBα 생성
➡ NF-κB 억제
➡ uterin wall: smooth muscle ▶ inflammation 억제

아교 Glycine / Proline / Hydroxyproline / Alanine

➡ collagen 주요 아미노산
➡ 근육 합성 촉진

당귀 decurcin ➡ erythrocyte protein kinase C inhibitor
➡ adducin-spectrin-actin complex 유지시킴.

작약 paeoniflorin ➡ superoxide scavenger

천궁 cnidilide ➡ α-adrenergic receptor blocker

애엽 cineol ➡ vasoconstriction

건지황 catalpol, 약리 추측 ➡ CD133+ CFU-GEMM (+) modulator
➡ hematopoietic stem cell 분화 촉진
➡ erythrocyte 생성 촉진

구감초탕 (炙甘草湯)

원문 傷寒 脈 結代，心 動悸, 炙甘草湯 主之。, 脈 按 之 來 緩，時 一 止 復 來 者，名 曰 結。又 脈 來動 而 中止，更 來 小數，中 有 還 者 反 動，名 曰 結，陰 也。脈 來 動 而 中止，不能 自還，因 而 復 動 者，名 曰 代， 陰 也。得 此 脈 者，必 難治。

원문 해설 세포병변성 감염증에서 맥이 결대한 경우 구감초탕을 쓴다. 맥이 늦고 한번 멈추었

다가 다시 뛰는 것을 "결"이라고 부른다. 맥이 뛰다가 멈춘 후 다시 뛸 때는 약간 빠르게 뛰고 순환하는 반동이 있는 것을 "결"이라 하고 음(부교감신경)이 원인임 맥이 뛰다가 멈춘 후 순환하는 형태 없이 다시 뛰는 것을 "대"라고 부르며 음(부교감신경)이 원인이고 치료하기 어렵다.

적응증 Chagas disease (샤가스 병)

병태 & 증상

Chagas disease

➡ heart parasympathetic neuron: Trypanosoma cruzi 부착

➡ lysosome: 세포 표면으로 이동하여 T. cruzi 융합

➡ T. cruzi infected macrophage: prostaglandin *I2* 분비

➡ T. cruzi 과 융합된 lysosome membrane 안정화

➡ 안정화된 lysosome: T. cruzi 활동성 감소되어 복제되기 전에 세포밖으로 유출 억제됨

➡ lysosome disruption

➡ 세포질: T. cruzi replication

➡ T. cruzi: Trypomastigotes 형태로 전환

➡ 세포밖 전파

➡ parasympathetic neuronal endings on the heart & myocardiocyte

: Trypomastigotes infection

➡ heart parasympathetic neuron 파괴 & myocardial fiber 손상

➡ 심장 전기전도계 손상

➡ sinoatrial (SA) node 자극 ↓ : P wave 소실: 結脈

➡ First-degree AV (atrioventricular) block

➡ atrioventricular (AV) node 자극 ↓ : T wave 변형: 代脈

➡ Second-degree AV block

➡ 심실 수축 ↓

➡ 관상동맥 혈류 감소

➡ myocardium ischemia

처방 목표 macrophage에서 prostaglandin *I2* 분비 억제 / 세포질: T. cruzi replication 억제 / heart parasympathetic neuron 재생 / myocardiocyte 재생 / myocardium ischemia 교정

처방 구성 炙甘草 四兩 / 生薑 三兩 / 人參 二兩 / 生地黃 一斤 / 桂枝 二兩 / 阿膠 二兩 / 麥門冬 半斤 / 麻仁 半升 / 大棗 十二枚

처방 약리

마자인 α-Linolenic acid (omega-3)

➡ 세포막 조성 변화
➡ arachidonic acid 감소
➡ prostaglandin I2 합성 억제

맥문동 ophiopogonin, 약리 추측 ➡ T. cruzi transcription inhibitor
➡ T. cruzi growth 억제

인삼 panax ginsenoside
➡ Transforming growth factor β (TGF-β) (+) modulator
➡ cell proliferation 촉진
➡ heart parasympathetic neuron & myocardiocyte 재생

구감초 18β-24-Hydroxyglycyrrhetinic acid
➡ HSD11B2 inhibitor
➡ cortisol 분해 억제
➡ mineralocorticoid receptors 자극 지속
➡ 재생된 heart parasympathetic neuron & myocardiocyte
➡ Na+/ K+ pumps 활성화

생지황 catalpol
➡ 약리추측: CD133+ circulating endothelial cell progenitor (+) modulator
➡ vessel bud formation
➡ 재생된 heart parasympathetic neuron & myocardiocyte 성숙

아교 Glycine / Proline / Hydroxyproline / Alanine
➡ myocardial fiber biosynthesis 촉진

생강 gingerol ➡ hydrogen peroxide scavenger
➡ 심근허혈 손상 억제

계지 cinnamic acid ➡ lactate oxidizer
➡ pyruvate 전환 촉진

대조 c-AMP ➡ 심근 ATP 합성 촉진

규자복령산 (葵子茯苓散)

원문 妊娠 有 水氣, 身重 `小便 不利, 洒 淅 惡寒, 起 即 頭眩, 葵子茯苓散 主之。

원문 해설 임신 중에 수분정체감이 있고, 몸이 무거우며 소변이 불편하고 술기운이 있는 것처럼 춥고, 일어서면 어지럼증이 있는 경우에는 규자복령산을 쓴다.

적응증 Deep venous thrombosis in pregnancy (임신부 심부정맥혈전증)

병태 & 증상

Pregnancy venous thrombosis

➡ 임신 first trimester: 자궁 커짐
➡ 장골 정맥 압박
➡ May-Thurner syndrome
➡ vein endothelium damage: IL-6 --> chills
➡ IL-6: platelet activation
➡ platelet: arachidonic acid metabolism ↑
➡ platelet aggregation
➡ deep venous thrombosis
➡ venous thromboembolism
➡ 정맥허혈, 폐동맥색전증: edema, dizziness

처방 목표 platelet: arachidonic acid metabolism 억제 / thrombus 억제

처방 구성 葵子 一斤 / 茯苓 三兩

처방 약리

규자 palmitic acid ➡ arachidonic acid-induced platelet aggregation inhibitor

복령 pachymic acid ➡ glycoprotein IIb/IIIa (gpIIb/IIIa) (-) modulator
➡ thrombus formation 억제

귤지강탕 (橘枳薑湯)

원문 胸 痹, 胸中 氣塞, 短氣, 茯苓杏仁甘草湯 主之; 橘枳薑湯 亦 主之。

원문 해설 심장부위가 저리고 막히는 느낌이 있으면서 호흡이 짧아지는 경우에는 복령행인감초탕이나 귤지강탕을 쓴다.

적응증 Chylothorax (유미흉증)

병태 & 증상

Chylothorax

➡ 우심부전, 가슴정맥 혈전
➡ thoracic duct 폐쇄
➡ lymphatic duct 폐쇄
➡ lymphatic duct: lymphocyte 침윤
➡ lymphocyte: calcium influx ↑ ▶ phospholipase C 활성화 ▶ IP3 활성화
▶ endoplasmic reticulum: calcium efflux ↑
▶ hydrogen peroxide ↑
▶ matrix metalloproteinases 전사 촉진
➡ thoracic duct 손상
➡ thoracic duct: protein plaque 형성
➡ 흉강: 유미 (chyle) 축적 ▶ dyspnoea

처방 목표 lymphocyte: hydrogen peroxide 제거 / lymphocyte: matrix metalloproteinases 차단 / thoracic duct: protein plaque 제거

처방 구성 橘皮 一斤 / 枳實 三兩 / 生薑 半斤

처방 약리

생강 gingerol ➡ hydrogen peroxide scavenger

지실 auraptene ➡ matrix metalloproteinase (MMP) blocker
귤피 rutin ➡ proteolytic activator
➡ protein plaque 제거

귤피죽여탕 (橘皮竹茹湯)

원문 噦 逆 者 , 橘皮竹茹湯 主之 。

원문 해설 난치성 딸꾹질이 있는 경우에는 귤피죽여탕을 쓴다.

적응증 Multiple sclerosis

병태 & 증상

Multiple sclerosis

➡ virus linked multiple sclerosis
: hunan herpes virus / varicella zoster virus / Epstein Barr virus / endogenous retrovirus / etc
➡ myelin oligodendrocyte glycoprotein & virus protein
➡ molecular mimicry response
➡ myelin oligodendrocyte glycoprotein: IgG & complement 부착
➡ oligodendrocyte: membrane attack complex 형성
➡ oligodendrocyte H_2O_2 ↑
➡ oligodendrocyte loss
➡ axon nerve: demyelination
➡ myelin plaque 생성
➡ multiple sclerosis
➡ nerve conduction disorders
➡ 주로 침범되는 부위: 시신경 / 뇌간 (severe hiccup) / 소뇌 / 척수

처방 목표 myelin oligodendrocyte glycoprotein: IgG 생성 억제 / oligodendrocyte H_2O_2 제거 / oligodendrocyte 재생 촉진 / myelin plaque 제거 / nerve conduction 촉진

처방 구성 橘皮 二升 / 竹茹 二升 / 大棗 三十枚 / 人參 一兩 / 生薑 半斤 / 甘草 五兩

처방 약리

감초 glycyrrhetinic acid
➡ 11-beta-hydroxysteroid dehydrogenase1 (HSD11B1) inhibitor
➡ glucocorticoid 작용
➡ IκBα 생성

➡ NF-κB 억제
➡ 항체 생성 억제

생강 gingerol ➡ hydrogen peroxide scavenger

인삼 panax ginsenoside
➡ Transforming growth factor β (TGF-β) (+) modulator
➡ SVZ neuronal progenitors: TGF-β (+) modulation
➡ oligodendrocyte proliferation 촉진

대조 c-AMP ➡ protein kinase A avtivator
➡ ATP 생성 촉진
➡ cell cycle ↑

귤피 rutin ➡ proteolytic activator
➡ myelin plaque 제거

죽여 Tyrosine ➡ Dopamine / Norepinephrine / Epinephrine biosynthesis

귤피탕 (橘皮湯)

원문 乾嘔 噦, 若 手足 厥 者, 橘皮湯 主之。

원문 해설 마른 구역과 딸꾹질이 있는데 손발까지 감각이상이 있는 경우에는 귤피탕을 쓴다.

적응증 Myelitis (척수염)

병태 & 증상

Myelitis

➡ myelin basic protein & EBV capsid, papilloma virus L2, etc
➡ molecular mimicry response
➡ spinal cord: myelin basic protein ▶ IgG & complement 부착
➡ myelin basic protein: membrane attack complex 형성

➡ myelin basic protein: H_2O_2 ↑
➡ spinal cord myelitis
➡ myelin plaque 생성
➡ nerve conduction disorders
: 목척수신경 / 가슴척수신경 / 허리척수신경 / 엉치척수신경
➡ 운동장애 (hiccup) & 감각장애 (cold & tingling hands and feet)

처방 목표 myelin basic protein: H_2O_2 제거 / myelin plaque 제거

처방 구성 橘皮 四兩 / 生薑 半斤

처방 약리

생강 gingerol ➡ hydrogen peroxide scavenger

귤피 rutin ➡ proteolytic activator
➡ myelin plaque 제거

기초역황환 (己椒藶黃丸)

원문 腹滿 , 口舌 乾燥 , 此 腸間 有 水氣 , 己椒藶黃丸 主之 。
稍增 , 口中 有 津液 。

원문 해설 복부가 팽창되고 구강과 혀가 건조해지는 것은 장간에 수분이 있기 때문이다. 기초역황환을 쓴다.

적응증 Mesenteric lymphoma (장간막 림프종)

병태 & 증상

Mesenteric lymphoma

➡ chronic infection
➡ mesenteric lymph nodes: persistent antigenic stimulation
➡ B cell: genetic alteration
➡ B cell: neoplastic transformation

➡ mesenteric lymphoma
➡ mesenteric lymphadenopathy
➡ 장정맥 조직액: 장간막 림프절 유입 실패 ▶ dry mouth
➡ 장정맥 울혈
➡ 장폐쇄

처방 목표 mesenteric lymphoma apoptosis 유도 / 장정맥 확장 유도 / 심장 수축력 강화 / 장경련 유도 / 장관 수분 배출 촉진

처방 구성 防己 / 椒目 / 葶藶 / 大黃 各 一兩 / 渴者 加 芒硝 半兩

처방 약리

대황 emodin ➡ tyrosine kinase Rc blocker
➡ mesenteric lymphoma 성장 억제

방기 sinomenine ➡ prostaglandin I2 (+) modulator in venous endothelium
➡ venous vasodilation
➡ 정맥 울혈 해소

정력자 helveticoside ➡ 강심배당체
➡ 심장 수축을 짧고 강하게 유도해서 확장기 길어짐
➡ 대정맥 유입 혈액량 증가
➡ 정맥 울혈 해소

초목 xanthoxin ➡ 경련독
➡ 장폐쇄 개선

망초 Sodium Sulfate ➡ Intraluminal distention pressure 상승시킴
➡ 울혈 수분 제거

길경탕 (桔梗湯)

원문 少陰病 , 二 三 日 , 咽痛 者 , 可 與 甘草湯 ; 不 差 , 與 桔梗湯 。

원문 해설 항체매개 독성이 시작되고 2~3일후 인후통이 있는 경우에 감초탕을 썼는데 낫지 않으면 길경탕을 쓴다.

적응증 Bacterial pharyngitis

병태 & 증상

Bacterial pharyngitis

➡ pharynx: commensal bacteria
➡ staphylococcus aureus / streptococcus pyrogen: transformation
➡ MyD88 (TLR adaptor protein) 억제 단백질 분비
➡ 내피세포의 TLR signal 차단
➡ IL-1 & TNF-a 분비 감소
➡ staphylococcus aureus / streptococcus pyrogen: activation
➡ pharynx infection
➡ B cell: IgM 생성
➡ 보체 유도
➡ 보체의존성 세포용해
➡ pharyngitis

처방 목표 인두점막상피의 TLR signal 촉진 / IgM 항체 생성 억제시킴

처방 구성 桔梗 一兩 / 甘草 二兩

처방 약리

길경 platycodin ➡ toll like receptor (+) modulator
➡ TLR signal 활성화
➡ IL-1 & TNF-a
➡ staphylococcus aureus / streptococcus pyrogen: 병원성 억제

감초 glycyrrhetinic acid
➡ HSD11B1 inhibitor
➡ cortisol 분해 억제
➡ glucocorticoid receptors 자극 지속
➡ IκBα 생성
➡ NF-κB 억제
➡ B cell 대사 억제
➡ 항체 형성 감소

낭아탕 (狼牙湯)

원문 少陰脈 滑 而 數 者, 陰中 即 生瘡, 陰中 蝕瘡 爛 者, 狼牙湯 洗之。

원문 해설 소음맥으로 매끄럽고 빠르며, 자궁경부가 헐고 짓무르는 경우에는 낭아탕으로 씻어 준다.

적응증 Chlamydia

병태 & 증상

Chlamydia

➡ genital tract epithelium: Chlamydia trachomatis infection
➡ Chlamydia trachomatis LPXD: Lipid A 합성
➡ Chlamydia trachomatis: replication
➡ inclusion formation
➡ cell lysis: cervicitis
➡ elementary body: extracellular spread

처방 목표 Chlamydia trachomatis LPXD 억제

처방 구성 狼牙 三兩

처방 약리

낭아 (선학초) luteolin, 약리 추측
➡ UDP-3-O-acyl-glucosamine N-acyltransferase (LPXD) inhibitor

당귀사역가오수유생강탕 (當歸四逆加吳茱萸生薑湯)

원문 手足 厥寒, 脈 細 欲 絕 者, 當歸四逆湯 主 之。若 其 人 內 有 久 寒 者, 宜

當歸四逆加吳茱萸生薑湯 。

원문 해설 손발이 심하게 차갑고 맥이 가늘어 끊어질 것 같은 경우에 당귀사역탕을 쓰고, 그 환자가 수족냉증을 오래 앓을 경우에는 당귀사역가오수유생강탕을 쓴다.

적응증 Autoimmune hemolytic anemia-mediated pancreatitis
(자가면역 용혈성빈혈-매개 췌장염)

병태 & 증상

Autoimmune hemolytic anemia-mediated pancreatitis

➡ erythrocyte: autoantibody 생성
➡ complement 유도
➡ erythrocyte: protein kinase C 활성화
➡ adducin phosphorylation
➡ adducin-spectrin-actin complex: 분리됨
➡ erythrocyte membrane: 불안정해짐
➡ deformity erythrocyte
➡ Met hemoglobin 형성
➡ Methemoglobinemia
➡ tissue hypoxia
➡ intravascular hemolysis
➡ dimer hemoglobin 형성: 신장 독성
➡ Met hemoglobin: spleen homolysis ↑
➡ splenic vein congestion
➡ pancreas: 정맥 배액 ↓
➡ 췌장 선방세포의 직접적 손상 또는 췌관 손상
➡ 췌장 선방세포내 산성화
➡ low-affinity Cholecystokinine (CCK) receptor 자극
➡ phospholipase C 활성화
➡ diacylglycerol 생성
➡ hydrogen peroxide: Ca+2 / calmodulin ↑
➡ protein kinase C 활성화
➡ 선방세포 vacuole내 pro-enzyme 활성화
➡ 산성화 조건: 췌장 선방세포내 공포 깨짐
➡ pro-enzyme: 세포질로 방출
➡ 선방세포 자가분해됨
➡ pancreatitis

처방 목표 erythrocyte: protein kinase C 억제 / Met hemoglobin 환원 / tissue hypoxia 교정 / dimer hemoglobin 이뇨 촉진 / low-affinity CCK receptor 차단 / 선방세포 hydrogen peroxide 제거

처방 구성 當歸 三兩 / 芍藥 三兩 / 炙甘草 二兩 / 通草 二兩 / 桂枝 三兩 / 細辛 三兩 / 生薑 半斤 / 吳茱萸 二升 / 大棗 二十五枚

처방 약리

당귀 decurcin ➡ erythrocyte protein kinase C inhibitor
➡ adducin-spectrin-actin complex 유지시킴
➡ hemolysis 억제

세신 eugenol ➡ MetHb reducer

계지 cinnamic acid ➡ lactate oxidizer
➡ 허혈세포 lactate 교정

작약 paeoniflorin ➡ superoxide scavenger
➡ 허혈세포 superoxide 제거

구감초 18β-24-Hydroxyglycyrrhetinic acid -> HSD11B2 inhibitor
➡ cortisol 분해 억제되고 mineralocorticoid receptors 자극 지속됨
➡ 허혈세포 Na+/ K+ pumps 활성화

대조 c-AMP ➡ cAMP-dependent protein kinase인 protein kinase A avtivator
➡ 허혈세포 glycogenolysis 촉진

통초 hedegeragenin ➡ Diuretic action
➡ 신사구체에 축적된 dimer hemoglobin 배출

오수유 evodiamine ➡ low-affinity CCK receptor blocker
➡ vacuole내 pro-enzyme 활성화 억제

생강 gingerol ➡ hydrogen peroxide scavenger
➡ 허혈세포 hydrogen peroxide 제거 & 선방세포 protein kinase C 억제

당귀사역탕 (當歸四逆湯)

원문 手足 厥寒, 脈 細 欲 絕 者, 當歸四逆湯 主之 。

원문 해설 손발이 심하게 차갑고 맥이 가늘어 끊어질 것 같은 경우에는 당귀사역탕을 쓴다.

적응증 Autoimmune hemolytic anemia (자가면역 용혈성빈혈)

병태 & 증상

Autoimmune hemolytic anemia

➡ erythrocyte: autoantibody 생성
➡ complement 유도
➡ erythrocyte: protein kinase C 활성화
➡ adducin phosphorylation
➡ adducin-spectrin-actin complex: 분리됨
➡ erythrocyte membrane: 불안정해짐
➡ deformity erythrocyte
➡ Met hemoglobin 형성
➡ Methemoglobinemia
➡ tissue hypoxia
➡ intravascular hemolysis
➡ dimer hemoglobin 형성
➡ dimer hemoglobin: heptoglobin 결합 ▶ 비장 & 간: 운반되어 분해됨
➡ heptoglobin 부족: dimer hemoglobin
▶ 신사구체 축적
▶ 핍뇨성 신부전 발생

처방 목표 erythrocyte: protein kinase C 억제 / Met hemoglobin 환원 / tissue hypoxia 개선 / dimer hemoglobin 이뇨 촉진

처방 구성 當歸 三兩 / 桂枝 三兩 / 芍藥 三兩 / 細辛 三兩 / 炙甘草 二兩 / 通草 二兩 / 大棗 二十五枚

처방 약리

당귀 decurcin ➡ erythrocyte protein kinase C inhibitor
➡ adducin-spectrin-actin complex 유지시킴
➡ hemolysis 억제

세신 eugenol ➡ MetHb reducer

계지 cinnamic acid ➡ lactate oxidizer ➡ pyruvate 전환

작약 paeoniflorin ➡ superoxide scavenger
➡ 허혈세포 superoxide 제거

구감초 18β-24-Hydroxyglycyrrhetinic acid
➡ HSD11B2 inhibitor
➡ cortisol 분해 억제
➡ mineralocorticoid receptors 자극 지속
➡ 허혈세포 Na+/ K+ pumps 활성화

대조 c-AMP ➡ protein kinase A avtivator
➡ ATP 생산 촉진

통초 hedegeragenin ➡ Diuretic action
➡ 신사구체에 축적된 dimer hemoglobin 배출

당귀산 (當歸散)

원문 婦人 妊娠，宜 常 服 當歸散 主之。日 再 服，妊娠 常服 即 易 產，胎 無 苦 疾，產後 百病 悉 主之。

원문 해설 임신 중에 당귀산을 매일 복용하면 태아가 건강해지고 순산하며 산후병도 예방한다.

적응증 Pregnancy essential supplements

병태 & 증상

➡ pregnancy
➡ 혈액량 & 적혈구 증가
➡ Iron deficiency & vitB 12 deficiency
➡ 적혈구 골격단백질 결함
➡ deformity erythrocyte 생성
➡ 산소포화도 감소
➡ umbilical artery endothelium 허혈: superoxide 생성
➡ 혈관평활근: α-adrenergic Rc Ca channel 자극
➡ 혈관평활근 경련
➡ 태반 동맥 허혈 ↑
➡ erythrocyte: s-nitrosothiol 분비
➡ superoxide + s-nitrosothiol: peroxynitrite 생성
➡ umbilical artery: VCAM-1 발현: monocyte 부착

처방 목표 적혈구 골격단백질 유지 / superoxide 제거 / α-adrenergic Rc 차단 / peroxynitrite 제거 / VCAM-1 차단

처방 구성 當歸 / 黃芩 / 芍藥 / 芎藭 各 一斤 / 白朮 半斤

처방 약리

당귀 decurcin ➡ erythrocyte protein kinase C inhibitor
➡ adducin-spectrin-actin complex 유지시킴

작약 paeoniflorin ➡ superoxide scavenger

천궁 cnidilide ➡ α-adrenergic receptor blocker

황금 baicalin ➡ peroxynitrite ($ONOO^-$) scavenger

백출 atractylon ➡ vascular cell adhesion molecule-1 (VCAM-1) blocker

당귀생강양육탕 (當歸生薑羊肉湯)

원문 寒疝 腹中痛，及 脅痛 裡急 者。產後 腹中痛，當歸生薑羊肉湯主之，并 治 腹中 寒疝，虛勞 不足。若 寒多 者，加 生薑 成 一斤 ；痛多 而 嘔 者，加 橘皮 二兩, 白朮 一兩。

원문 해설 허리와 아랫배가 차가우면서 아프고, 복부 통증이 있으면서, 옆구리가 땅기고 아픈 경우와 산후 복통에 당귀생강양육탕을 쓴다.

적응증 Spherocytosis (원형적혈구증)

병태 & 증상

Spherocytosis

➡ 선천성 구상적혈구증 / 온난자가면역성용혈성빈혈 / 수혈부작용 / 신생아의 ABO 용혈성질환 / Clostridium welchii 패혈증 / 열 / 인산 결핍에 의한 적혈구 ATP 저하 / etc

➡ erythrocyte: intracellular hydrogen peroxide ↑

➡ erythrocyte: protein kinase c 활성화

➡ adducin+spectrin+actin complex 분리

➡ spectrin 결손

➡ spherocyte 전환

➡ reticuloendothelial system (RES): liver & spleen

➡ spherocyte hemolysis

➡ RES macrophage: TNF-α 분비 ▶ chills

➡ RES endothelium: VCAM-1 발현

➡ monocyte 이동: spherocyte hemolysis ↑

➡ hepatomegaly & splenomegary: side abdominal pain

➡ monocyte repiratory burst

➡ reticular fiber 손상

➡ protein plaque 형성

처방 목표 erythrocyte intracellular hydrogen peroxide 제거 / erythrocyte: protein kinase c 억제 / spectrin 합성 촉진 / RES endothelium: VCAM-1 차단 / protein plaque 제거

처방 구성 當歸 三兩 / 生薑 五兩 / 羊肉 一斤 / 橘皮二兩 / 白朮 一兩

처방 약리

생강 gingerol ➡ hydrogen peroxide scavenger

당귀 decurcin ➡ erythrocyte protein kinase C inhibitor
➡ adducin-spectrin-actin complex 유지시킴

양육 tryptophan ➡ spectrin biosynthesis
➡ spherocyte 형성 억제

백출 atractylon ➡ vascular cell adhesion molecule-1 (VCAM-1) blocker

귤피 rutin ➡ proteolytic activator
➡ reticular fiber plaque 제거

당귀작약산 (當歸芍藥散)

원문 婦人 懷妊 , 腹 中 絞 痛 , 當歸芍藥散 主之 。

원문 해설 임신 중에 배가 꼬이듯이 아픈 경우에는 당귀작약산을 쓴다.

적응증 Pregnancy hypertention (임신고혈압)

병태 & 증상

Pregnancy hypertention

➡ pregnancy
➡ 혈액량 & 적혈구 증가
➡ Iron deficiency & vitB 12 deficiency
➡ 적혈구 골격단백질 결함
➡ deformity erythrocyte 생성
➡ 산소포화도 감소
➡ erythrocyte: s-nitrosothiol 소진

➡ 혈관 수축
➡ 조직 저산소증
➡ renin-angiotensin system 작동
➡ blood: angiotensin II ↑
➡ umbilical artery: vascular smooth muscle
➡ vcam-1 expression via type 1 ANG II receptor
➡ leukocyte & monocyte adhesion
➡ 혈관내피하 공간: leukocyte & monocyte 이동
➡ 혈관내피 손상
➡ 혈소판 응집: thrombus formation
➡ umbilical artery endothelium: 허혈
➡ umbilical artery endothelium: superoxide 생성
➡ vascular smooth muscle: α-adrenergic Rc Ca channel 자극
➡ umbilical artery spasm
➡ 탯줄 꼬임

처방 목표 적혈구 골격단백질 유지 / vcam-1 차단 / type 1 ANG II receptor 차단 / thrombus 제거 / superoxide 제거 / α-adrenergic Rc 차단

처방 구성 當歸 三兩 / 芍藥 一斤 / 茯苓 四兩 / 白朮 四兩 / 澤瀉 半斤 / 芎藭 半斤

처방 약리

당귀 decurcin ➡ erythrocyte protein kinase C inhibitor
➡ adducin-spectrin-actin complex 유지시킴

백출 atractylon ➡ vascular cell adhesion molecule-1 (VCAM-1) blocker

택사 alisol ➡ angiotensin II receptor blocker

복령 pachymic acid ➡ glycoprotein IIb/IIIa (gpIIb/IIIa) (-) modulator
➡ thrombus formation 억제

작약 paeoniflorin ➡ superoxide scavenger

천궁 cnidilide ➡ α-adrenergic receptor blocker

당귀패모고삼환 (當歸貝母苦參丸)

원문 妊娠，小便難，飮食 如 故，當歸貝母苦參丸 主之。

원문 해설 임신 중에 소변 보기 힘들고 음식은 평소와 같을 때는 당귀패모고삼환을 쓴다.

적응증 Pregnancy trichomonasis (임신부 트리코모나스증)

병태 & 증상

Pregnancy trichomoniasis

➡ pregnancy
➡ 혈액량 & 적혈구 증가
➡ Iron deficiency & vitB 12 deficiency
➡ 적혈구 골격단백질 결합
➡ deformity erythrocyte 생성
➡ 산소포화도 감소
➡ 무증상 trichomonas vaginalis: 영양불량
➡ gene transformation: tyrosinase 활성화
➡ 이동에 필요한 actin cytoskeleton 형성
➡ 편모 운동성 증가
➡ 병원성 전환
➡ trichomonasis: 방광염 / 미숙한 태막의 파열 / 임신초기의 조산 / 자궁내부 성장지연

처방 목표 적혈구 골격단백질 유지 / tyrosinase 활성화 억제 / trichomonas vaginalis 대사 억제

처방 구성 當歸 四兩 / 貝母 四兩 / 苦參 四兩 / 男子 加 滑石 半兩。

처방 약리

당귀 decurcin ➡ erythrocyte protein kinase C inhibitor
➡ adducin-spectrin-actin complex 유지시킴

고삼 trifolirhizin ➡ protozoa tyrosinase (-) modulator

패모 verticine ➡ calcium ATPase blocker
➡ Trichomonas vaginalis: calcium ATPase 차단
➡ Trichomonas vaginalis 대사 감소: 균독성 약화됨

대건중탕 (大建中湯)

원문 心胸 中 寒 痛, 嘔 不能 飮食, 腹 中 滿, 上衝 皮 起, 出 見 有 頭 足, 上下 痛 而 不可 觸 近, 大建中湯 主之。

원문 해설 오한이 들며, 구토가 나서 음식을 먹지 못하고, 복부팽만감이 있으며 위쪽으로 상충감이 들고, 복부에 오르락내리락 거리는 형태가 보이며 아파서 만지지도 못하게 하는 경우에는 대건중탕을 쓴다.

적응증 Intussusception (장 중첩)

병태 & 증상

Intussusception

➡ commensal bacteria: Salmonella typhimurium & Escherichia coli
➡ maltose receptor: bacteriophage infection
➡ Salmonella typhi & E coli: transformation
➡ pathogenic bacteria 전환
➡ Peyer's patch epithelium: IL-8 분비
➡ neutrophil 유도
➡ neutrophil phagocytosis
➡ HClO 분비 via H2O2
➡ Peyer's patch destruction
➡ ileocecum: colon으로 말려들어감 ▶ chills
➡ intussusception: vomitting, intense abdominal pain

처방 목표 Salmonella typhimurium & E coli: maltose receptor 차단 / HClO 분비 억제 / Peyer's patch 재생 촉진 / ileocecum 운동 억제

처방 구성 蜀椒 二合 / 乾薑 四兩 / 人參 二兩 / 膠飴 一升

처방 약리

교이 maltose ➡ Salmonella typhi & E coli: maltose receptor 부착
➡ bacteriophage 부착 차단

건강 shogaol ➡ neutrophil H2O2 scavenger
➡ HClO 분비 억제

촉초 sanshool ➡ potassium leak channel blocker
➡ intestinal smooth muscle cell 마비

인삼 panax ginsenoside
➡ Transforming growth factor β (TGF-β) (+) modulator
➡ Peyer's patch epithelium: proliferation 촉진

대반하탕 (大半夏湯)

원문 胃反 嘔吐 者, 大半夏湯 主之。

원문 해설 음식물이 내려가지 않고 모두 토하는 경우에는 대반하탕을 쓴다.

적응증 Pyloric stenosis in Behcet's Disease (베체트 유문협착증)

병태 & 증상

Pyloric stenosis in Behcet's Disease

➡ streptococcus infection
➡ streptococcus surface protein & 유문부 세동맥 pericyte desmin
: molecular mimicry
➡ streptococcus surface protein: antibody 생성
➡ pericyte desmin: antibody 부착
➡ antibody-dependent cell-mediated cytotoxicity: macrophage 유도
➡ pericyte 손상
➡ 혈관내피 부종
➡ 유문부 상피세포: 허혈
➡ heparan sulfate 탈락
➡ anion charge 소실
➡ pyloric stenosis
➡ gastric outlet obstruction: vomiting

처방 목표 pericyte 증식 촉진 / heparan sulfate 생성 촉진

처방 구성 半夏 二升 / 人參 三兩 / 白蜜 一升

처방 약리

인삼 panax ginsenoside
➡ Transforming growth factor β (TGF-β) (+) modulator
➡ pericyte 증식 촉진
백밀 (꿀) xylose & galactose ➡ heparan sulfate 구성 단당류

반하 triterpenoid ($C_{30}H_{48}O_7S$)
➡ Rho GTPase family transcription promotor
➡ heparan sulfate 생성 촉진

대승기탕 (大承氣湯)

원문 二陽 并病，太陽證 罷，但 發 潮熱，手足 濈然 汗出, 大便 難 而 譫語 者, 下之 則 愈，宜 大承氣湯 。傷寒，若 吐 若 下 後，不解，不 大便 五 六 日，上至 十餘日, 日晡 所 發 潮熱，不惡寒，獨語 如 見 鬼狀，若 劇者，發 則 不 識人, 循 衣 摸 床，惕 而 不安，微 喘 直視，脈 弦 者 生，澀 者 死； 微 者, 但 發熱 譫語 者，大承氣湯 主 之 。

원문 해설 림프절과 점막연관림프절 감염증이 같이 생긴 뒤, 림프감염증은 낫고, 단지 조수가 반복되는 듯한 열이 있으면서 손발에서 찜찜하게 땀이 나고, 대변이 힘들면서 헛소리를 하는 경우에는 병소를 빼내야 되며 대승기탕을 쓴다. 세포병변성 감염병에서 토하거나 설사한 후에도 낫지 않고, 5~6일 동안 대변이 없고, 10여일이 지나서는 해가 저물 때 조열이 생기며, 오한은 없고, 귀신을 본 사람처럼 혼잣말을 하며, 심한 경우에는 사람을 못 알아 보고, 옷이나 침상을 더듬으며, 무서워하고 불안해하며, 약간 호흡곤란이 있고, 눈을 똑바로 뜨는데, 맥이 울리는 경우에는 살고, 막히는 경우에는 죽는다. 심하지 않은 경우에는 단지 발열하고 헛소리를 하게 되며 대승기탕을 쓴다.

적응증 Diffuse large B cell lymphoma of small intestine MALT
(소장 점막림프조직의 미만성 B세포 림프종)

병태 & 증상

Diffuse large B cell lymphoma of small intestine MALT

➡ small intestine MALT lymphoma
➡ VEGF autocrine
➡ diffuse large B cell lymphoma 형성
➡ diffuse large B cell lymphoma: growth factor autocrine
➡ tyrosine kinase Rc: diffuse large B cell lymphoma 성장
➡ diffuse large B cell: matrix metalloproteinases (MMP) 분비
➡ lymph node: destruction
➡ diffuse large B cell: dissemination
➡ 주로 brain: diffuse large B cell lymphoma 침투
▶ nonsense, clouded consciousness
➡ IL-1 분비: fever, sweating

처방 목표 VEGF Rc 차단 ➡ B cell transformation 억제 / tyrosine kinase Rc 차단 / matrix metalloproteinases (MMP) 차단 / Peyer`s patch: B cell clones 장관 배출

처방 구성 大黃 四兩 / 厚朴 半斤 (炙) / 枳實 五枚 (炙) / 芒硝 三合

처방 약리

대황 emodin ➡ tyrosine kinase Rc blocker
➡ diffuse large B cell lymphoma 성장 억제

후박 honokiol ➡ VEGF receptor blocker
➡ B cell lymphoma transformation 억제

지실 auraptene ➡ matrix metalloproteinases (MMPs) blocker
➡ diffuse large B cell 전이 억제

망초 Sodium Sulfate ➡ Intraluminal distention pressure 상승시킴
➡ submucosa: leaking
➡ Peyer`s patch: B cell clones 장관 배출

대시호탕 (大柴胡湯)

원문 太陽病，過經 十餘日，反 二 三 下 之，後 四 五 日，柴胡證 仍 在 者, 先 與 小柴胡 ; 嘔 不止，心 下 急， 鬱鬱 微煩 者，為 未 解 也，與 大柴胡湯 下 之 則 愈 。傷寒 發熱，汗出 不解，心 中 痞 硬， 嘔吐 而 下利 者, 大柴胡湯 主 之 。

원문 해설 림프절 감염병이 10 여일이 지나 2~3회 치료한 후 4~5일이 지나도 시호증이아직 있는 것이므로 소시호탕을 쓴다. 구역이 계속되고, 흉부 아래로 편치 않고, 우울한 감이 있으면서 괴로운 증상이 있으면 아직 낫지 않은 것이므로 대시호탕을 쓴다. 세포병변성 감염병에서 발열하고 땀 흘린 뒤에도 낫지 않고, 흉부가 결리면서 딱딱한 감이 있으며, 구토와 설사를 하는 경우에는 대시호탕을 쓴다.

적응증 Hepatocellular carcinoma (간암)

병태 & 증상

Hepatocellular carcinoma

➡ chronic hepatitis B virus & hepatitis C virus infection
➡ virus replicon RNAs
➡ NOS2 gene expression ↑
➡ nitric oxide + superoxide
➡ peroxynitrite ($ONOO^-$) ↑
➡ HBV gene & HCV RNA: mutation
➡ HBV gene & HCV RNA: mutant protein 생산
➡ mutant protein: p53 binding
➡ p53 inactivation
➡ hepatocyte apoptosis & cell-growth control: 실패
➡ oncogenic hepatocyte: 출현
➡ oncogenic hepatocyte: PDGF 분비
➡ hepatic stellate cell (HSC): 활성화
➡ HSC: matrix metalloproteinases (MMP) 분비
➡ HSC: integrin 분해
➡ HSC: 기저막에서 분리
➡ HSC: oncogenic hepatocyte 쪽으로 이동 via hydrogen peroxide & calcium
➡ HSC: hepatocyte growth factor 분비

➡ tyrosine kinase 활성화

➡ oncogenic hepatocyte: proliferation

➡ hepatocellular carcinoma

처방 목표 virus replicon RNAs 제거 / superoxide 제거 / peroxynitrite ($ONOO^-$) 제거 / matrix metalloproteinases 차단 / integrin 복구 / HSC hydrogen peroxide 제거 / HSC calcium 감소 / tyrosine kinase 차단

처방 구성 柴胡 半斤 / 黃芩 三兩 / 芍藥 三兩 / 半夏 半升 / 生薑 五兩 / 枳實 四枚(炙) / 大棗 十二枚 / 大黃 二兩

처방 약리

시호 saikosaponin, 약리추측 ➡ small interfering RNA (siRNA) (+) modulator
➡ hepatitis virus RNA replication inhibition

작약 paeoniflorin ➡ superoxide scavenger

황금 baicalin ➡ peroxynitrite ($ONOO^-$) scavenger

지실 auraptene ➡ matrix metalloproteinases (MMP) blocker

반하 triterpenoid ($C_{30}H_{48}O_7S$)
➡ Rho GTPase family transcription promotor
➡ integrin 합성 촉진

생강 gingerol ➡ hydrogen peroxide scavenger

대조 c-AMP ➡ Inhibition of granular organelles phosphorylation
➡ calcium efflux 차단

대황 emodin ➡ tyrosine kinase blocker

대오두전 (大烏頭煎)

원문 寒疝 繞臍痛, 若發則白汗出, 手足厥冷, 其脈沉緊者, 大烏頭煎主之。

원문 해설 오한이 들면서 배가 아픈데, 배꼽을 뱅 둘러서 통증이 있고, 심해지면 땀이 저절로 나며, 손발이 몹시 차가워지고, 맥은 가라앉고 굵은 경우에는 대오두전을 쓴다.

적응증 Volvulus (장꼬임증)

병태 & 증상

Volvulus

➡ mesenteric lymph nodes: macrophage

▶ intracellular-bacteria infection

➡ intracellular-bacteria: activation

➡ macrophage: protease 분비

➡ lymph nodes matrix: degradation

➡ macrophage: cytokine

➡ tissue remodeling

➡ mesenteric lymph nodes: calcification

➡ mesentery & bowel: adhesion

➡ volvulus

➡ bowel obstruction: TNF-α ▶ sweating, cold hands and feet

처방 목표 macrophage: cytokine 분비 억제 / mesentery & retroperitoneum: adhesion 억제

처방 구성 烏頭 大者 五枚 / 蜜 二升

처방 약리

오두 hypaconitine, 약리 추측

➡ tissue macrophage: Voltage-gated proton channels blocker

➡ Voltage-gated proton channels 차단

➡ 조직 대식세포내 수소이온 축적

➡ tissue macrophage 대사 억제

➡ cytokine 분비 억제

밀 (꿀): xylose & galactose ➡ heparan sulfate 구성 단당류

➡ 장간막 & 후복막 유착 억제

대청룡탕 (大青龍湯)

원문 太陽 中風, 脈 浮緊, 發熱 惡寒, 身疼痛, 不汗出 而 煩躁者, 大青龍湯 主之, 若 脈 微弱, 汗出 惡風者, 不可 服之, 服之 則 厥逆, 筋惕肉瞤, 此 為逆也。 傷寒, 脈 浮緩, 身不疼, 但 重, 乍 有輕時, 無 少陰證者, 大青龍湯 發之。

원문 해설 림프절 감염병으로 Hypothalamic set point가 상승되어 있고, 맥이 뜨면서 딴딴하고 발열과 오한이 있고 동통이 생기며, 땀은 없고, 마음이 괴롭고 초조한 경우에는 대청룡탕을 쓴다. 만약 맥이 약하면서, 땀이 나며 추위를 타는 경우에는 복용하지 않는다. 만약 복용하면 손발이 차가워지고 근육이 부들거리며 떨리게 되는데 역이 된 것이다. 세포병변성 바이러스 감염병에서 맥이 뜨면서 느리고, 동통 없이 단지 몸이 무겁고 증상이 잠깐 가벼워지는 때가 있으며 자가면역성 증상이 없는 경우에는 대청룡탕을 쓴다.

적응증 IFN-γ resistant viral infection

병태 & 증상

Virus infection

➡ dendritic cell: virus phagocytosis
➡ IFN-α 분비
➡ Natural killer cell 유도
➡ Natural killer cell: degranulation
➡ IFN-γ 분비
➡ 만약, *IFN-γ*: 회피 바이러스인 경우
➡ IFN-γ 지속
➡ virus infected cell: MHC class I molecules 발현 ↑
➡ CD8+ T cell activation
➡ CD8+ T cell: TNF-α 분비: fever / chills / no sweating
➡ virus infected cell: FAS 작동

▶ 당대사 급격한 증가
▶ lactate
▶ mitochondria ROS ↑
▶ mitochondria dysfunction
▶ apoptosis

➡ lactatemia: discomfort / ache
➡ NKc-generated hydroxyl radical 유출
➡ tissue damage

처방 목표 Natural killer cell: degranulation 억제 / CD8+ T cell activation 억제 / mature CD8+ T cell apoptosis 유도 / lactatemia 교정 / hydroxyl radical 제거

처방 구성 麻黃 六兩 / 桂枝 二兩 / 炙甘草 二兩 / 杏仁 四十枚 / 生薑 三兩 / 大棗 十枚 / 石膏 如 雞子大

처방 약리

마황 ephedrine ➡ Epinephrine receptors agonist
➡ adenylate cyclase 활성화
➡ cAMP ↑
➡ NKc secretion 억제

생강 gingerol ➡ H2O2 scavenger
➡ T cell p56kk 억제
➡ T cell 활성화 억제

대조 cAMP ➡ T cell: Inhibition of granular organelles phosphorylation
➡ endoplasmic reticulum: calcium 분비 억제됨
➡ T cell 활성화 억제

석고 CaSO4 ➡ calcium mediated T-cell apoptosis 유도

계지 cinnamic acid ➡ lactate oxidizer
➡ Cori cycle: lactate 대사 촉진
➡ lactatemia 개선

구감초 18β-24-Hydroxyglycyrrhetinic acid -〉 HSD11B2 inhibitor
➡ cortisol 분해 억제
➡ mineralocorticoid receptors 자극 지속
➡ aldosterone 작용 동일
➡ H+ secretion
➡ lactatemia 개선

행인 benzoic acid ➡ hydroxyl radical scavenger

대함흉탕 (大陷胸湯)

원문 太陽病, 脈 浮 而 動數, 浮 則 為風, 數 則 為熱, 動 則 為痛, 數 則 為 虛 。, 客 氣 動 膈 , 短氣 躁煩, 心中 懊憹 , 陽氣 內 陷 , 心 下 因 硬 , 則 為 結胸, 大陷 胸湯 主之 。若 不 結胸, 但 頭汗出 , 餘 處 無汗 , 劑頸 而 還 , 小便 不利 , 身 必 發黃 。傷寒 六 七 日 , 結胸 熱實 , 脈 沉而緊 , 心下痛 , 按之 石硬 者, 大陷胸 湯 主之。結胸證 , 其 脈 浮 大 者 , 不可 下 , 下 之 則 死 。結胸證 悉 具 , 煩 躁 者 亦 死 。

원문 해설 림프절 감염증으로 맥이 뜨고 요동치고 빠르다. 뜨는 것은 풍이 된 것으로 근육대사가 촉진된 것이며, 빠른 것은 발열되고 궤양이 된 것이며, 요동치는 것은 통증이 된 것이며 , 염증이 복막에 있는 것으로 호흡이 얕아지며 초조해지며, 마음이 굉장히 괴로워진다, 백혈구가 천공을 일으켜서 복부가 딱딱해지는 것을 결흉이라 하며 대함흉탕으로 치료한다. 만약, 천공이 낫지 않으면 소장 폐쇄로 혈 중에 간접형 빌리루빈이 증가되어 황달이 되고 소변보기가 불편해짐. 세포병변성 감염증 6~7일 뒤 복부가 딱딱해지고 열감이 있으면서 복부에 막히는 느낌이 있고, 복부통이 있으면서 만지면 더욱더 복부강직이 되면 대함흉탕을 쓴다. 복부강직이 있으면서 맥이 뜨면서 큰 것은, 백혈구가 복막에 유출된 삼출물을 탐식하고 있는 것이므로 사하제로 림프구를 배출시키면 안 된다. 만약 림프구를 배출시키면 (패혈증으로) 죽는다. 복부강직이 있고 기타 천공증상이 전부 있으면서 번조감(박테리아혈증)이 있으면 죽는다.

적응증 Intestine MALT lymphoma-complicated perforation
(소장 점막림프종에 의한 천공)

병태 & 증상

Intestine MALT lymphoma complicated perforation

➡ lymphoma cell
➡ perforin & granzyme 분비
➡ tissue destruction
➡ perforation
➡ 복막 자극
➡ 반사성 경련: 복부경직
➡ 마비성 장폐쇄: 소장액 축적
➡ 소장액 유출되면 복막염 될 수 있음

처방 목표 lymphoma cell: apoptosis 시킴 / Peyer`s patch: lymphoma cell clones 장관 배출 / 소장액 제거

처방 구성 大黃 六兩 / 芒硝 一升 / 甘遂 一錢七

처방 약리

대황 emodin ➡ tyrosine kinase blocker
➡ lymphoma cell 성장 정지시킴

망초 Sodium Sulfate ➡ Intraluminal distention pressure 상승시킴
➡ submucosa: leacking
➡ Peyer`s patch: lymphoma cell clones 장관 배출

감수 Tirucallol ➡ aldosterone receptor blocker
➡ body fluid volume 감소시킴
➡ 소장액 감소

대함흉환 (大陷胸丸)

원문 病 發 於 陽, 而 反 下 之, 熱 入 因 作 結胸。病 發 於 陰, 而 反 下 之, 因 作 痞 也。所 以 成 結胸 者, 以 下 之 太 早 故也。結胸 者, 項 亦 強, 如 柔痓 狀, 下 之 則 和, 宜 大陷胸丸。

원문 해설 백혈구의 식균작용이 관여하는 병인 경우, 거꾸로 백혈구를 배출시키면 제거되지 않은 병원미생물로 인해 림프구가 악성전환되어 천공이 된다 영양부족으로 정상세균이 병원성세균으로 형질전환되어 생긴 병인 경우, 거꾸로 백혈구를 배출시키면 세균의 병독성인자에 의해 속 쓰림이 생긴다 이런 이유로 천공이 되는 경우는 너무 빨리 백혈구를 배출시키는 게 원인이다 천공이 된 경우에는 목 부위에 강직감이 오고 각궁반장과 같은 형상이 되며 이때는 원인이 되는 악성림프구를 배출시켜야 된다. 대함흉환을 쓴다.

적응증 Post-perforation peritonitis (천공 후 복막염)

병태 & 증상

Post-perforation peritonitis

➡ 복막에 장액 유출
➡ 염증성 삼출물 형성
➡ 복막염
➡ 반사성 경련 심해짐: 나무판 같은 복부경직

처방 목표 lymphoma cell: apoptosis 시킴 / Peyer`s patch: lymphoma cell clones 장관 배출 / 소장액 제거 / 복막에 형성된 삼출물을 정맥 배액 촉진 / 삼출물의 산화 억제시킴 / 천공된 부위와 복막의 유착을 억제시킴

처방 구성 大黃 半斤 / 葶藶子 半斤 / 芒硝 半斤 / 杏仁 半升 / 甘遂 末 一錢七 / 白蜜 二合

처방 약리

대황 emodin ➡ tyrosine kinase blocker: lymphoma cell 성장 정지시킴

망초 Sodium Sulfate ➡ Intraluminal distention pressure 상승시킴
➡ submucosa: leacking
➡ Peyer`s patch: lymphoma cell clones 배출

감수 Tirucallol ➡ aldosterone receptor blocker
➡ body fluid volume 감소시킴

정력자 helveticoside ➡ 강심배당체
➡ 대정맥을 통해 유입되는 혈액량이 증가
➡ 정맥 배액 촉진됨

행인 benzoic acid ➡ hydroxyl radical scavenger
➡ 삼출물 산패 억제

백밀(꿀) xylose & galactose ➡ heparan sulfate biosynthesis
➡ 천공부위와 복막의 유착은 상피세포끼리의 heparan sulfate 손실이 원인임
➡ heparan sulfate의 합성 촉진
➡ 천공부위와 복막의 유착 억제

대황감수탕 (大黃甘遂湯)

원문 婦人 少腹滿 如 敦 狀, 小便 微 難 而 不渴, 生 後 者, 此 為 水 與 血 俱 結 血 室 也, 大黃甘遂湯 主之。

원문 해설 부인 아랫배가 쟁반대처럼 불러 있고, 소변이 약간 불편하며 갈증이 없는 것은 생리(배란) 후에 난소에서 수분과 혈액이 찬 낭종이 생긴 것으로 대황감수탕을 쓴다.

적응증 Ovarian cancer (난소암)

병태 & 증상

Ovarian cancer

➡ ovulation
➡ ovulation-induced reactive oxidants 생성
➡ ovarian surface epithelium: damage
➡ damage-repair responses 반복
➡ ovarian surface epithelium: DNA damage
➡ ovarian surface epithelium: oncogenesis
➡ EGF autocrine
➡ EGF-Rc & tyrosine kinase domain: 활성화
➡ ovarian cancer: cyst formation
➡ utero-ovarian ligament: shortening
➡ ovarian torsion

처방 목표 tyrosine kinase 차단 / cyst 제거 / utero-ovarian ligament 재생

처방 구성 大黃 四兩 / 甘遂 二兩 / 阿膠 二兩

처방 약리

대황 emodin ➡ tyrosine kinase blocker

감수 tirucallol ➡ aldosterone receptor blocker
➡ body fluid volume 감소시킴
➡ cyst 제거

아교 Glycine / Proline / Hydroxyproline / Alanine

➡ collagen의 주요 아미노산

➡ utero-ovarian ligament 재생

대황감초탕 (大黃甘草湯)

원문 食 已 即 吐 者，大黃甘草湯 主之。

원문 해설 식 후에 바로 토하는 경우에는 대황감초탕을 쓴다.

적응증 Barrett`s esophagus (바렛 식도)

병태 & 증상

Barrett`s esophagus

➡ acid reflux disease / candida, herpes simplex, cytomegalovirus infection / alcohol

➡ esophageal: mucosal cell injury (esophagitis)

➡ esophagitis 반복

➡ mucosa cell: NF-κB activation

➡ growth factor 전사 활성: autocrine, paracrine

➡ tyrosine kinase 활성화

➡ hyperplasia: vomiting after meals

처방 목표 NF-κB 억제 / tyrosine kinase Rc 차단

처방 구성 大黃 四兩 / 甘草 一兩

처방 약리

감초 glycyrrhetinic acid

➡ 11-beta-hydroxysteroid dehydrogenase1 (HSD11B1) inhibitor

➡ IκBα 생성

➡ NF-κB 억제

대황 emodin ➡ tyrosine kinase Rc blocker

대황목단탕 (大黃牡丹湯)

원문 腸癰者, 少腹腫痞, 按之即痛如淋, 小便自調, 時時發熱, 自汗出, 復惡寒, 其脈遲緊者, 膿未成, 可下之, 當有血。
脈洪數者, 膿已成, 不可下也, 大黃牡丹湯主之。

원문 해설 장옹은 아랫배에 종기가 있어 저릿저릿하고 누르면 임질 같은 염증성 통증이 있으며, 소변이 저절로 나오고 때 때로 발열하며 땀 흘린 뒤 오한이 난다. 맥이 느리고 팽팽하면 아직 농이 성하지 않은 것으로 망초로 사하시켜야 되며 반드시 변혈이 있을 것이다. 맥이 넓고 잦으면 농이 이미 성해 있는 것으로 망초 같은 사하제만 써서는 안 되며 대황목단탕을 쓴다.

적응증 Diverticulitis (게실염)

병태 & 증상

Diverticulitis

➡ 대장근육 약화
➡ 점막 & 점막하층: 근육층으로 돌출
➡ 혈관 눌림
➡ 혈관 퇴행
➡ arteriovenous malformation (동정맥 기형) via tyrosine kinase
➡ 장평활근: 허혈 손상
➡ 평활근 수축력 저하
➡ 장내 압력에 대한 장근육의 지탱력 저하
➡ 점막 & 점막하층: 돌출 진행
➡ 돌출된 epithelium: estrogen mediated cell growth
➡ diverticulosis (게실주머니 형성)
➡ diverticula (게실): inspisated stool & water 축적
➡ inspisated stool & water: G- bacteria 증식 환경 제공
➡ G- bacteria: 증식
➡ diverticula necrosis
➡ diverticulitis

처방 목표 arteriovenous tyrosine kinase 차단 / 장평활근: 허혈 손상 억제 / diverticula epithelium: estrogen 차단 / diverticula: inspisated stool & water 배출 / diverticula: G- bacteria 항균

처방 구성 大黃 四兩 / 牡丹 一兩 / 桃仁 五十枚 / 瓜子 半升 / 芒硝 三合

처방 약리

대황 emodin ➡ tyrosine kinase blocker
➡ arteriovenous 성장 정지

목단피 β-Sitosterol
➡ manganese superoxide dismutase & glutathione peroxidase (+) modulator
➡ 장평활근 허혈 손상의 원인이 되는 활성산소를 제거시킴

도인 amygdalin
➡ 체내 활성 성분: thiocyanate (amygdalin metabolite)
➡ 4S estrogen receptor (ER) ▶ 5S estrogen receptor 전환 억제
(4S monomer: estrogen 저친화성, 5S dimer: estrogen 고친화성)

망초 Sodium Sulfate ➡ Intraluminal distention pressure 상승시킴
➡ submucosa: leacking
➡ diverticula 내의 inspisated stool & water 배출

동과자 urea ➡ 알카리환경 G- bacteria 세포막 파괴

대황부자탕 (大黃附子湯)

원문 脅下 偏 痛，發熱，其 脈 緊 弦，此 寒 也，以 溫 藥 下之，宜 大黃附子湯 。

원문 해설 갈빗대 한쪽 밑이 아프고 발열하며, 맥은 팽팽하고 울리는 경우는, 막혀서 생긴 병이므로 따뜻한 약을 쓴다. 대황부자탕을 쓴다.

적응증 Distal extrahepatic cholangiocarcinoma (원위부 간외담관암)

병태 & 생리

Distal extrahepatic cholangiocarcinoma

➡ peripheral blood: met-hemoglobin ↑

➡ intravascular hemolysis

➡ liver: bilirubin influx ↑
➡ bilirubin oversaturated bile 생산
➡ distal extrahepatic bile duct: bilirubin crystal 형성
➡ plasma-protein coated crystal: neutrophil 유도
➡ neutrophil HOCl 분비
➡ bilirubin crystal oxidation
➡ bilirubin crystal 음전하 ↑
➡ calcium binding
➡ calcium bilirubinate 형성
➡ bile duct endothelium: injury & repair 반복
➡ bile duct endothelium: adenomatous hyperplasia
➡ adenomatous cholangiocyte: EGF autocrine
➡ tyrosine kinase domain 활성화
➡ distal extrahepatic cholangiocarcinoma 형성
➡ mucin overproducing
➡ mucin + calcium bilirubinate
➡ pigment gallstone 형성

처방 목표 peripheral blood: met-hemoglobin 환원 / neutrophil HOCl 분비 억제 / tyrosine kinase 차단

처방 구성 大黃 三兩 / 炮附子 三枚 / 細辛 二兩

처방 약리

세신 eugenol ➡ MetHb reducer

포부자 aconitine

➡ 약리추측: neutrophil` Voltage-gated proton channels blocker
(식균작용에 의해 증가된 세포내 proton을 세포외로 방출시키는 채널)
➡ Voltage-gated proton channels 차단
➡ 호중구내 수소이온 축적
➡ neutrophil 대사 억제

대황 emodin ➡ tyrosine kinase blocker

대황자충환 (大黃蟅蟲丸)

원문 五勞虛極羸瘦，腹滿不能飮食，食傷、憂傷、飮傷、房室傷、飢傷，勞傷、經絡營衛氣傷，內有乾血，肌膚甲錯，兩目黯黑，緩中補虛，大黃蟅蟲丸主之。

원문 해설 오장의 기능이 극도로 약해져서 핏기가 없이 마르게 되면, 복부가 팽만하여 음식을 먹지 못하게 되는데, 이것은 기아 / 근심 / 노동 / 성생활 / 음주 등의 원인으로 체내에 출혈판이 생긴 것으로, 피부는 딱딱하고 거칠어지며, 눈자위는 흐릿하면서 까매지게 되는데, 병소를 천천히 제거해야 하며 대황자충환을 쓴다.

적응증 Kaposi sarcoma (카포시 육종)

병태 & 증상

Kaposi's sarcoma

➡ lymphatic endothelium: Human herpesvirus 8 (HHV8) infection

➡ HHV8 infected endothelium: mitogen-activated protein kinase 활성화

➡ AP-1 유도: IL-6 전사 활성

➡ IL-6 분비

➡ HHV8 infected endothelium: superoxide ↑

▶ Ras gene signal 활성화 ▶ cell growth ↑

➡ HHV8 infected endothelium: hydroxyl radical ↑

▶ p53 gene: mutation ▶ apoptosis 억제

➡ HHV8 infected endothelium: hyperplasia

➡ peritumoral & intratumoral angiogenesis

➡ hyperplasia endothelium: erythrocyte 유입

➡ spindle cell 형성

➡ spindle cell: mannose receptor 발현

➡ macrophage 유도

➡ macrophage: phagocytosis

➡ extracellular peroxynitrite ($ONOO^-$) ↑

➡ lymph vessel barrier: destruction

➡ HHV8 infected endothelium: IL-6

➡ fibroblast: NF-κB 활성화 ▶ estrogen receptor 발현 ↑

▶ proliferation ↑
▶ fibrosarcoma cell 전환

➡ fibrosarcoma cell: fibroblast growth factor 분비
➡ spindle cell: tyrosine kinase domain 활성화
➡ spindle cell: proliferation & migration
➡ Kaposi's sarcoma 형성
➡ 이동 조직: skin / mouth / respiratory tract / gastrointestinal tract
➡ Kaposi's sarcoma: lysis
➡ hemorrhagic patches
➡ 합병증: obstruction / organ perforation / sepsis

처방 목표 HHV8 infected endothelium: superoxide 제거 / HHV8 infected endothelium: hydroxyl radical 제거 / extracellular peroxynitrite ($ONOO^-$) 제거 / fibroblast: NF-κB 억제 / fibroblast: estrogen receptor 차단 / fibrosarcoma cell: apoptosis 유도 / spindle cell: tyrosine kinase domain 차단 / hemorrhagic patches 제거 / 조혈 촉진

처방 구성 大黃 十分 / 黃芩 二兩 / 甘草 三兩 / 桃仁 一升 / 杏仁 一升 / 芍藥 四兩 / 乾地黃 十兩 / 乾漆 一兩 / 虻蟲一升 / 水蛭 百枚 / 蠐螬 一升 / 蟅蟲 半升

처방 약리

작약 paeoniflorin ➡ Superoxide scavenger
➡ HHV8 infected endothelium: Ras gene signal 활성화 억제
➡ cell growth ↓

행인 benzoic acid ➡ Hydroxyl radical scavenger
➡ HHV8 infected endothelium: p53 gene mutation 억제
➡ apoptosis 유도
➡ HHV8 infected endothelium: hyperplasia 억제

황금 baicalin ➡ Peroxynitrite ($ONOO^-$) scavenger
➡ extracellular peroxynitrite ($ONOO^-$) ↓
➡ lymph vessel barrier: destruction 억제

감초 glycyrrhetinic acid
➡ 11-beta-hydroxysteroid dehydrogenase1 (HSD11B1) inhibitor

➡ glucocorticoid 작용
➡ IκBα 생성
➡ NF-κB 억제
➡ fibroblast: estrogen receptor 발현 억제
➡ fibroblast: proliferation 억제
➡ fibroblast: fibrosarcoma cell 전환 억제

도인 amygdalin
➡ 체내 활성 성분: thiocyanate (amygdalin metabolite)
➡ 4S estrogen receptor (ER) ▶ 5S estrogen receptor 전환 억제
(4S monomer: estrogen 저친화성, 5S dimer: estrogen 고친화성)
➡ fibroblast: estrogen receptor
▶ 5S dimer 전환 억제
➡ fibroblast: proliferation 억제

건칠 urishiol ➡ Fibrosarcoma cell p27 (+) modulator
➡ fibrosarcoma apoptosis

대황 emodin ➡ Tyrosine kinase blocker
➡ spindle cell: tyrosine kinase domain 차단
➡ spindle cell: proliferation & migration 억제
➡ Kaposi's sarcoma 형성 억제

맹충 (등에) anophelin ➡ Thrombin esterase blocker
➡ hemorrhagic patches 생성 억제

수질 (거머리) hirudin ➡ Thrombolytic activator
➡ hemorrhagic patches 생성 억제

제조 (굼벵이) fibrinolytic serine protease ➡ Fibrinolysis
➡ hemorrhagic patches 생성 억제

자충 (흙바퀴) ESW extraction, 약리 추측
➡ Erythrocyte C3b receptor (+) modulator
➡ macrophage: hemorrhagic patches 식균 촉진

건지황 catalpol, 약리 추측 ➡ CD133+ CFU-GEMM (+) modulator
➡ 조혈 촉진

대황초석탕 (大黃硝石湯)

원문 黃疸 腹滿，小便不利 而 赤，自汗出，此 為 表和 裡實，當 下 之，宜 大黃硝石湯 。

원문 해설 황달과 복부팽만감이 있고 소변이 불편하고 붉으며, 땀이 흐르는 것은 체표에는 독성물질이 흐르고 장부에는 종양이 있기 때문이다. 병소를 빼내야 하며 대황초석탕을 쓴다.

적응증 Klatskin tumor (간문부 담관암)

병태 & 증상

Klatskin tumor

➡ hilar bile duct cholangiocyte: Gut bacterial translocation
➡ chronic cholangitis
➡ cholangiocyte: adenomatous hyperplasia
➡ adenomatous cholangiocyte : EGF autocrine
➡ tyrosine kinase domain 활성화 ▶ 세포 증식
➡ hilar bile duct: cholangiocarcinoma
➡ hilar bile duct: 압력 상승
➡ diconjugated bilirubin: 혈 중 역류 ▶ urine bilirubin
▶ 혈 중 unconjugated bilirubin ↑ ▶ jaundice
& translocated bacteria: 혈류 이동 ▶ sepsis

처방 목표 Gut bacterial translocation 억제 / tyrosine kinase 차단 / 혈 중 unconjugated bilirubin 환원 / sepsis 억제

처방 구성 大黃 四兩 / 黃柏 四兩 / 硝石 四兩 / 梔子 十五枚

처방 약리

망초 Sodium Sulfate ➡ Intraluminal distention pressure 상승시킴
➡ submucosa: leacking
➡ lymphatic drainage 배액
➡ Gut bacteria 제거

대황 emodin ➡ tyrosine kinase Rc blocker

치자 crocin ➡ unconjugated bilirubin antioxidant

황백 phellodendrine, 약리 추측 ➡ CD14 blocker ➡ sepsis 차단

패혈증 ➡ 혈액내 Monocyte / Macrophage / Neutrophil CD14
➡ 세균 LPS 및 항원 인식
➡ cytokine 분비
➡ T cell 분화
➡ TNF-α 분비
➡ multi-organ failure

대황황련사심탕 (大黃黃連瀉心湯)

원문 心下痞，按 之 濡，其 脈 關上 浮 者，大黃黃連瀉心湯 主之。傷寒 大 下 後，復 發汗，心下痞, 惡寒 者, 表 未解也, 不可 攻 痞，當 先 解表，表 解 乃 可 攻 痞, 解表 宜 桂枝湯，攻 痞 宜 大黃黃連瀉心湯 。

원문 해설 명치 밑이 쓰리고, 누르면 연한 느낌이 있고, 관상맥이 떠있는 경우에는 대황황련사심탕을 쓴다. 세포병변성 감염병으로 크게 고생한 후, 다시 땀이 나며, 명치 밑이 쓰리고 오한이 있으면 아직 표증이 풀리지 않은 것이므로 병소를 제거시키기 전에 표증을 풀어줘야 하므로 먼저 계지탕을 쓴 뒤, 대황황련사심탕으로 병소를 제거시킨다.

적응증 Gastric MALT lympoma (위장 점막림프종)

병태 & 증상

Gastric MALT lympoma

➡ H. pylori: persistent infection
➡ B cell infiltration
➡ B cell clones formation
➡ <u>H. pylori: persistent antigenic stimulation</u>

➡ B cell: genetic alteration
➡ B cell: neoplastic transformation

처방 목표 H. pylori 항원성 억제 / neoplastic B cell: apoptosis시킴

처방 구성 大黃 二兩 / 黃連 一兩

처방 약리

황련 berberine ➡ sortase inhibitor
➡ H. pylori: peptidoglycan 합성 억제
➡ 항원성 감소되어 면역반응 억제됨

대황 emodin ➡ tyrosine kinase blocker
➡ neoplastic B cell 성장 정지시킴

도핵승기탕 (桃核承氣湯)

원문 太陽病 不解，熱 結 膀胱，其人 如 狂，血 自下，下 者 愈。其 外 不解 者，尚 未 可 攻，當 先 解 其 外。外 解 已，但 少腹 急結 者，乃 可 攻 之， 宜 桃核承氣湯。

원문 해설 림프절 감염병이 낫지 않고 방광부위에 열감이 있어서 환자가 안절부절하여 미친 듯이 보이는데, 하혈로 병소가 배출되면 낫는다. 표증이 풀리지 않으면 병소를 공격할 수 없으므로 먼저 표증을 낫게 해야 한다 표증이 나은 후, 아랫배에 땅기면서 엉기는 증상이 있는 경우에는 병소를 공격해야 되며 도핵승기탕을 쓴다.

적응증 Cervical cancer (자궁암)

병태 & 증상

Cervical cancer

➡ cervical squamous epithelium: human papillomavirus (HPV) infection
➡ cervical squamous epithelium: oncogenic change
➡ EGF autocrine

➡ EGF-Rc & tyrosine kinase domain: 활성화
➡ squamous epithelium: hyperplasia
➡ squamous cell carcinoma
➡ 배란기: estrogen ↑
➡ glycogen 축적 ▶ glycogenolysis ↑
➡ mucin 분비
➡ lactate ↑↑
➡ squamous cell carcinoma 주위: acidity ↑
➡ squamous cell carcinoma: IL-8 분비 --> AP-1 & NF-κB
➡ squamous cell carcinoma: aggressive (침윤형) type 전환
➡ lymphatic drainage: metastasis

치료 목표 tyrosine kinase 차단 / estrogen 차단 / lactate 제거 / acidity 교정 / lymphatic drainage 배액

처방 구성 桃仁 五十個 / 大黃 四兩 / 桂枝 二兩 / 炙甘草 二兩 / 芒硝 二兩

처방 약리

대황 emodin ➡ tyrosine kinase blocker

도인 amygdalin
➡ 체내 활성 성분: thiocyanate (amygdalin metabolite)
➡ 4S estrogen receptor (ER) ▶ 5S estrogen receptor 전환 억제
(4S monomer: estrogen 저친화성, 5S dimer: estrogen 고친화성)

계지 cinnamic acid ➡ lactate oxidizer
➡ pyruvate 전환 촉진

구감초 18β-24-Hydroxyglycyrrhetinic acid
➡ 11-beta-hydroxysteroid dehydrogenase2 (HSD11B2) inhibitor
➡ aldosterone 생리작용과 동일
➡ H+ secretion
➡ acidity 교정

망초 Sodium Sulfate ➡ Intraluminal distention pressure 상승시킴
➡ submucosa: leacking
➡ lymphatic drainage 배액
➡ squamous cell carcinoma 전이 억제

도화탕 (桃花湯)

원문 少陰病，下利 便膿血 者, 桃花湯 主之。少陰病，二 三 日 至 四 五 日，腹痛，小便 不利，下利 不止，便膿血 者, 桃花湯 主之。

원문 해설 항체매개 감염병에서 설사하고 농혈변을 보는 경우에는 도화탕을 쓴다. 항체매개 감염병이 2~3일이 지나고 4~5일째 복통이 있고 소변이 불편하며 설사가 계속 되고 농혈변을 보는 경우에는 도화탕을 쓴다.

적응증 Ulcerative colitis (궤양성대장염)

병태 & 증상

Ulcerative colitis

➡ colon mucosa: capillary endothelial cells
➡ cytomegalovirus (CMV) reactivation
➡ specific CMV antibody 출현
➡ Fc receptor: neutrophil 유도
➡ neutrophil phagocytosis
➡ HClO 분비 via H_2O_2
➡ mucosa cell & capillary endothelial cells: necrosis
➡ bleeding
➡ dead neutrophil + dead mucosa cell: protein-rich fluid
➡ pus 생성
➡ 수분 흡수 불량: diarrhea

처방 목표 HClO 분비 억제 / mucosa cell 재생 촉진 / pus 제거

처방 구성 赤石脂 一斤 / 乾薑 一兩 / 粳米 一升

처방 약리

건강 shogaol ➡ neutrophil H_2O_2 scavenger
➡ HClO 분비 억제

경미 magnesium ➡ DNA replication cofactor

적석지 Al_2O_3, $2SiO_2 \cdot 4H_2O$ ➡ Cation absorbent
➡ pus 주성분인 양이온 단백성분을 흡착하여 제거시킴

두풍마산 (頭風摩散)

원문 寸口脈 沉 而 弱 , 沉 即 主 骨 , 弱 即 主 筋 , 沉 即 為 腎, 弱 即 為 肝 。汗出 入 水 中 , 如 水 傷 心 , 歷節 黃 汗出 , 故 曰 歷節 。趺陽脈 浮 而 滑 , 滑 則 穀氣 實 , 浮 則 汗自出 。少陰脈 浮而弱 , 弱 則 血不足 , 浮 則 為 風 , 風 血 相搏, 即 疼痛 如掣 。盛人 脈 澀 小 , 短氣 , 自汗出 , 歷節痛 , 不可 屈伸 , 此 皆 飮酒 汗出 當 風 所 致 。

원문 해설 촌구맥이 가라앉아 있는 것은, 뼈에 병소가 있고, 콩팥이 원인이 된 것이고, 떠있는 것은 근육에 병소가 있고, 간이 원인이 된 것이다. 땀을 흘릴 때, 물속에 들어가면 교감신경이 손상되어, 관절염과 황한병이 생긴다. 부양맥이 떠있는 것은 발한이 있는 것이고, 매끈한 것은 열량이 넘치는 것이다. 소음맥이 떠있는 것은 염증성 반응이 있는 것이고, 약한 것은 빈혈이 있는 것으로, 관절염이 될 수 있다. 성인의 맥이 껄끄럽고 작으며, 호흡이 짧고, 땀을 흘리면서 관절염이 있는 것은 알코올성 간염이 원인이다.

적응증 IL-1 mediated arthritis

병태 & 증상

IL-1 mediated arthritis

many infection: macrophage ▶ IL-1
& obesity: adipocyte ▶ IL-1
& autoimmune disease: macrophage ▶ IL-1 ▶ iron 결핍 ▶ anemia
& alcoholic hepatitis: hepatocyte ▶ IL-1

➡ synoviocyte IL-1 Rc: IL-1 축적
➡ synoviocyte: NF-κB 활성화
➡ synoviocyte inflammation: IL-8 분비
➡ neutrophil 유도
➡ neutrophil: elastase 분비
➡ hyaluronate destruction
➡ synovitis

처방 목표 neutrophil: elastase 분비 억제

처방 구성 炮大附子 一枚 / 鹽 等分

처방 약리

포부자 aconitine

➡ 약리추측: neutrophil` Voltage-gated proton channels blocker
(식균작용에 의해 증가된 세포내 proton을 세포외로 방출시키는 채널)
➡ Voltage-gated proton channels 차단
➡ 호중구내 수소이온 축적
➡ neutrophil 대사 억제
➡ elastase 분비 억제

령감오미가강신반하행인탕 (苓甘五味加薑辛半夏杏仁湯)

원문 水 去 嘔 止，其 人 形 腫 者，加 杏仁 主之。其 證 應 內 麻黃，以 其 人 遂 痺，故 不 內 之。若 逆 而 內 之 者，必 厥，所 以 然 者，以 其 人 血虛，麻 黃 發 其陽 故也, 苓甘五味加薑辛半夏杏仁湯 主之。

원문 해설 폐포간질에 수분이 제거되고 갈증이 없어졌는데, 전체적으로 부은 것 같으면 행인을 가한다, 증상으로는 당연히 마황을 써야 되지만, 마비감이 없으므로 마황을 쓰지 않으며, 마황을 쓰면 잘못된 치료가 된다, 위에 열거한 증상은 혈허증이므로 마황을 쓰지 않고 령감오미가강신반하행인탕을 쓴다.

적응증 Chronic left heart failure-mediated alveolitis (만성좌심부전-매개 폐포염)

병태 & 증상

Chronic left heart failure-mediated alveolitis

➡ 만성좌심부전
➡ 폐포 모세혈관 울혈
➡ 폐포 손상
➡ 폐포환기량 저하
➡ pulmonary artery pressure ↑

➡ 좌심실: out flow ↓
➡ 좌심실 심첨부: thrombus formation
➡ 폐포 모세혈관 울혈
➡ alveolar macrophage: IL-8
➡ 폐포 간질: neutrophil 유도
➡ neutrophil phagocytosis
➡ HClO 분비 via H2O2
➡ alveolar-capillary barrier: damage
➡ 폐포 간질: erythrocyte 유입
➡ Met hemoglobin 형성 ▶ 혈관 수축
➡ HClO + ferrous ion ▶ hydroxyl radical 생성
➡ 폐포 간질 inflammation & alveolitis
➡ 폐포 간질: fibroblast ▶ collagen 분비: thirsty, neusea
▶ alveolar-capillary barrier 복구

처방 목표 폐포환기량 증가 / 좌심실 심첨부: thrombus 억제 / alveolar macrophage 대사 억제 / HClO 분비 억제 / Met hemoglobin 환원 / hydroxyl radical 제거 / 폐포 세포 상환 촉진

처방 구성 茯苓 四兩 / 甘草 三兩 / 五味 半升 / 乾薑 三兩 / 細辛 三兩 / 半夏 半升 / 杏仁 半升

처방 약리

오미자 schizandrin ➡ acetylcholinesterase inhibitor
➡ 횡격막근 수축 강화

복령 pachymic acid ➡ glycoprotein IIb/IIIa (gpIIb/IIIa) (-) modulator
➡ thrombus formation 억제

감초 glycyrrhetinic acid
➡ 11-beta-hydroxysteroid dehydrogenase1 (HSD11B1) inhibitor
➡ glucocorticoid 작용
➡ IκBα 생성
➡ NF-κB 억제
➡ alveolar macrophage 대사 억제

건강 shogaol ➡ neutrophil H2O2 scavenger
➡ HClO 분비 억제

세신 eugenol ➡ MetHb reducer

행인 benzoic acid ➡ hydroxyl radical scavenger

반하 triterpenoid ($C_{30}H_{48}O_7S$)
➡ Rho GTPase family transcription promotor
➡ focal adhesion 생성
➡ 폐포 세포 상환 촉진

령감오미가강신반행대황탕 (苓甘五味加薑辛半杏大黃湯)

원문 若 面熱 如 醉，此 為 胃熱 上衝 熏 其 面，加 大黃 以 利之。

원문 해설 만약 얼굴에 술 취한 듯한 열이 있으면, 위열로 인한 것이므로 대황을 가한다

적응증 Chronic left heart failure-mediated alveolar carcinoma

병태 & 증상

Chronic left heart failure-mediated alveolar carcinoma (만성좌심부전-매개 폐포암)

➡ pneumonia
➡ 폐포 손상
➡ 폐포환기량 저하
➡ pulmonary artery pressure ↑
➡ 좌심실: out flow ↓
➡ 좌심실 심첨부: thrombus formation
➡ alveolar macrophage: IL-8
➡ 폐포 간질: neutrophil 유도
➡ neutrophil phagocytosis
➡ HClO 분비 via H_2O_2
➡ alveolar-capillary barrier: damage
➡ 폐포 간질: erythrocyte 유입

➡ erythrocyte oxidation
➡ Met hemoglobin 형성
➡ 폐포 간질: fibroblast 이동 ▶ collagen 분비: thirsty, neusea
➡ alveolar-capillary barrier: 복구
➡ HClO + ferrous ion ▶ hydroxyl radical 생성
➡ alveolitis
➡ 발암물질 축적
➡ alveolar carcinoma

처방 목표 폐포환기량 증가 / 좌심실 심첨부: thrombus 억제 / alveolar macrophage 대사 억제 / HClO 분비 억제/ Met hemoglobin 환원 / 폐포 간질: fibroblast 이동 촉진 / hydroxyl radical 제거 / alveolar carcinoma 성장 억제

처방 구성 茯苓 四兩 / 甘草 三兩 / 五味 半升 / 乾薑 三兩 / 細辛 三兩 / 半夏 半升 / 杏仁 半升 / 大黃 三兩

처방 약리

오미자 schizandrin ➡ acetylcholinesterase inhibitor
➡ 횡격막근 수축 강화

복령 pachymic acid ➡ glycoprotein IIb/IIIa (gpIIb/IIIa) (-) modulator
➡ thrombus formation 억제

감초 glycyrrhetinic acid
➡ 11-beta-hydroxysteroid dehydrogenase1 (HSD11B1) inhibitor
➡ glucocorticoid 작용
➡ IκBα 생성
➡ NF-κB 억제
➡ alveolar macrophage 대사 억제

건강 shogaol ➡ neutrophil H2O2 scavenger
➡ HClO 분비 억제

세신 eugenol ➡ MetHb reducer

반하 triterpenoid (C30H48O7S)
➡ Rho GTPase family transcription promotor

➡ focal adhesion 생성
➡ fibroblast 이동 촉진

행인 benzoic acid ➡ hydroxyl radical scavenger

대황 emodin ➡ tyrosine kinase blocker
➡ alveolar carcinoma 성장 억제

령감오미강신탕 (苓甘五味薑辛湯)

원문 衝 氣 即 低 , 而 反 更 咳 `胸滿 者 , 用 桂苓五味甘草湯去桂加乾薑細辛, 以 治 其 咳 滿 。

원문 해설 젖산혈증으로 인한 심장독성이 가라앉고서, 반대로 기침을 하며, 심장부위에 그득한 증상이 있는 경우에는 계령오미감초탕에서 계지를 빼고 건강과 세신을 추가하여 써서 기침과 심장부위의 팽만감을 치료한다.

적응증 Chronic left heart failure-mediated alveolar-capillary barrier damage
(만성좌심부전-매개 폐포-모세혈관 장벽 손상)

병태 & 증상

Chronic left heart failure-mediated alveolar-capillary barrier damage

➡ 만성 좌심부전
➡ 폐포 모세혈관 울혈
➡ 폐포 손상
➡ 폐포환기량 저하
➡ pulmonary artery pressure ↑
➡ 좌심실: out flow ↓
➡ 좌심실 심첨부: thrombus formation
➡ 폐포 모세혈관 울혈
➡ alveolar macrophage: IL-8
➡ 폐포 간질: neutrophil 유도
➡ neutrophil phagocytosis

➡ HClO 분비 via H2O2
➡ alveolar-capillary barrier: damage
➡ 폐포 간질: erythrocyte 유입
➡ Met hemoglobin 형성

처방 목표 폐포환기량 증가 / 좌심실 심첨부: thrombus 억제 / alveolar macrophage 대사 억제 / HClO 분비 억제 / Met hemoglobin 환원

처방 구성 茯苓 四兩 / 甘草 三兩 / 乾薑 三兩 / 細辛 三兩 / 五味子 半升

처방 약리

오미자 schizandrin ➡ acetylcholinesterase inhibitor
➡ 횡격막근 수축 강화

복령 pachymic acid ➡ glycoprotein IIb/IIIa (gpIIb/IIIa) (-) modulator
➡ thrombus formation 억제

감초 glycyrrhetinic acid
➡ 11-beta-hydroxysteroid dehydrogenase1 (HSD11B1) inhibitor
➡ glucocorticoid 작용
➡ IκBα 생성
➡ NF-κB 억제
➡ alveolar macrophage 대사 억제

건강 shogaol ➡ neutrophil H2O2 scavenger
➡ HClO 분비 억제

세신 eugenol ➡ MetHb reducer

마자인환 (麻子仁丸)

원문 趺陽脈 浮 而 澀, 浮 則 胃氣強, 澀 則 小便數, 浮 澀 相 搏, 大便 則 堅, 其 脾 為 約, 麻子仁丸 主之。

원문 해설 부양맥이 떠있고 막히는 감이 있는 경우, 떠있는 것은 위장관이 강직되어 있는 것이고, 막히는 감이 있는 것은 빈뇨가 있는 것이다, 위장관의 강직과 빈뇨가 같이 있을 때는, 뒤이어 대변이 굳어지게 되는데, 이는 위장관이 꽉 막혀 있어서 생기는 증상으로 마자인환을 쓴다.

적응증 Colon cancer (대장암)

병태 & 증상

Colon cancer

➡ high fat diets
➡ bile acids 분비 ↑
➡ colon mucosa: deoxycholic acid (DCA) & lithocholic acid (LCA) 접촉 ↑
➡ DCA & LCA mediated cytotoxicity
➡ adenomatous polyposis coli (APC) gene: mutation
➡ colon mucosa: cancerous cell 전환
➡ colon mucosa: EGF receptor tyrosine kinase ↑ ▶ 증식
VEGF 발현 ▶ angiogenesis ▶ 성장
matrix metalloproteinase 분비 ▶ 침윤
➡ adenomatous polyp 형성
➡ adenomatous polyp: amphiregulin (EGF family) 발현
▶ prostaglandin 생성 촉진 ▶ TK-dependent signal ↑
▶ cell division
➡ adenomatous polyp: superoxide ↑
▶ Ras gene signal 활성화 ▶ cell growth ↑
➡ adenomatous polyp: hydroxyl radical ↑
▶ p53 gene: mutation ▶ apoptosis 억제
➡ colon cancer 형성: constipation, bladder pressure

처방 목표 tyrosine kinase Rc 차단 / VEGF Rc 차단 / matrix metalloproteinase 차단 / prostaglandin 생성 억제 / superoxide 제거 / hydroxyl radical 제거

처방 구성 麻子仁 二升 / 芍藥 半斤 / 枳實 一斤 / 大黃 一斤 / 厚朴 一尺 / 杏仁 一升

대황 emodin ➡ tyrosine kinase blocker

후박 honokiol ➡ VEGF receptor blocker

지실 auraptene ➡ matrix metalloproteinase (MMP) blocker

마자인 α-Linolenic acid (omega-3)

➡ 대장암 세포의 세포막 지방산 조성 변화 유도
➡ α-Linoleic acid (omega-6) ▶ α-Linolenic acid (omega-3)
➡ eicosanoid & diacylglycerol 감소
➡ prostaglandin 생성 억제

작약 paeoniflorin ➡ superoxide scavenger

행인 benzoic acid ➡ hydroxyl radical scavenger

마황가출탕 (麻黃加朮湯)

원문 濕家 身 煩疼，可 與 麻黃加朮湯 發 其汗 為 宜，愼 不可 以 火攻 之。

원문 해설 습병이 생기면 몸이 괴로우면서 쑤시고 아프게 되는데, 마황가출탕으로 땀을 나게 해서 치료하며, 온침이나 뜸으로 치료하는 것은 삼가야 한다.

적응증 Immune complexes-mediated vasculitis (면역복합체-매개 혈관염)

병태 & 증상

Immune complexes-mediated vasculitis

➡ circulating immune complexes
➡ small vessel: circulating immune complexes 침착
➡ natural killer cell FcR III: immune complexes 부착
➡ natural killer cell: maturation

➡ natural killer cell: TNF-α degranulation
➡ vascular endothelium: VCAM-1 발현
➡ vascular endothelium: leukocyte 부착
➡ tissue: leukocyte transmigration
➡ leukocyte: reactive oxygen species
➡ tissue inflammation
➡ NKc-generated hydroxyl radical: 혈관 유출
➡ vasculitis
➡ tissue hypoxia
➡ lactatemia

처방 목표 natural killer cell: degranulation 억제 / vascular endothelium: VCAM-1 차단 / hydroxyl radical 제거 / lactatemia 교정

처방 구성 麻黃 三兩 / 桂枝 二兩 / 炙甘草 二兩 / 杏仁 七十個 / 白朮 四兩

처방 약리

마황 ephedrine ➡ Epinephrine receptors agonist
➡ adenylate cyclase 활성화
➡ cAMP ↑
➡ Natural killer cell: degranulation & secretion 억제

백출 atractylon ➡ vascular cell adhesion molecule-1 (VCAM-1) blocker

행인 benzoic acid ➡ hydroxyl radical scavenger

계지 cinnamic acid ➡ lactate oxidizer
➡ Cori cycle: lactate 대사 촉진
➡ lactatemia 개선

구감초 18β-24-Hydroxyglycyrrhetinic acid
➡ 11-beta-hydroxysteroid dehydrogenase2 (HSD11B2) inhibitor
➡ aldosterone 작용 동일
➡ H+ secretion

마황부자감초탕 (麻黃附子甘草湯)

원문 少陰病，得 之 二 三 日，麻黃附子甘草湯 微 發汗，以 二 三 日 無 證, 故 微 發汗 也。

원문 해설 항체매개 독성병이 생기고 2~3일 후 마황부자감초탕으로 약하게 땀을 내주면 2~3일 후 낫는다.

적응증 Early autoimmune response in tissue

병태 & 증상

Early autoimmune response in tissue

➡ target cell: autoantigen 발현
➡ antidody 부착
➡ target cell: antibody coating
➡ natural killer cell FcR III: antibody coated cell 부착
➡ natural killer cell: IFN-γ 분비
➡ neutrophil 유도
➡ neutrophil: IL-12
➡ natural killer cell: 활성화
➡ natural killer cell: IFN-γ 분비 촉진: fever
➡ antibody coated cell: IFN-γ R에 binding
➡ antibody coated cell: 세포막의 FAS 작동
➡ Na+/ K+ pump 손상
➡ 세포부종 & 세포손상
➡ antibody coated cell: apoptosis

처방 목표 neutrophil: IL-12 분비 억제 / natural killer cell: secretion 억제 / Na+/ K+ pump 활성화

처방 구성 麻黃 二兩 / 炙甘草 二兩 / 炮附子 一枚

처방 약리

포부자 aconitine

➡ 약리추측: neutrophil` Voltage-gated proton channels blocker

(식균작용에 의해 증가된 세포내 proton을 세포외로 방출시키는 채널)
➡ Voltage-gated proton channels 차단
➡ 호중구내 수소이온 축적
➡ neutrophil 대사 억제
➡ IL-12 분비 억제

마황 ephedrine ➡ Epinephrine receptors agonist
➡ adenylate cyclase 활성화
➡ cAMP ↑
➡ NKc secretion 억제

구감초 18β-24-Hydroxyglycyrrhetinic acid
➡ HSD11B2 inhibitor
➡ cortisol 분해 억제
➡ mineralocorticoid receptors 자극 지속
➡ Na+/ K+ pumps 전사 촉진

마황세신부자탕 (麻黃細辛附子湯)

원문 少陰病，始 得 之，反 發熱，脈 沉 者, 麻黃細辛附子湯 主之。

원문 해설 항체매개 독성병은 원래 수족냉증이 생기는데, 반대로 발열하고 맥이 가라앉아 있으면 마황부자세신탕을 쓴다.

적응증 Early autoimmune response in erythrocyte

병태 & 증상

Early autoimmune response in erythrocyte

➡ erythrocyte: C3b coated immune complex 부착
➡ natural killer cell FcR III: erythrocyte 부착
➡ natural killer cell: IFN-γ 분비
➡ neutrophil 유도
➡ neutrophil: IL-12

➡ natural killer cell: 활성화
➡ natural killer cell: IFN-γ 분비 촉진: fever
➡ erythrocyte 손상
➡ erythrocyte hemoglobin: Met hemoglobin 전환

처방 목표 neutrophil: IL-12 분비 억제 / natural killer cell: secretion 억제 / Met hemoglobin 환원

처방 구성 麻黄 二兩 / 細辛 二兩 / 炮附子 一枚

처방 약리

포부자 aconitine
➡ 약리추측: neutrophil` Voltage-gated proton channels blocker
(식균작용에 의해 증가된 세포내 proton을 세포외로 방출시키는 채널)
➡ Voltage-gated proton channels 차단
➡ 호중구내 수소이온 축적
➡ neutrophil 대사 억제
➡ IL-12 분비 억제

마황 ephedrine ➡ Epinephrine receptors agonist
➡ adenylate cyclase 활성화
➡ cAMP ↑
➡ NKc secretion 억제

세신 eugenol ➡ Met-hemoglobin reducer

마황승마탕 (麻黃升麻湯)

원문 傷寒 六 七 日, 大 下 後, 寸 脈 沉 而 遲, 手足 厥逆, 下 部 脈 不 至, 喉 咽 不 利, 唾 膿 血, 泄利 不 止 者, 為 難 治, 麻黃升麻湯 主之。

원문 해설 세포병변성 감염증으로 6~7일 동안 크게 앓고 나은 뒤에, 촌맥이 가라앉고 느리며 손발이 몹시 차갑고, 척맥이 잡히지 않으며 인후가 불편하고 침에 농혈이 섞여 있으며, 설사가 그치지 않는 경우는 치료하기 힘들며 마황승마탕을 쓴다.

적응증 Infectious mononucleosis (전염성 단핵구증)

병태 & 증상

Infectious mononucleosis

➡ lymphatic tissue: EBV infected latent B cell
➡ EBV infected latent B cell: adenovirus combination
➡ EBV infected latent B cell: transformation
➡ EBV infected latent B cell: p53 phoshorylation 억제 ▶ cell cycle 지속
& Bcl-2 activation ▶ apoptosis 억제
➡ EBV infected latent B cell: uncontrolled proliferation
➡ EBV infected latent B cell: IL-12 분비
➡ natural killer cell 유도
➡ natural killer cell: IFN-γ 분비
➡ EBV infected latent B cell: MHC class II 발현 촉진
➡ cytotoxic T cell 유도
➡ EBV infected latent B cell: cell lysis ▶ sore throat, swollen lymph node
➡ EBV virion & naked DNA: blood transmission
➡ tissue 이동
➡ EBV gp350: tissue epithelium CR2 부착
➡ tissue epithelium: EBV endocytosis
➡ EBV replication: cell lysis
▶ ulcerative colitis (diarrhea) / pneumonitis / uveitis
/ pericarditis / hepatitis. etc

➡ cytotoxic T cell: hyperplasia
➡ hemophagocytic lymphohistiocytosis
▶ pancytopenia / thrombocytopenia / neutropenia
➡ phagocytosis: extracellular peroxynitrite ($ONOO^-$) ↑
➡ peroxynitrite: 혈관내피 VCAM-1 발현
➡ leukocyte 침윤
➡ vasculitis (thrombus formation)
➡ tissue ischemia: lactate ↑ & superoxide ↑ & Na+/ K+ pumps ↓
▶ cold hands & feet
➡ tissue necrosis

처방 목표 p53 phoshorylation 촉진 / Bcl-2 억제 / natural killer cell: IFN-γ 분비 억제 /

cytotoxic T cell apoptosis 유도 / tissue epithelium CR2 차단 / pancytopenia 개선 / neutropenia 개선 / extracellular peroxynitrite ($ONOO^-$) 제거 / VCAM-1 차단 / thrombus 제거 / lactate ↑ & superoxide ↑ & Na+/ K+ pumps ↓ 교정 / tissue 분화 & 재생

처방 구성 麻黃 二兩半 / 升麻 一兩 一分 / 當歸 一兩 一分 / 知母 十八銖 / 黃芩 十八銖 / 萎蕤 十八銖 (一作 菖蒲) / 芍藥 六銖 / 天門冬 六銖 / 桂枝 六銖 / 茯苓 六銖 / 炙甘草 六銖 / 石膏 六銖 / 白朮 六銖 / 乾薑 六銖

처방 약리

승마 cimigenol, 약리 추측 ➡ p53 phoshorylation activator

천문동 smilagenin, 약리 추측 ➡ Bcl-2 (-) modulator

마황 ephedrine ➡ Epinephrine receptors agonist
➡ adenylate cyclase 활성화
➡ cAMP ↑
➡ Natural killer cell: degranulation & secretion 억제

석고 $CaSO_4$ ➡ calcium mediated T-cell apoptosis 유도

위유 (둥글레): convallamarin, 약리 추측 ➡ CR2 blocker

당귀 decurcin ➡ erythrocyte protein kinase C inhibitor
➡ adducin-spectrin-actin complex 유지시킴
➡ erythrocyte 수명 연장

건강 shogaol ➡ neutrophil H_2O_2 scavenger
➡ neutrophil 수명 연장

황금 baicalin ➡ peroxynitrite ($ONOO^-$) scavenger

백출 atractylon ➡ vascular cell adhesion molecule-1 (VCAM-1) blocker

복령 pachymic acid ➡ glycoprotein IIb/IIIa (gpIIb/IIIa) (-) modulator
➡ thrombus formation 억제

계지 cinnamic acid ➡ lactate oxidizer
➡ Cori cycle: pyruvate 전환 촉진

작약 paeoniflorin -> superoxide scavenger

구감초 18β-24-Hydroxyglycyrrhetinic acid
➡ HSD11B2 inhibitor
➡ cortisol 분해 억제
➡ mineralocorticoid receptors 자극 지속
➡ Na+/ K+ pumps 전사 촉진

지모 timosaponin ➡ nestin (+) modulator
➡ multi-differentiation 세포에서 발현되는 단백질
➡ 조직특수성 분화 유도

마황연교적소두탕 (麻黃連軺赤小豆湯)

원문 傷寒 瘀 熱 在 裡, 身 必 黃, 麻黃連軺赤小豆湯 主之。

원문 해설 세포병변성 감염증에서 체열이 지속되면 반드시 황달이 생긴다. 마황연교적소두탕을 쓴다.

적응증 Warm autoantibody-mediated hemolytic anemia (온난자가항체-매개 용혈성빈혈)

병태 & 증상

Warm autoantibody-mediated hemolytic anemia

➡ bone marrow B-cell: Epstein-Barr virus infection
➡ Myeloid DCs: IL-12 분비
➡ natural killer cell 유도
➡ natural killer cell: IFN-γ 분비
➡ B-cell proliferation
➡ NKc-generated hydroxyl radical 유출
➡ B-cell: mutation

➡ B-cell: malignant proliferation
➡ B-cell lymphoproliferative disorders
➡ bone marrow: acidity ↓ ▶ bone marrow injury
➡ B-cell CD20: antigen binding
➡ warm & cold autoantibody 분비
➡ erythrocyte FcR: warm autoantibody (IgG) 부착
➡ IgG coated erythrocyte: macrophage phagocytosis
➡ hemolysis ↑ : jaundice

처방 목표 natural killer cell: degranulation 억제 / NKc-generated hydroxyl radical 제거 / B-cell: malignant proliferation 억제 / bone marrow: acidity 교정 / B-cell CD20 차단 / IgG Fc region 차단

처방 구성 麻黃 二兩 / 連軺 二兩 / 杏仁 四十個 / 赤小豆 一升 / 大棗 十二枚 生梓白皮 一升 / 生薑 二兩 / 炙甘草 二兩

처방 약리

마황 ephedrine ➡ Epinephrine receptors agonist
➡ adenylate cyclase 활성화
➡ cAMP ↑
➡ Natural killer cell: degranulation 억제

행인 benzoic acid ➡ hydroxyl radical scavenger

생재백피 β-lapachone ➡ AMPK phosphorylation activator
➡ AKT/mTOR pathway inhibition
➡ B-cell: malignant proliferation 억제

대조 cAMP ➡ AMPK (+) modulator
➡ B-cell: malignant proliferation 억제

생강 gingerol ➡ hydrogen peroxide scavenger
➡ calmodulin 활성화
➡ AMPK 활성화
➡ B-cell: malignant proliferation 억제

구감초 18β-24-Hydroxyglycyrrhetinic acid

➡ 11-beta-hydroxysteroid dehydrogenase2 (HSD11B2) inhibitor
➡ aldosterone 생리작용과 동일
➡ H+ secretion
➡ acidity 교정

연교 forsythiaside, 약리 추측 ➡ B-cell CD20 blocker

적소두 (팥) albumin, 약리추측 ➡ immunoglobulin Fc region binder
➡ IgG Fc region: erythrocyte FcR 부착 억제

마황탕 (麻黃湯)

원문 太陽病, 頭痛, 發熱, 身疼, 腰痛, 骨節 疼痛, 惡風, 無汗 而 喘 者, 麻黃湯 主之 。

원문 해설 림프절 감염증으로 두통, 발열, 동통, 요통, 관절통이 있으며 추위를 타고 땀은 없으면서 숨이 찬 경우에는 마황탕을 쓴다.

적응증 heat shock protein & IFN-a resistant viral infection

병태 & 증상

Virus infection

➡ lymph node immune cell: virus infection
➡ lymph node immune cell: virus infection ➡ IL-1 분비 ➡ 발열 유도
➡ lymph node immune cell: heat shock protein 활성화 ▶ virus replication 억제
➡ heat shock protein & IFN-a: 회피 바이러스인 경우
➡ IL-1 지속
➡ B cell proliferation
➡ 중화 항체 최고조 ▶ virus activity
➡ virus infected cell: antibody 부착
➡ mature Natural killer cell 유도
➡ mature Natural killer cell: secretion & degranulation
➡ TRAIL / granule / TNF-α : headache / fever / coldness / no sweating / dry cough

➡ antibody coated virus infected cell: TRAIL & FAS & granule 작동

▶ 당대사 급격한 증가

▶ lactate ↑

▶ mitochondria ROS ↑

▶ mitochondria dysfunction

▶ apoptosis

➡ lactatemia: ache / back pain / arthralgia

➡ NKc-generated hydroxyl radical 유출

➡ tissue damage

처방 목표 mature Natural killer cell: degranulation & secretion 억제 / lactatemia 교정 / hydroxyl radical 제거

처방 구성 麻黃 三兩 / 桂枝 二兩 / 炙甘草 一兩 / 杏仁 七十個

처방 약리

마황 ephedrine ➡ Epinephrine receptors agonist

➡ adenylate cyclase 활성화

➡ cAMP ↑

➡ Natural killer cell: degranulation & secretion 억제

계지 cinnamic acid ➡ lactate oxidizer

➡ Cori cycle: lactate 대사 촉진

➡ lactatemia 개선

구감초 18β-24-Hydroxyglycyrrhetinic acid

➡ 11-beta-hydroxysteroid dehydrogenase2 (HSD11B2) inhibitor

➡ aldosterone 작용 동일

➡ H+ secretion

➡ lactatemia 개선

행인 benzoic acid ➡ hydroxyl radical scavenger

마황행인감초석고탕 (麻黃杏仁甘草石膏湯)

원문 發汗 後, 不可 更行 桂枝湯, 汗出 而 喘, 無大熱 者, 可與 麻黃杏仁甘草石膏湯.

원문 해설 IL-1 매개 감염증(발한) 후에는 계지탕을 다시 쓰지 않으며, 땀나면서 숨이 가쁘고 큰열이 없는 경우에는 마황행인감초석고탕을 쓴다.

적응증 Asthma (천식)

병태 & 증상

Asthma

➡ bronchial endothelium: allergen attack
➡ dendritic cell: antigen 제시
➡ immature T cell: antigen 전달 받음
➡ immature T cell: T-helper type 2 (Th2) cells 분화
➡ Th2 cells: chemokine 분비: sweating
➡ eosinophil 유도
➡ eosinophil granule 활성화
: degranulation & eosinophil peroxidase (EPO) 활성화
➡ EPO generated hydroxyl radical 생성
➡ extracellular matrix: hydroxyl radical 유출
➡ bronchial endothelium: Na+/ K+ pumps 손상
➡ bronchitis

처방 목표 T-helper type 2 cells apoptosis 유도 / eosinophil degranulation 억제 / extracellular matrix: hydroxyl radical 제거 / bronchial endothelium: Na+/ K+ pumps 활성화

처방 구성 麻黃 四兩 / 杏仁 五十個 / 炙甘草 二兩 / 石膏 半斤

처방 약리

석고 $CaSO_4$ ➡ calcium mediated T cell apoptosis 유도

마황 ephedrine ➡ Epinephrine receptors agonist
➡ adenylate cyclase 활성화

➡ cAMP ↑
➡ eosinophil degranulation 억제됨

행인 benzoic acid ➡ hydroxyl radical scavenger

구감초 18β-24-Hydroxyglycyrrhetinic acid ➡ HSD11B2 inhibitor
➡ cortisol 분해 억제
➡ mineralocorticoid receptors 자극 지속
➡ aldosterone 작용 동일
➡ Na+/ K+ pumps 활성화

마황행인의이감초탕 (痲黃杏仁薏苡甘草湯)

원문 病 者 一身 盡 疼, 發熱 , 日晡 所 劇 者 , 名 風濕 。此病 傷 於 汗出 當 風 , 或 久傷 取 冷 所 致 也, 可 與 痲黃杏仁薏苡甘草湯 。

원문 해설 환자의 온몸이 다 쑤시고 발열하며, 해질 무렵에 통증이 심해지는 것을 풍습이라 부른다. 이것은 땀이 난 뒤(감염병을 앓은 후) 풍을 받아 (항체매개 독성) 생기거나, 감염부위가 차갑게 노출되어 생기며, 마황행인의이감초탕을 쓴다.

적응증 Reactive arthritis (반응성 관절염)

병태 & 증상

Reactive arthritis

➡ genital, urinary, gastrointestinal tract: bacterial infection
➡ Chlamydia trachomotis / Ureaoplasma urealyticum / Salmonella spp / Shigella spp / Yersinia spp / Campylobacter spp
➡ bacteria antibody 출현
➡ joint synoviocyte: HLA-B27 (MHC class I allele) 발현
➡ molecular mimic response
➡ HLA-B27: bacteria antibody 부착
➡ antibody-dependent cellular cytotoxicity
➡ Natural killer cell (NKc) 유도

➡ NKc: TRAIL-dependent secretion

➡ antibody coated synoviocyte: TRAIL 작동

▶ 당대사 급격한 증가

▶ mitochondria ROS ↑

▶ mitochondria dysfunction

▶ synovitis

➡ NKc-generated hydroxyl radical 유출

➡ synoviocyte: Na+/ K+ pumps 손상

➡ synovitis

처방 목표 joint synoviocyte: HLA-B27 (MHC class I allele) 발현 억제 / NKc secretion 억제 / hydroxyl radical 제거 / synoviocyte: Na+/ K+ pumps 활성화

처방 구성 麻黃 半兩 / 炙甘草 一兩 / 薏苡仁 半兩 / 杏仁 十個

처방 약리

의이인 stigmasterol, 약리 추측 ➡ MHC class I molecule (-) modulator

마황 ephedrine ➡ Epinephrine receptors agonist

➡ adenylate cyclase 활성화

➡ cAMP ↑

➡ Natural killer cell: secretion 억제

행인 benzoic acid ➡ hydroxyl radical scavenger

구감초 18β-24-Hydroxyglycyrrhetinic acid

➡ 11-beta-hydroxysteroid dehydrogenase2 (HSD11B2) inhibitor

➡ aldosterone 작용 동일

➡ Na+/ K+ pumps 전사 촉진

맥문동탕 (麥門冬湯)

원문 大逆 上氣， 咽喉 不利， 止逆 下氣 者, 麥門冬湯 主之。

원문 해설 숨이 넘어갈 정도로 심한 기침을 하고 목구멍이 아프고 기침이 멈추면 몸이 처지는 경우에는 맥문동탕을 쓴다.

적응증 Pulmonary tuberculosis (폐결핵)

병태 & 증상

Pulmonary tuberculosis

➡ lung macrophage: M. tuberculosis ➡ persistent infection
➡ starvation & low oxygen pressure
➡ M. tuberculosis: thehalose dimycolate 합성
➡ macrophage: focal adhesion kinase 활성화
➡ macrophage fusion 형성
➡ blood macrophage 유도됨
➡ macrophage fusion 증가
➡ granuloma formation
➡ M. tuberculosis: SigF overexpression
➡ M. tuberculosis: intracellular growth
➡ M. tuberculosis: hydrolytic enzyme 분비
➡ macrophage necrosis
➡ cavity formation
➡ 심한 기침이 유발되고 몸 밖으로 M. tuberculosis 전파됨

처방 목표 macrophage 대사 & 이동 억제시킴 / M. tuberculosis growth 억제시킴 / cavity 복구시킴

처방 구성 麥門冬 七升 / 半夏 一升 / 人參 三兩 / 甘草 二兩 / 粳米 三合 / 大棗 十二枚

처방 약리

감초 glycyrrhetinic acid ➡ HSD11B1 inhibitor
➡ cortisol 분해 억제

➡ glucocorticoid receptors 자극 지속
➡ IκBα 생성
➡ NF-κB 억제
➡ macrophage 대사 & 이동에 필요한 cytokine 생성 억제

맥문동 ophiopogonin, 약리 추측 ➡ M. tuberculosis` SigF transcription inhibitor
➡ M. tuberculosis growth 억제됨

인삼 panax ginsenoside
➡ Transforming growth factor β (TGF-β) (+) modulator
➡ cell proliferation 촉진

반하 triterpenoid (C30H48O7S)
➡ Rho GTPase family transcription promotor
➡ focal adhesion 생성
➡ 상피세포 이동 촉진

경미 magnesium ➡ DNA replication cofactor

대조 c-AMP ➡ protein kinase A avtivator
➡ ATP 생산 촉진
➡ cell cycle

모려택사탕 (牡蠣澤瀉散)

원문 大 病 差 後, 從 腰以下 有 水氣 者 , 牡蠣澤瀉散 主之 。

원문 해설 큰병을 앓은 후에, 허리 아래로 부종이 있는 경우에는 모려택사탕을 쓴다.

적응증 Lymphatic filariasis (림프사상충증)

병태 & 증상

Lymphatic filariasis

➡ severe disease
➡ malnutrition
➡ protein breakdown
➡ antibody 감소
➡ filarial parasite infection: Brugia malayi, Wuchereria bancrofti, Brugia timori
➡ adult filaria: microfilaria 생산
➡ adult filaria: collagen encoding gene 발현
▶ collagen synthesis
▶ sheath 생성
➡ sheathed microfilaria 출현
➡ 이동: lymphatic vessels
➡ lymphatic vessels: obstruction
➡ tissue: accumulation of protein-rich fluid ▶ edema
➡ fibroblast 활성화: collagen 분비
➡ fibrosclerosis
➡ edema tissue: water accumulation
➡ hyponatremia
➡ 세포외액이 세포내부로 이동
➡ lymphedema ↑

처방 목표 adult filaria: collagen synthesis 억제 / fibroblast: collagen 분비 억제 / hyponatremia 교정 / lymphedema 교정

처방 구성 牡蠣 / 澤瀉 / 蜀漆 / 葶藶子 / 商陸根 / 海藻 / 栝蔞根 各 等分

처방 약리

촉칠 halofuginone ➡ ring-collagen synthesis inhibitor

과루근 trichosanthin ➡ Ribosome inactivating protein
➡ collagen synthesis 억제

모려 NaCl ➡ saline solution
➡ hyponatremia 교정

택사 alisol ➡ Angiotensin II receptor blocker
➡ lymphedema 교정

해조 (바닷말): mannitol ➡ 삼투성 이뇨제
➡ lymphedema 교정

정력자 helveticoside ➡ Cardiac glycoside
➡ 정맥 배액 촉진

상륙근 KNO3 ➡ Potassium supplements
➡ 세포내 수분 교정

목방기탕 (木防己湯)

원문 膈間 支飮，其人 喘 滿，心下 痞堅，面色 黧黑，其脈 沉 緊，得 之 數 十 日，醫 吐 下 之 不 愈，木防己湯 主之。

원문 해설 흉막에 수분 축적이 있어서 호흡곤란과 뻐근함을 느끼며, 심장부위가 저리고 단단하며, 얼굴이 얼룩덜룩하고, 맥이 가라앉고 팽팽하다, 병이 생긴 지 수십 일이 지난 뒤, 최토법이나 사하법으로 낫지 않을 경우에는 목방기탕을 쓴다.

적응증 left heart failure-mediated pulmonary venous congestion
좌심부전-매개 폐정맥 울혈)

병태 & 증상

Pulmonary venous congestion

➡ myocardial infarction
➡ left heart failure
➡ ischemic cardiomyopathy
➡ 불완전경색
➡ myocardiocyte: lactate ↑
➡ myocardiocyte damage: 간질세포로 전환
➡ 좌심실근 수축력 저하
➡ 만성 좌심부전
➡ 좌심방: out flow ↓
➡ pulmonary venous congestion
➡ pulmonary capillary congestion: dyspnea, cyanosis of face
➡ 림프관 배액

처방 목표 myocardiocyte: lactate 교정 / myocardiocyte 재생: 심근수축력 회복 / 폐정맥 울혈 해소 / 림프관 배액 촉진

처방 구성 木防己 三兩 / 石膏 十二枚 雞子大 / 桂枝 三兩 / 人參 四兩

처방 약리

계지 cinnamic acid ➡ lactate oxidizer
➡ pyruvate 전환 촉진

인삼 panax ginsenoside
➡ Transforming growth factor β (TGF-β) (+) modulator
➡ cell proliferation 촉진
➡ myocardiocyte 재생

방기 sinomenine ➡ prostaglandin I2 (+) modulator in venous endothelium
➡ venous vasodilation
➡ 폐정맥 울혈 감소

석고 $CaSO_4$ ➡ calcium-mediated T cell apoptosis
➡ lymph node: mature T cell apoptosis
➡ 림프관 배액을 위한 공간 확보됨

목방기탕거석고가복령망초탕 (木防己湯去石膏加茯苓芒硝湯)

원문 膈間 支飮, 其人 喘 滿, 心下 痞堅, 面色 黧黑, 其脈 沉 緊, 得 之 數 十 日, 醫 吐 下 之 不 愈, 木防己湯 主之。虛 者 即 愈, 實 者 三日 復發, 復 與 不 愈 者, 宜 木防己湯去石膏加茯苓芒硝湯 主之。

원문 해설 흉막에 수분 축적이 있어서 호흡곤란과 뻐근함을 느끼며, 심장부위가 저리고 단단하며, 얼굴이 얼룩덜룩하고, 맥이 가라앉고 팽팽하다, 병이 생긴 지 수십 일이 지난 뒤, 최토법이나 사하법으로 낫지 않을 경우에는 목방기탕을 쓴다. 만성 좌심부전인 경우는 낫고, 좌심실근 기능이 급격히 나빠져 3일 만에 재발 한 후 목방기탕으로 낫지 않는 경우에는 목방기탕거석고가복령망초탕을 쓴다.

적응증 Left heart failure-mediated pleural effusion (좌심부전-매개 흉막삼출)

pleural effusion (흉막 삼출)

➡ myocardial infarction
➡ left heart failure
➡ ischemic cardiomyopathy
➡ 불완전경색
➡ myocardiocyte: lactate ↑
➡ myocardiocyte damage: 간질세포로 전환
➡ 좌심실근 수축력 저하
➡ 좌심실: out flow ↓
➡ 좌심실 심첨부: thrombus formation
➡ pulmonary venous congestion
➡ pulmonary capillary congestion: dyspnea, cyanosis of face
➡ pulmonary capillary pressure 25mmHg ↑
➡ 흉막벽쪽 모세혈관으로 배액
➡ 흉막에 물 고임

처방 목표 myocardiocyte: lactate 교정 / myocardiocyte 재생: 심근수축력 회복 / thrombus 억제 / 폐정맥 울혈 해소 / 흉막 림프관 배액 촉진

처방 구성 木防已 二兩 / 桂枝 二兩 / 人參 四兩 / 芒硝 三合 / 茯苓 四兩

처방 약리

계지 cinnamic acid ➡ lactate oxidizer
➡ Cori cycle: pyruvate 전환 촉진

인삼 panax ginsenoside
➡ Transforming growth factor β (TGF-β) (+) modulator
➡ cell proliferation 촉진
➡ myocardiocyte 재생

복령 pachymic acid ➡ glycoprotein IIb/IIIa (gpIIb/IIIa) (-) modulator
➡ thrombus formation 억제

방기 sinomenine ➡ prostaglandin I2 (+) modulator in venous endothelium
➡ venous vasodilation
➡ 폐정맥 울혈 감소

망초 Sodium Sulfate ➡ Intraluminal distention pressure 상승시킴
➡ 삼투압성 수분 배출 촉진
➡ 흉막 림프관 배액 촉진

문합산 (文蛤散)

원문 渴欲飮水不止者，文蛤散主之，文蛤五兩，杵為散，以沸湯五合，和服方寸匕。

원문 해설 갈증이 나서 물을 마시지만, 갈증이 해소되지 않는 경우에는 문합산을 쓴다. 문합 5량 (187.5g)을 찧어서 가루로 만든 뒤, 끓는 물 900ml에 담갔다가 꺼내어 작은 숟가락으로 먹는다.

적응증 Isonatremic dehydration (등장성 탈수)

병태 & 증상

Isonatremic dehydration

➡ 심한 발한 & 구토 & 설사
➡ 체액 소실
➡ 맹물 (저장성용액) 섭취
➡ 탈수가 교정되기 전에 혈장 Na 농도가 정상화 됨 (135-145 mEq/L)
➡ 등장성 탈수: thirst
➡ 계속 맹물을 마시면 저나트륨혈증 발생

처방 목표 Na 공급 (수액요법: 0.9% saline)

처방 구성 文蛤 五兩

처방 약리

문합 (대합조개): 염분농도가 약간 낮은 내만의 모래바닥에서 서식
➡ NaCl 보충

문합탕 (文蛤湯)

원문 吐 後 `渴 欲 得水 而 貪飲 者, 文蛤湯 主之, 兼 主 微風 `脈緊 `頭痛。
七味, 以 水 六升, 煮 取 二升, 溫服 一升, 汗出 即 愈。

원문 해설 토한 후에 갈증이 나서 물을 마셔도 계속 해서 물을 찾게 되는 경우에는 문합탕을 쓴다. 갈증과 겸해 약간 춥고 맥이 굵으며 머리 아픈 것도 치료한다.

적응증 Chronic obstructive pulmonary disease (COPD)-mediated hyponatremia
(만성폐쇄성 폐질환-매개 저나트륨혈증)

병태 & 증상

COPD-mediated hyponatremia

➡ smoking / noxious particles & gas
➡ large airway: bronchitis
➡ highly susceptible to viral infection
➡ large airway brochial epithelium: virus infection 반복
➡ virus infected epithelium: IFN-a 분비 지속
➡ natural killer cell 유도
➡ natural killer cell: IFN-γ 분비 ▶ chills, headache
➡ Th1 cell 유도: IFN-γ, IL-2 분비
➡ macrophage 유도
➡ macrophage: 대사 촉진 ▶ endoplasmic reticulum calcium efflux ↑
▶ hydrogen peroxide ↑ ▶ NF-κB 활성화
▶ inflammatory gene expression
➡ chronic bronchitis
➡ NKc-generated hydroxyl radical 유출
➡ chronic bronchitis
➡ goblet cell & mucous gland: hyperplasia
➡ large airway: chronic obstruction
➡ respiration volume ↓
➡ 동맥혈 PaO2 ↓
➡ renin-angiotensin-aldosterone system 활성화
➡ arginine vasopressin (AVP)
➡ hypervolemic hyponatremia (보통, Na 125-135 mEq/L): vomitting

처방 목표 natural killer cell: IFN-γ 분비 억제 / Th1 cell apoptosis 유도 / macrophage: endoplasmic reticulum calcium efflux 억제 / macrophage ▶ hydrogen peroxide 제거 / macrophage ▶ NF-κB 억제 / Na 공급 (수액요법: 0.9% saline)

처방 구성 文蛤 五兩 / 麻黃 三兩 / 甘草 三兩 / 生薑 三兩 / 石膏 五兩 / 杏仁 五十枚 / 大棗 十二枚

처방 약리

마황 ephedrine ➡ Epinephrine receptors agonist
➡ adenylate cyclase 활성화
➡ cAMP ↑
➡ NKc secretion 억제

석고 $CaSO_4$ ➡ calcium mediated Th cell apoptosis 유도

대조 cAMP ➡ macrophage: Inhibition of granular organelles phosphorylation
➡ endoplasmic reticulum: calcium efflux 억제

생강 gingerol ➡ hydrogen peroxide scavenger

감초 glycyrrhetinic acid
➡ 11-beta-hydroxysteroid dehydrogenase1 (HSD11B1) inhibitor
➡ glucocorticoid 작용
➡ IκBα 생성
➡ NF-κB 억제

문합 (대합조개): 염분농도가 약간 낮은 내만의 모래바닥에서 서식
➡ NaCl 보충

반석탕 (礬石湯)

원문 礬石湯, 治 脚氣 衝心

원문 해설 반석탕은 다리에 힘이 빠지는 것과, 심근독성병을 치료한다.

적응증 Beriberi (각기병)

병태 & 증상

Beriberi

➡ Thiamine (Vit B1) 결핍
➡ Thiamine pyrophosphate 감소
➡ pyruvate dehydrogenase complex ↓
& α-ketoglutarate dehydrogenase complex ↓
➡ pyruvate: mitochondria entry 실패
➡ lactate 축적
➡ ATP ↓
➡ Na+/ K+ pumps 약화
➡ Na+세포내 유입
➡ H2O 유입
➡ 세포 부종
➡ Thiamine 결핍에 민감한 세포
➡ 심근: 심근 부종 ▶ 심부전
& 말초신경: 신경세포 부종 ▶ 근위축

처방 목표 심근세포 & 말초신경 세포내 수분 제거

처방 구성 礬石 二兩

처방 약리

반석 $KAl(SO_4)_2 \cdot 12H_2O$ (aluminium potassium sulfate = Alum)
➡ astringent (수렴제)
➡ 세포내 수분 수렴

반석환 (礬石丸)

원문 婦人 經水閉 不利，臟 堅癖 不止，中 有 乾血，下 白物，礬石丸 主之 。

원문 해설 생리가 나오지 않거나 불순하며, 딱딱한 덩어리가 없어지지 않는 것은, 자궁내막에

마른 혈종이 있는 것으로서 흰색 질 분비물이 나오게 되며 반석환을 쓴다.

적응증 Endometrium grandular polyp (자궁내막 용종)

병태 & 증상

Endometrium grandular polyp

➡ menstrual cycle & early prognancy

➡ mid-secretory phase & embryonic development

➡ endometrium glandular epithelium: superoxide ↑

➡ SOD 고갈: hydrogen peroxide ↑

➡ hydrogen peroxide + copper

➡ hydroxyl radical 생성

➡ endometrium glandular epithelium

▶ p53 gene: mutation ▶ apoptosis 억제

➡ endometrium glandular epithelium: hyperplasia

➡ secretion ↑ ▶ superficial edema: vaginal dischage

처방 목표 hydroxyl radical 제거 / superficial edema 제거

처방 구성 礬石 三分 / 杏仁 一分

처방 약리

반석 KAl(SO4)2·12H2O (aluminium potassium sulfate = Alum)

➡ astringent (수렴제)

행인 benzoic acid ➡ hydroxyl radical scavenger

반하건강산 (半夏乾薑散)

원문 乾嘔, 吐逆, 吐 涎 沫, 半夏乾薑散 主之。

원문 해설 구역기가 있고 음식물을 토하려 하며 신물이 넘어 오면 반하건강산을 쓴다.

적응증 Cytomegalovirus esophagitis (사이토메가로바이러스 식도염)

병태 & 증상

Cytomegalovirus esophagitis

➡ esophageal mucosal cell: cytomegalovirus infection
➡ CMV specific antibody 출현
➡ Fc receptor: neutrophil 유도
➡ neutrophil phagocytosis
➡ HClO 분비 via H2O2
➡ mucosa cell: necrosis

처방 목표 HClO 분비 억제 / mucosa cell 세포상환 촉진

처방 구성 半夏 / 乾薑 等分

처방 약리

건강 shogaol ➡ neutrophil H2O2 scavenger
➡ HClO 분비 억제

반하 triterpenoid (C30H48O7S)
➡ Rho GTPase family transcription promotor
➡ focal adhesion 생성
➡ 상피세포 이동 촉진

반하마황환 (半夏麻黃丸)

원문 心 下 悸 者 , 半夏麻黃丸 主之 。

원문 해설 명치 밑이 떨리는 경우에는 반하마황환을 쓴다.

적응증 Eosinophilic gastroenteritis (호산구성 위장관염)

병태 & 증상

Eosinophilic gastroenteritis

➡ Food hypersensitivity
➡ gastrointestinal tract mucosa: eosinophil 침윤
➡ food specific IgE ↑
➡ eosinophil degranulation
➡ gastroenteritis

처방 목표 eosinophil degranulation 억제 / 위장관 점막상피 상환 촉진

처방 구성 半夏 / 麻黄 等分

처방 약리

마황 ephedrine ➡ Epinephrine receptors agonist
➡ adenylate cyclase 활성화
➡ cAMP ↑
➡ eosinophil degranulation 억제

반하 triterpenoid (C30H48O7S)
➡ Rho GTPase family transcription promotor
➡ focal adhesion 생성
➡ 상피세포 이동 촉진

반하사심탕 (半夏瀉心湯)

원문 傷寒 五 六 日 , 嘔 而 發熱 者 , 柴胡湯 證 具 , 而 以 他藥 下 之, 柴胡證 仍 在 者, 復 與 柴胡湯 。
此 雖 已 下 之 , 不為 逆 , 必 蒸 蒸 而 振, 卻 發熱 汗出 而 解 。
若 心下滿 而 硬痛 者 , 此 為 結胸 也 , 大陷胸湯 主之 。
, 但 滿 而 不痛 者 , 此為 痞 , 柴胡 不 中 與 之 , 宜 半夏瀉心湯 。

원문 해설 세포병변성 감염증이 5~6일 경과 된 후 구역하고 발열하면 시호탕을 쓰고, 사하제를 쓴 뒤에라도 시호증이 있으면 다시 시호탕을 쓴다. 사하제를 쓴 뒤 시호탕을 써

도 잘못된 방법은 아니다. 찌는 듯이 떨리는데 발열하고 땀나면 낫는다. 만약 명치 밑이 팽만하고 딴딴한 통증이 있으면 결흉이라 부르며 대함흉탕을 쓴다. 단지 팽만감과 속 쓰림만 있고 통증이 없다면 시호제가 아니라 반하사심탕을 쓴다.

적응증 Gastric ulcer (위궤양)

병태 & 증상

Gastric ulcer

➡ Helicobacter pylori in Stomach body & antrum
➡ Helicobacter pylori: 병원성 균으로 형질전환
➡ Helicobacter pylori: Cag pathogenicity island (Cag PAI) 유전자 활동
➡ H. pylori peptidoglycan: type IV secretion system 형성
➡ peptidoglycan: macrophage 유도
➡ extracellular peroxynitrite ($ONOO^-$)
➡ 상피세포 & 점막세포 손상
➡ mucin 분비 ↓ : heartburn
➡ Helicobacter pylori: CagE gene
➡ epithelial cell: IL-8 분비
➡ neutrophil 유도
➡ neutrophil phagocytosis
➡ HClO 분비 via H2O2
➡ 점막근층 손상
➡ Gastric ulcer

처방 목표 H. pylori: peptidoglycan 합성 억제 / extracellular $ONOO^-$ 제거 / 손상된 상피 & 점막세포가 정상 상피로 덮이도록 세포 상환 촉진 시킴 / 상피 & 점막세포 증식 촉진 / HClO 분비 억제 / 위산 분비 억제시킴

처방 구성 半夏 半升 / 黃芩 / 乾薑 / 人參 / 炙甘草 各 三兩 / 黃連 一兩 / 大棗 十二枚

처방 약리

황련 berberine ➡ sortase inhibitor
➡ H. pylori peptidoglycan 합성 억제
➡ 병독성 감소됨

황금 baicalin ➡ peroxynitrite ($ONOO^-$) scavenger

반하 triterpenoid (C30H48O7S)

➡ Rho GTPase family transcription promotor

➡ focal adhesion 생성

➡ 상피 & 점막세포 이동 촉진

인삼 panax ginsenoside

➡ Transforming growth factor beta (TGF-β) (+) modulator

➡ 상피 & 점막세포 증식 촉진

대조 c-AMP ➡ Protein kinase A avtivator

➡ ATP 생성 촉진

➡ cell cycle ↑

건강 shogaol ➡ neutrophil H_2O_2 scavenger

➡ HClO 분비 억제

구감초 18β-24-Hydroxyglycyrrhetinic acid

➡ 11-beta-hydroxysteroid dehydrogenase2 (HSD11B2) inhibitor

➡ aldosterone 생리작용과 동일

➡ H+ secretion

➡ 위산 분비 억제

반하산급탕 (半夏散及湯)

원문 少陰病，咽 中 痛, 半夏散及湯 主之。

원문 해설 항체매개 독성병으로 목구멍이 아픈 경우에는 반하산급탕을 쓴다.

적응증 Soft palate ulcer (연구개염)

병태 & 증상

Soft palate ulcer

➡ soft palate: coxsackie virus infection
(연구개: 음식물이 코로 역류하지 않도록 하는 목젖 부위의 림프성 근육조직)
➡ coxsackie virus: cytolytic virus
➡ muscular palate에서 증식 후 세포막 뚫고 나옴
➡ muscular palate: intracellular lactate ↑
➡ ATP ↓
➡ Na+/ K+ pumps 손상
➡ Soft palate ulcer: sore throat

처방 목표 연구개 상피 상환 촉진 / intracellular lactate 교정 / Na+/ K+ pumps 활성화

처방 구성 半夏 / 桂枝 / 炙甘草 等分

처방 약리

반하 triterpenoid (C30H48O7S)
➡ Rho GTPase family transcription promotor
➡ focal adhesion 생성
➡ 상피세포 이동 촉진

계지 cinnamic acid ➡ lactate oxidizer
➡ pyruvate 전환 촉진

구감초 18β-24-Hydroxyglycyrrhetinic acid
➡ HSD11B2 inhibitor
➡ cortisol 분해 억제
➡ mineralocorticoid receptors 자극 지속
➡ Na+/ K+ pumps 전사 촉진

반하후박탕 (半夏厚朴湯)

원문 婦人 咽中 如 有 炙臠 , 半夏厚朴湯 主之 。
作 胸滿 , 心 下 堅 , 咽中 帖 帖 , 如 有 炙肉 , 吐 之 不 出 , 吞 之 不 下 。

원문 해설 부인의 목구멍에 구운 고깃점이 있는 것 같은 경우에는 반하후박탕을 쓴다. 흉부가 그득하고 명치가 단단하며 목구멍이 촘촘하여 구운 고깃점이 걸려 있는 것 같고 토해서 빼내려 해도 나오지 않으며 삼켜도 내려가지 않는 증상에 쓴다.

적응증 Inferior pharyngeal stenosis in Behcet's Disease
(베체트 하인두 협착증)

병태 & 증상

Inferior pharyngeal stenosis in Behcet's Disease

➡ streptococcus infection
➡ streptococcus surface protein & 하인두 정맥 epithelium: molecular mimicry
➡ streptococcus surface protein: antibody 생성
➡ 하인두 정맥 epithelium: antibody 부착
➡ antibody-dependent cell-mediated cytotoxicity: macrophage 유도
➡ 하인두 정맥 epithelium: vasculitis
➡ thrombus formation
➡ vein occlusion
➡ angiogenesis
➡ 신생혈관 출혈
➡ inferior pharynx squamous cell: necrosis
➡ inferior pharyngeal stenosis: feeling of irritation

처방 목표 thrombus 제거 / angiogenesis 억제 / 편평세포 분열 촉진 / 편평세포 상환 촉진

처방 구성 半夏 一升 / 厚朴 三兩 / 茯苓 四兩 / 生薑 五兩 / 乾蘇葉 二兩

처방 약리

복령 pachymic acid ➡ glycoprotein IIb/IIIa (gpIIb/IIIa) (-) modulator
➡ thrombus formation 억제

후박 honokiol ➡ VEGF receptor blocker ➡ 혈관신생 억제

소엽 linoleic acid ➡ estrogen receptor alpha (ERα) agonist
➡ squamous cell division 촉진

반하 triterpenoid (C30H48O7S)

➡ Rho GTPase family transcription promotor
➡ focal adhesion 생성
➡ 편평세포 이동 촉진

생강 gingerol ➡ hydrogen peroxide scavenger
➡ focal adhesion kinase 활성화
➡ 편평세포의 입체적 이동 촉진

방기복령탕 (防己茯苓湯)

원문 皮水 為 病，四肢 腫，水氣 在 皮膚中，四肢 聶聶 動 者，防己茯苓湯 主之。

원문 해설 피부 속에 물이 고이는 병에 걸리면, 팔다리에 부종이 생기는데, 찰랑찰랑 움직이는 부종인 경우에는 방기복령탕을 쓴다.

적응증 Chronic right heart failure-mediated systemic congestion
(만성우심부전-매개 전신울혈)

병태 & 증상

Chronic right heart failure-mediated systemic congestion

➡ 우심실근 수축력 ↓ : lactate 축적
➡ 우심실: out flow ↓
➡ 우심실 심첨부: thrombus formation
➡ systemic venous congestion ↑
➡ capillary: physical damage
➡ capillaritis
➡ fibrin clot 형성
➡ fluid accumulation: edema under the skin
➡ monocyte infiltration
➡ skin inflammation

처방 목표 우심실근 lactate 교정 / thrombus 억제 / systemic venous congestion 해소 / fibrin clot 제거 / monocyte 대사 억제

처방 구성 防己 三兩 / 黃耆 三兩 / 桂枝 三兩 / 茯苓 六兩 / 甘草 二兩

처방 약리

계지 cinnamic acid ➡ lactate oxidizer
➡ pyruvate 전환
➡ intracellular lactate 교정

복령 pachymic acid ➡ glycoprotein IIb/IIIa (gpIIb/IIIa) (-) modulator
➡ thrombus formation 억제

방기 sinomenine ➡ prostaglandin I2 (+) modulator in venous endothelium
➡ venous vasodilation
➡ 정맥 울혈 감소

황기 astragaloside ➡ Tissue plasminogen activator (+) modulator
➡ fibrinolysis

감초 glycyrrhetinic acid
➡ 11-beta-hydroxysteroid dehydrogenase1 (HSD11B1) inhibitor
➡ glucocorticoid 작용
➡ IκBα 생성
➡ NF-κB 억제
➡ monocyte 대사 억제

방기지황탕 (防己地黃湯)

원문 防己地黃湯, 治 病 如 狂 狀 , 妄行 , 獨語 不 休 , 無 寒熱 , 其 脈 浮 。

원문 해설 방기황기탕은 미친 것 같은 증상을 치료한다. 안절부절하고 혼잣말을 계속 하며 오한과 발열 없이 맥이 뜬 경우에 쓴다.

적응증 Cerebral venous sinus thrombosis (뇌 정맥동 혈전증)

병태 & 증상

➡ 결체조직 질환, 혈액응고 장애, 감염
➡ cerebral venous sinus thrombosis
➡ focal ischemia
➡ 허혈 뇌세포: 세포질 lactate ↑
➡ 허혈 주변부 뇌세포: calcium influx ↑
▶ arachidonic acid 대사 증가
▶ cyclooxygenase-2 mediated prostaglandins 생성
➡ prostaglandin E2
➡ blood-brain barrier breakdown
➡ intraparenchymal: leukocyte infiltration
➡ intracranial pressure ↑: chaos consciousness

처방 구성 cerebral venous sinus 확장 / 허혈 뇌세포: 세포질 lactate 교정 / cyclooxygenase-2 억제 / blood-brain barrier 재생 / leukocyte infiltration 억제

처방 구성 防己 一錢 / 桂枝 三錢 / 防風 三錢 / 甘草 二錢 / 生地黃 二斤

처방 약리

방기 sinomenine ➡ prostaglandin I2 (+) modulator in venous endothelium
➡ venous vasodilation

계지 cinnamic acid ➡ lactate oxidizer
➡ pyruvate 전환

방풍 deltoin ➡ cyclooxygenase-2 blocker

생지황 catalpol, 약리추측
➡ CD133+ circulating endothelial cell progenitor (+) modulator
➡ vessel bud formation
➡ angiogenesis
➡ blood-brain barrier 재생

감초 glycyrrhetinic acid
➡ 11-beta-hydroxysteroid dehydrogenase1 (HSD11B1) inhibitor
➡ glucocorticoid 작용

➡ IκBα 생성
➡ NF-κB 억제
➡ leukocyte 이동 억제

방기황기탕 (防己黃耆湯)

원문 風濕, 脈 浮 身 重, 汗出 惡風 者, 防己黃耆湯 主之。

원문 해설 체액이 저류되고 맥이 뜨며 몸이 무거워지고, 땀이 나면서 추위를 타는 경우에는 방기황기탕을 쓴다.

적응증 Right heart failure-mediated venous congestion (우심부전-매개 정맥울혈)

병태 & 증상

Right heart failure-mediated venous congestion

➡ venous congestion: ankles / legs / abdomen / liver / lung / heart
➡ tissue hypoxia
➡ capillary endothelium: VCAM-1 발현
➡ monocyte adhesion
➡ monocyte ROS burst
➡ capillaritis: IL-8 ↑ ▶ sweating, coldness
➡ fibrin clot 형성

처방 목표 venous congestion 해소 / capillary endothelium: VCAM-1 차단 / monocyte ROS burst 억제 / fibrin clot 제거

처방 구성 防己 一兩 / 甘草 半兩 / 白朮 七錢半 / 黃耆 一兩 一分 / 生薑 四片 / 大棗 一枚 喘 者 加 麻黃 半兩 胃中 不和 者 加 芍藥 三分 氣上衝 者 加 桂枝 三分 下有 陳寒 者 加 細辛 三分

처방 약리

방기 sinomenine ➡ prostaglandin I2 (+) modulator in venous endothelium
➡ venous vasodilation
➡ 정맥 울혈 해소

백출 atractylon ➡ vascular cell adhesion molecule-1 (VCAM-1) blocker

감초 glycyrrhetinic acid
➡ 11-beta-hydroxysteroid dehydrogenase1 (HSD11B1) inhibitor
➡ glucocorticoid 작용
➡ IκBα 생성
➡ NF-κB 억제
➡ monocyte 대사 억제

황기 astragaloside ➡ Tissue plasminogen activator (+) modulator
➡ fibrinolysis

배농산 (排膿散)

원문 瘡癰 腸癰 浸淫病 脈證 并治

적응증 Impetigo (농가진)

병태 & 증상

Impetigo

➡ skin commensal bacteria
: staphylococcus aureus, streptococcus pyrogens
➡ skin injury
➡ staphylococcus aureus, streptococcus pyrogens: TCPs protein 분비
➡ skin endothelium: Myd88 protein blocking
➡ skin endothelium: toll like receptor signal 차단
➡ IL-1 / TNF-α ↓
➡ commensal bacteria ▶ pathogen bacteria 전환
➡ pathogen bacteria 대사 ↑: superoxide ↑
➡ matrix metalloproteinases (MMPs) 분비
➡ dermis matrix 분해
➡ dermis ulcer

처방 목표 TLR signal 활성화 / superoxide 제거 / matrix metalloproteinases 차단

처방 구성 枳實 十六枚 / 芍藥 六分 / 桔梗 二分

처방 약리

길경 platycodin ➡ toll like receptor (+) modulator

작약 paeoniflorin ➡ superoxide scavenger

지실auraptene ➡ matrix metalloproteinases (MMPs) blocker

배농탕 (排膿湯)

원문 瘡癰 腸癰 浸淫病 脈證 并治, 浸 淫 瘡 , 從 口 流 向 四肢 者 , 可 治 ; 從 四 肢 流 來 入口 者 , 不可 治

원문 해설 깊이 파고든 종기가 입에서 팔다리 쪽으로 퍼지면 치료가 가능하고 팔다리에서 입 쪽으로 퍼지면 치료가 불가능하다.

적응증 Erysipelas (단독)

병태 & 증상

Erysipelas

➡ skin dermis commensal bacteria: streptococcus pyrogens
➡ skin dermis injury
➡ streptococcus pyrogens: TCPs protein 분비
➡ skin endothelium: Myd88 protein blocking
➡ skin endothelium: toll like receptor signal 차단
➡ IL-1 / TNF-α ↓
➡ commensal bacteria ▶ pathogen bacteria 전환
➡ lymph node: necrosis
➡ bacteremia: tissue spreading
➡ macrophage TLR: streptococcus pyrogens 인식

➡ macrophage: Rac 1 활성화
➡ PI3K 활성화 via Calcium
➡ AKT protein 활성화 via low hydrogen peroxide
➡ NF-κB 활성화
➡ inflammatory response
➡ tissue inflammation

처방 목표 toll like receptor signal 활성화 / macrophage Calcium signal 차단 / macrophage hydrogen peroxide 제거 / macrophage NF-κB 억제

처방 구성 甘草 二兩 / 桔梗 三兩 / 生薑 一兩 / 大棗 十枚

처방 약리

길경 platycodin ➡ toll like receptor (+) modulator

대조 cAMP ➡ inhibition of granular organelles phosphorylation
➡ macrophage ` endoplasmic reticulum: calcium 분비 억제

생강 gingerol ➡ hydrogen peroxide scavenger

감초 glycyrrhetinic acid
➡ 11-beta-hydroxysteroid dehydrogenase1 (HSD11B1) inhibitor
➡ glucocorticoid 작용
➡ IκBα 생성
➡ NF-κB 억제

백두옹가감초아교탕 (白頭翁加甘草阿膠湯)

원문 產後 下利 虛 極, 白頭翁加甘草阿膠湯 主之 。

원문 해설 산후에 몸이 약해져서 설사를 심하게 하는 경우에는 백두옹가감초아교탕을 쓴다.

적응증 Postpartum Crohn's disease (산 후 크론병)

병태 & 증상

Postpartum Crohn's disease

➡ postpatum: Th2 cell-mediated immune response
➡ 체액성 면역력 ↓
➡ Mycobacterium, other pathogenic bacteria: 활성화
➡ unusual peptidoglycan 생성
➡ 상피세포 NOD2 gene mutation
(NOD2: nucleotide-binding oligomerization domain 2)
➡ Mycobacterium, other pathogenic bacteria: 면역반응 시작됨
➡ 상피세포 NF-kB pathway
➡ IL-32 발현
➡ microvascular에서 ICAM 발현
➡ macrophage 침착
➡ macrophage granuloma 형성
➡ TNF-α: fever
➡ 소장상피세포 & 술잔세포 & 근육층 & Mycobacterium, other pathogenic bacteria
: apoptosis
➡ granulomatous colitis
➡ 합병증: Mycobacterium, other pathogenic bacteria ▶ LPS-induced sepsis
& 장막층까지 macrophage 이동 ▶ 혈관손상

처방 목표 unusual peptidoglycan 생성 억제 / NOD2 gene mutation 억제 / 상피세포 NF-kB pathway 차단 / LPS-induced sepsis 억제 / 장막층까지 macrophage 이동 억제 / 근육 재생 촉진

처방 구성 白頭翁 二兩 / 甘草 二兩 / 阿膠 二兩 / 秦皮 三兩 / 黃連 三兩 / 柏皮 三兩

처방 약리

황련 berberine ➡ sortase inhibitor: peptidoglycan 합성 억제

진피 aesculetin ➡ NOD2 gene mutation inhibitor in Intestinal epithelial cells

백두옹 anemonin ➡ NF-kB blocker in Intestinal epithelial cells

황백 phellodendrine
➡ 약리 추측: Monocyte / Macrophage / Neutrophil 의 CD14 blocker

패혈증 ➡ 혈액내 Monocyte / Macrophage / Neutrophil CD14
➡ LPS 및 세균 항원 부착
➡ T cell 전달
➡ T cell 분화
➡ TNF-α 분비
➡ multi-organ failure

감초 glycyrrhetinic acid
➡ 11-beta-hydroxysteroid dehydrogenase1 (HSD11B1) inhibitor
➡ glucocorticoid 작용
➡ IκBα 생성
➡ NF-κB 억제
➡ macrophage 이동 억제됨

아교 Glycine / Proline / Hydroxyproline / Alanine
➡ collagen 주요 아미노산
➡ collagen 합성 촉진

백두옹탕 (白頭翁湯)

원문 熱利 下重 者, 下利 欲 飮水 者, 以 有熱 故 也, 白頭翁湯 主 之。

원문 해설 열이 있으면서 설사하고 설사해도 개운하지 않으며 갈증이 나서 물을 마시는 경우에는 백두옹탕을 쓴다.

적응증 Crohn's disease (크론병)

병태 & 증상

Crohn's disease

➡ small intestine epithelial cell
: Mycobacterium, other pathogenic bacteria 융합
➡ Mycobacterium, other pathogenic bacteria
: unusual peptidoglycan 생성

➡ 상피세포 NOD2 gene mutation
(NOD2: nucleotide-binding oligomerization domain 2)
➡ Mycobacterium, other pathogenic bacteria: 면역반응 시작됨
➡ 상피세포 NF-kB pathway
➡ IL-32 발현
➡ microvascular에서 ICAM 발현
➡ macrophage 침착
➡ macrophage granuloma 형성
➡ TNF-α: fever
➡ 소장상피세포 & 술잔세포 & 근육층 & Mycobacterium, other pathogenic bacteria
: apoptosis
(손상된 근육 재생 -> hydroxy group 소모 ➡ thirsty)
➡ granulomatous colitis
➡ 합병증: Mycobacterium, other pathogenic bacteria ▶ LPS-induced sepsis

처방 목표 unusual peptidoglycan 생성 억제 / NOD2 gene mutation 억제 / 상피세포 NF-kB pathway 차단 / LPS-induced sepsis 억제

처방 구성 白頭翁 二兩 / 黃蘗 三兩 / 黃連 三兩 / 秦皮 三兩

처방 약리

황련 berberine ➡ sortase inhibitor
➡ Mycobacterium, other pathogenic bacteria: peptidoglycan 합성 억제

진피 aesculetin ➡ NOD2 gene mutation inhibitor in Intestinal epithelial cells

백두옹 anemonin ➡ NF-kB blocker in Intestinal epithelial cells

황백 phellodendrine
➡ 약리 추측: Monocyte / Macrophage / Neutrophil 의 CD14 blocker

패혈증 ➡ 혈액내 Monocyte / Macrophage / Neutrophil CD14

➡ LPS 및 세균 항원 부착
➡ T cell 전달
➡ T cell 분화
➡ TNF-α 분비
➡ multi-organ failure

백엽탕 (柏葉湯)

원문 吐血 不止 者, 柏葉湯 主之。

원문 해설 토혈이 그치지 않는 경우에는 백엽탕을 쓴다.

적응증 Esophageal varices bleeding (식도정맥류 출혈)

병태 & 증상

Esophageal varices bleeding

➡ liver cirrhosis
➡ portal hypertension
➡ esophageal veins: congestion
➡ 식도 모세혈관 내피: 허혈
➡ 식도 모세혈관 내피: selectin 발현
➡ neutrophil 유도
➡ neutrophil phagocytosis
➡ HClO 분비 via H2O2
➡ esophageal varices bleeding: hematemesis

처방 목표 HClO 분비 억제 / 지혈

처방 구성 柏葉 三兩 / 乾薑 三兩 / 艾 三把

처방 약리

건강 shogaol ➡ neutrophil H2O2 scavenger
➡ HClO 분비 억제

백엽 tannin ➡ coagulant acid
➡ tannin hydroxyl group: 혈관 콜라겐의 아미노기와 결합
➡ 파열된 콜라겐층 고정화

애엽 cineol ➡ vasoconstriction

백출부자탕 (白朮附子湯)

원문 傷寒 八 九 日, 風濕 相搏, 身體 疼煩, 不能 自 轉側, 不嘔 不渴, 脈 浮 虛 而 澀 者, 桂枝附子湯 主之; 若 大便 堅, 小便 自利 者, 去桂加白朮湯 (白朮附子湯) 主之。

원문 해설 세포병변성 감염증이 8~9째 백혈구 공격으로 세포내부종이 발생하여 몸이 쑤시고 아프며 움직일 수 없게 된 경우, 구역과 갈증이 없으며 맥이 뜨면서 부족하고 막히는 맥상이면 계지부자탕으로 치료한다. 만약 대변이 굳고 소변이 저절로 나오면 거계가백출탕을 쓴다.

적응증 Myoglobin-mediated renal failure

병태 & 증상

Myoglobin-mediated renal failure

➡ myositis
➡ myoglobinemia
➡ renal tubular cell: myoglobin endocytosis
➡ MAP kinase 활성화 ▶ AP-1 & NF-κB ▶ tubular cell inflammation
& c-src kinase 활성화 ▶ VCAM-1 발현
➡ renal parenchyma: neutrophil 유도
➡ neutrophil: elastase 분비
➡ renal parenchyma: injury

처방 목표 renal tubular cell: myoglobin 분비시킴 / renal tubular cell: VCAM-1 차단 / neutrophil: elastase 분비 억제

처방 구성 白朮 二兩 / 炮附子 一枚半 / 炙甘草 一兩 / 生薑 一兩半 / 大棗 六枚

처방 약리

구감초 18β-24-Hydroxyglycyrrhetinic acid
➡ HSD11B2 inhibitor
➡ cortisol 분해 억제
➡ mineralocorticoid receptors 자극 지속
➡ Na+/ K+ pumps 전사 촉진

➡ renal tubular cell: myoglobin secretion 촉진

대조 cAMP ➡ intracellular cAMP level ↑
➡ renal tubular cell: myoglobin endocytosis 억제

생강 gingerol ➡ hydrogen peroxide scavenger
➡ renal tubular cell: myoglobin endocytosis 억제

백출 atractylon ➡ vascular cell adhesion molecule-1 (VCAM-1) blocker

포부자 aconitine
➡ 약리추측: neutrophil` Voltage-gated proton channels blocker
(식균작용에 의해 증가된 세포내 proton을 세포외로 방출시키는 채널)
➡ Voltage-gated proton channels 차단
➡ 호중구내 수소이온 축적
➡ neutrophil 대사 억제
➡ elastase 분비 억제

백통가저담즙탕 (白通加豬膽汁湯)

원문 少陰病，下利，脈微者，與白通湯。利不止，厥逆無脈，乾嘔煩者，白通加豬膽汁湯主之。服湯脈暴出者死，微續者生。

원문 해설 항체매개 감염증으로 설사하고 맥이 약한 경우에는 백통탕을 쓴다. 설사가 계속 되고 맥은 일체 잡히지 않으며 건구역질을 하고 괴로운 경우에는 백통가저담즙즙탕을 쓴다. 복용 후 맥이 갑자기 뛰면 죽고, 약하게 차차 살아나면 산다.

적응증 Henoch-Schonlein purpura associated colitis & paralytic ileus
(헤노호-쉐라인 자반증에 연관된 대장염 & 장마비)

병태 & 증상

➡ GI tract (주로: 공장 & 회장): small arterioles & venules
➡ circulating IgA deposition

➡ antibody-dependent cell-mediated cytotoxicity (ADCC)
➡ macrophage 유도
➡ IL-8 분비
➡ neutrophil 유도
➡ neutrophil phagocytosis
➡ HClO 분비 via H2O2
➡ small arterioles & venules: endothelium 손상
➡ extrinsic pathway: prothrombin 활성화 via factor VII, IX, X
➡ thrombin 생성
➡ 장허혈
➡ fibrin clot
➡ paralytic ileus

처방 목표 macrophage: IL-8 분비 억제 / HClO 분비 억제 / factor VII, IX, X 흡착 제거 / fibrin clot 분해 / paralytic ileus 개선

처방 구성 葱白 四莖 / 乾薑 一兩 / 附子 一枚 / 人尿 五合 / 豬膽汁 一合

처방 약리

부자 hypaconitine
➡ 약리 추측: macrophage` Voltage-gated proton channels blocker
(식균작용에 의해 증가된 세포내 proton을 세포외로 방출시키는 채널)
➡ proton 방출 억제
➡ 세포내 pH ↓
➡ macrophage 대사 억제
➡ IL-8 분비 억제

건강 shogaol ➡ neutrophil H2O2 scavenger
➡ HClO 분비 억제

총백 allicin ➡ factor VII, IX, X 흡착
➡ thrombin 형성 억제

사람 오줌 urokinase ➡ plaminogen 활성화
➡ plasmin 생성
➡ fibrin clot 분해

돼지 담즙 장운동 촉진시킴

백통탕 (白通湯)

원문 少陰病 , 下利, 白通湯 主之 。

원문 해설 항체매개 감염병으로 발생된 설사에는 백통탕을 쓴다.

적응증 Henoch-Schonlein purpura associated colitis
(헤노호-쉐라인 자반증에 연관된 대장염)

병태 & 증상

Henoch-Sch-nlein purpura-associated colitis

➡ GI tract (주로: 공장 & 회장): small arterioles & venules
➡ circulating IgA deposition
➡ antibody-dependent cell-mediated cytotoxicity (ADCC)
➡ macrophage 유도
➡ IL-8 분비
➡ neutrophil 유도
➡ neutrophil phagocytosis
➡ HClO 분비 via H2O2
➡ small arterioles & venules: endothelium 손상
➡ extrinsic pathway: prothrombin 활성화 via factor VII, IX, X
➡ thrombin 생성
➡ 장허혈

처방 목표 macrophage: IL-8 분비 억제 / HClO 분비 억제 / factor VII, IX, X 흡착 제거

처방 구성 蔥白 四莖 / 乾薑 一兩 / 附子 一枚

처방 약리

부자 hypaconitine
➡ 약리 추측: macrophage` Voltage-gated proton channels blocker
(식균작용에 의해 증가된 세포내 proton을 세포외로 방출시키는 채널)
➡ proton 방출 억제
➡ 세포내 pH ↓

➡ macrophage 대사 억제
➡ IL-8 분비 억제
건강 shogaol ➡ neutrophil H_2O_2 scavenger
➡ HClO 분비 억제

총백 allicin ➡ factor VII, IX, X 흡착
➡ thrombin 형성 억제

백합계자황 (百合雞子湯)

원문 百合病，吐 之 後 者，用 後 方 主之。

원문 해설 백합병에서 구토 증세가 있으면 백합계자탕을 쓴다.

적응증 Bornavirus vagus-nerve infection

병태 & 증상

Bornavirus vagus-nerve infection

➡ 미주신경 연접 조직: bornavirus infection
➡ interneuron: replication
➡ 1차 axoplasmic transport
➡ vagus-nerve: bornavirus infection ▶ vomiting
➡ 2차 axoplasmic transport

처방 목표 vagus-nerve acetylcholine 분비 촉진
➡ acetylcholine: interneuron cAMP 합성 방해
➡ protein kinase A 억제
➡ axoplasmic transport 억제

처방 구성 百合 七枚 / 雞子黃 一枚

처방 약리

계자황 (계란노른자): lecithin ➡ acetylcholine 원료

백합 colchicine ➡ microtubule polymerization inhibitor
➡ axoplasmic transport 억제

백합세방 (百合洗方)

원문 百合病 一 月 不 解，變 成 渴 者，百合洗方 主之。洗已，食 煮 餠，勿 以 鹽 豉 也。

원문 해설 백합병이 1개월을 지나도록 낫지 않고 갈증이 심해지면 백합세방을 쓴다. 백합물로 씻은 뒤에는 밀가루 음식을 먹을 때 소금과 콩소스를 먹지 않는다. 소금은 혈압을 올려서 축삭이동을 촉진하고, 콩소스는 산화질소를 생성시켜 축삭이동을 촉진하므로 먹지 않는다.

적응증 Bornavirus monocyte infection

병태 & 증상

Bornavirus monocyte infection

➡ bornavirus infected monocyte: collagenase
➡ extracellular matrix 분해 ▶ collagen synthesis ▶ hydroxyl group 소모
▶ thirst
➡ peripheral nerve: bornavirus transmigration
➡ axoplasmic transport toward CNS

처방 목표 axoplasmic transport 차단

처방 구성 百合 一升，以 水 一斗，漬 之 一 宿，以 洗 身。

처방 약리

백합 colchicine ➡ microtubule polymerization inhibitor
➡ axoplasmic transport 억제

백합지모탕 (百合知母湯)

원문 百合病 者, 百 脈 一 宗, 悉 致 其 病 也。意 欲 食 復 不 能 食, 常 默 默, 欲 臥 不能 臥, 欲 行 不能 行, 欲 飮 食, 或 有 美 時, 或 有 不用 聞 食臭 時, 如 寒 無 寒, 如 熱 無 熱, 口苦, 小便 赤, 諸 藥 不能 治, 得 藥 則 劇 吐 利, 如 有 神靈 者, 身 形 如 和, 其 脈 微 數。每 溺 時 頭 痛 者, 六十日 乃 愈 ;若 溺 時 頭 不 痛, 淅然 者, 四十日 愈 : 若 溺 快 然, 但 頭 眩 者, 二十日 愈。其 證 或 未 病 而 預 見, 或 病 四, 五 日 而 出, 或 病 二十日 或 一月 微見 者, 各 隨 證 治 之。百合病 發汗 後 者, 百合知母湯 主 之。

원문 해설 백합병에 걸리면 모든 맥이 다같이 영향을 받아 병증을 만든다. 음식을 먹고 싶어도 더 먹을 수 없고, 늘 말이 없으며, 눕고 싶어도 눕지 못하고 걸으려 해도 걸을 수 없고, 음식이 맛있다가도 냄새 맡기도 싫어지며, 추운 듯 보이지만 몸에 한기는 없으며 더운 듯 보이지만 몸에 열은 없고, 입이 쓰고 소변색이 붉어진다. 모든 약이 효과가 없고, 약을 먹으면 심하게 토하고 설사하게 된다. 마치 신 내린 것처럼 보이며 겉모습은 괜찮으며 맥은 가늘고 빠르다. 소변을 볼 때마다 두통이 있는 경우에는 60일이면 낫고, 소변 볼 때 두통은 없고 오싹하 게 추위를 타면 40일이면 낫고, 소변은 시원하게 보는데 단지 머리만 어지러울 때는 20일이면 낫는다. 병이 완전히 시작하지 않았는데 미리 증상이 보이기도 하며, 병이 시작한 후 증상이 4~5일 뒤에 나타날 수도 있으며, 혹은 20일이나 한 달이 지나서 증상이 약하게 나타날수도 있으므로 병증에 따라서 치료한다. 백합병에 걸린 뒤 땀을 흘린 경우에는 백합지모탕을 쓴다.

적응증 Bornavirus CNS infection

병태 & 증상

Bornavirus CNS infection

➡ bornavirus infected animal: droplet spread / excretion / blood
➡ human infection
➡ interneuron: bornavirus replication ▶ IL-1 : sweating
➡ axoplasmic transport toward CNS
➡ CNS infection
➡ CNS tropism: limbic system & hippocampus
➡ neuron degeneration
➡ psychiatric disorder: 행동장애, 정서장애, 기억장애

처방 목표 axoplasmic transport 차단 / neuron multi-differentiation 유도

처방 구성 百合 七枚 / 知母 三兩

처방 약리

백합 colchicine ➡ microtubule polymerization inhibitor
➡ axoplasmic transport 억제

지모 timosaponin ➡ nestin (+) modulator
➡ multi-differentiation 세포에서 발현되는 단백질
➡ 조직특수성 분화 유도

백합지황탕 (百合地黃湯)

원문 百合病，不 經 吐 `下 `發汗，病 形 如 初 者，百合地黃湯 主之。，大便 當 如 漆。

원문 해설 백합병에서 개재뉴런감염이나 적혈구감염, 림프절감염과 다른 경로의 감염을 일으켜 백합병 증상을 보이는 경우에는 백합지황탕을 쓴다. 약을 복용하면 옻처럼 까만 변이 나온다.

적응증 Bornavirus blood-brain barrier infection

병태 & 생리

Bornavirus blood-brain barrier infection

➡ monocyte: bornavirus infection
➡ monocyte activation
➡ brain microvascular endothelial cells: monocyte adhesion
➡ monocyte cytokine
➡ brain microvascular endothelial cells: damage
➡ monocyte: CNS transmigration
➡ blood brain barrier: breakdown
➡ neurological disorders

➡ axoplasmic transport

처방 목표 brain microvascular endothelial cells 재생 / axoplasmic transport 차단

처방 구성 百合 七枚 / 生地黃 汁 一升

처방 약리

생지황 catalpol, 약리추측

➡ CD133+ circulating endothelial progenitor cell (+) modulator

➡ vessel bud formation (혈관싹 형성)

➡ angiogenesis

백합 colchicine ➡ microtubule polymerization inhibitor

➡ axoplasmic transport 억제

백합활석산 (百合滑石散)

원문 百合病 變 發 熱 者, 一 作 發 寒 熱。百合滑石散 主之。 當 微 利 者, 止 服, 熱 則 除。

원문 해설 백합병에서 발열 하는 경우와 오한과 열이 같이 생기는 경우에는 백합활석산을 쓴다. 복용 후 설사하면 바이러스가 림프절에서 장관으로 배출되는 것이므로 복용을 중단한다.

적응증 Bornavirus gut-lymph monocytes infection

병태 & 증상

Bornavirus gut-lymph monocytes infection

➡ gut-lymph monocytes: bornavirus infection

➡ bornavirus infected monocyte: IL-1 ▶ fever

➡ activated monocyte: vascular endothelial cells adhesion

➡ vascular endothelial cells: damage ▶ IL-6: chills

➡ nervous site: 이동

➡ axoplasmic transport toward CNS

처방 목표 bornavirus RNA 흡착 제거 / axoplasmic transport 억제

처방 구성 百合 一兩 / 滑石 三兩

처방 약리

활석 $Mg_3(Si_4O_{10})(OH)_2$ ➡ ammonia & Nucleic acid absorbent
: bornavirus RNA 흡착

백합 colchicine ➡ microtubule polymerization inhibitor
➡ axoplasmic transport 억제

백호가계지탕 (白虎加桂枝湯)

원문 溫瘧者，其脈如平，身無寒但熱，骨節疼煩，時嘔，白虎加桂枝湯主之。

원문 해설 학질처럼 반복되는 발열이 있고, 맥은 정상이며, 한기는 없이 단지 열만 나면서, 뼈마디가 괴롭게 쑤시고, 약간 구역기가 있는 경우에는 백호가계지탕을 쓴다.

적응증 Viral thyroiditis (바이러스성 갑상선염)

병태 & 증상

Viral thyroiditis

➡ thyrocyte: coxsackie B4 virus infection
➡ thyrocyte: HLA-DR expression ↑
➡ HLA-DR: thyroperoxidase (TPO) 제시
➡ coxsackie B4 virus: antigen & thyrocyte: TPO
➡ molecular mimicry response
➡ TPO specific CD8+ T cell 출현
➡ CD8+ T cell: thyrocyte 공격
➡ thyrocyte apoptosis
➡ thyroid hormone 유출
➡ thyroid storm (1~2개월 지속)
➡ liver & muscle: metabolism ↑ ▶ fever 반복

➡ ATP ↑
➡ lactatemia
➡ urate 분비 ↓ ▶ hyperuricemia

처방 목표 CD8+ T cell apoptosis 유도 / thyrocyte 분화 유도 / lactatemia 교정

처방 구성 知母 六兩 / 炙甘草 二兩 / 石膏 一斤 / 粳米 二合 / 桂枝 三兩

처방 약리

석고CaSO4 ➡ calcium mediated T-cell apoptosis 유도

지모 timosaponin ➡ nestin (+) modulator
➡ multi-differentiation 세포에서 발현되는 단백질
➡ thyrocyte progenitor cell
➡ 조직특수성 분화 유도
➡ thyrocyte 분화

경미 magnesium ➡ DNA replication cofactor

계지 cinnamic acid ➡ lactate oxidizer
➡ Cori cycle: pyruvate 전환 촉진
➡ lactatemia 교정

구감초 18β-24-Hydroxyglycyrrhetinic acid
➡ 11-beta-hydroxysteroid dehydrogenase2 (HSD11B2) inhibitor
➡ aldosterone 생리작용과 동일
➡ H+ secretion
➡ lactatemia 교정

백호가인삼탕 (白虎加人參湯)

원문 服 桂枝湯，大汗出 後，大煩渴 不解， 脈 洪大 者, 白虎加人參湯主之。傷寒若汗若吐若下後, 七`八日不解, 熱結在裡, 表裡俱熱, 時時惡風, 大渴, 舌上乾燥 而煩, 欲飮水數升者, 白虎加參湯主之。傷寒無大熱, 口燥渴, 心煩, 背微惡

寒, 白虎加人參湯主之。傷寒脈浮, 發熱無汗, 其表不解, 不可與白虎湯; 渴欲飮水, 無表證者, 白虎加人參湯主之。

원문 해설 계지탕을 복용한 다음 땀이 크게 난 후 심한 갈증이 생겨서 해소되지 않고 맥이 넓고 큰 경우에는 백호가인삼탕을 쓴다. 세포병변성 감염증을 치료한 후 7~8일이 지나도 낫지 않고 속열이 있으면서 체표에도 열이 있고, 가끔씩 춥고 심한 갈증이 나면서 혀가 말라서 괴롭고, 물을 몇 리터씩 마시는 경우에는 백호가인삼탕을 쓴다. 세포병변성 감염증에서 큰열이 없고 기분이 편하지 않으면서 등에 오한이 나는 경우에는 백호가인삼탕을 쓴다. 세포병변성 감염증에서 발열하고 땀이 없는 것은 바이러스 증식이 계속 되고 있는 것이므로 백호탕은 보류하고, 물을 자꾸 마시려하고 열이 없는 경우에는 백호가인삼탕을 쓴다.

적응증 Coxsackie B4 virus-mediated Type 1 diabetes

병태 & 증상

Coxsackie B4 virus-mediated Type 1 diabetes

➡ β-cell: coxsackie B4 virus infection
➡-〉 β-cell: HLA-DR expression ↑
➡ HLA-DR: glutamic acid decarboxylase (GAD) 제시
➡ coxsackie B4 virus: 2C protein & β-cell: GAD
▶ molecular mimicry
➡ GAD specific CD8+ T cell 출현
➡ CD8+ T cell: β-cell 공격
➡ β-cell loss ↑
➡ severe β-cell deficiency: polydipsia
➡ Type 1 diabetes

처방 목표 CD8+ T cell: apoptosis 유도 / pancreatic duct: endothelial progenitor cell -〉 nestin 발현
➡ β-cell로 분화 촉진시킴 / pancreatic duct: endothelial progenitor cell 증식 촉진 / β-cell: DNA 복제 촉진 / 복제된 β-cell: Na+/ K+ pump 활성화시킴

처방 구성 知母 六兩 / 石膏 一斤 / 炙甘草 三兩 / 粳米 六合 / 人參 三兩

처방 약리

석고 CaSO4 ➡ calcium mediated T-cell apoptosis 유도

지모 timosaponin

➡ nestin (+) modulator

➡ multi-differentiation 세포에서 발현되는 단백질

➡ pancreatic duct: endothelial progenitor cell 조직특수성 분화 유도함

➡ β-cell로 분화

인삼 panax ginsenoside

➡ Transforming growth factor β (TGF-β) (+) modulator

➡ pancreatic duct: endothelial progenitor cell

➡ proliferation 촉진

경미 magnesium ➡ DNA replication cofactor

구감초 18β-24-Hydroxyglycyrrhetinic acid

➡ HSD11B2 inhibitor

➡ cortisol 분해 억제

➡ mineralocorticoid receptors 자극 지속

➡ 재생된 β-cell Na+/ K+ pumps 활성화

REFERENCE

J Hou, C Said, D Franchi, P Dockstader and N K Chatterjee. Antibodies to glutamic acid decarboxylase and P2-C peptides in sera from coxsackie virus B4-infected mice and IDDM patients. Diabetes October 1994 vol. 43 no. 10 1260-1266.

백호탕 (白虎湯)

원문 傷寒，脈 浮滑，此 表 有熱，裡 有寒，白虎湯 主之。三陽 合病，腹滿 身重，難 以 轉側，口 不仁 面 垢，譫語 遺尿，發汗 則 譫語，下 之 則 額上 生汗，手足 厥冷，若 自汗出 者，白虎湯 主之 。

원문 해설 세포병변성 감염증에서 맥이 뜨면서 매끄러우면 겉은 열이 있고 속은 냉기가 있는 것이므로 백호탕을 쓴다. 림프절 감염병 & 위장관 점막림프절 감염병 & 세망내피계-비장 감염병이 모두 관여하여, 복부팽만감이 오고 몸이 무거우며, 근육운동이 안 되고 말하기가 힘들며 얼굴이 때낀 것 같고, 헛소리를 하며 소변이 자주 나오는

데 발열하면 즉시 헛소리를 하고, 사하제를 쓰면 이마위에서 진땀이 흐르고 손발이 차가워지는데, 계속 땀나는 경우에는 백호탕을 쓴다.

적응증 IL-1 mediated Type 1 diabetes

병태 & 증상

IL-1 mediated Type 1 diabetes

➡ virus infection
➡ lymph node: 지속 감염
➡ macrophage: IL-1 분비 지속
➡ β-cell: iNOS ↑
➡ β-cell: oxidation of glucose to CO2 ↓
➡ Krebs cycle enzyme aconitase: activity ↓
➡ ATP levels ↓
➡ β-cell death
➡ β-cell-specific antigens 출현
➡ CD8+ T cell 활성화
➡ CD8+ T cell: β-cell 공격
➡ β-cell loss
➡ Type 1 diabetes
➡ hypoglycemia: feeling of warmth, coldness, sweating, pallor, paresthesias, stomach ache, paralysis, delirium

처방 목표 CD8+ T cell apoptosis 유도 / pancreatic duct: endothelial progenitor cell ➡ nestin 발현 ➡ β-cell로 분화 촉진시킴 / β-cell: DNA 복제 촉진 / 복제된 β-cell: Na+/ K+ pump 활성화시킴

처방 구성 知母 六兩 / 石膏 一斤 / 炙甘草 二兩 / 粳米 六合

처방 약리

석고 CaSO4 ➡ calcium mediated T-cell apoptosis 유도

지모 timosaponin
➡ nestin (+) modulator

➡ multi-differentiation 세포에서 발현되는 단백질
➡ pancreatic duct: endothelial progenitor cell 조직특수성 분화 유도함
➡ β-cell로 분화

경미 magnesium ➡ DNA replication cofactor

구감초 18β-24-Hydroxyglycyrrhetinic acid
➡ HSD11B2 inhibitor
➡ cortisol 분해 억제
➡ mineralocorticoid receptors 자극 지속
➡ 재생된 β-cell Na+/ K+ pumps 활성화

REFERENCE

Sarah A. Steer1, Anna L. Scarim1, Kari T. Chambers1, John A. Corbett1*. Interleukin-1 Stimulates β-Cell Necrosis and Release of the Immunological Adjuvant HMGB1. PLoS Med 3(2): e17.

별갑전환 (鱉甲煎丸)

원문 病瘧，以月一日發，當以十五日愈；設不差，當月盡解，如其不差，當云何？師曰：此結為癥瘕，名曰瘧母，急治之，宜鱉甲煎丸。

원문 해설 학질모기에 물려서, 발병되면 마땅히 15일(간세포 증식기, 14일)이면 낫는데 만약 낫지 않아도 발병한지 한 달 안에는 (적혈구 파열 & 항체) 나을 텐데 만약 이 때도 낫지 않는 경우는 어떤 이유입니까 ? 이것은 적혈구가 깨지지 않고 뭉쳐 있는 것이 원인이므로 급히 치료해야 한다. 별갑전환을 쓴다.

적응증 Plasmodium falciparum malaria (열대열원충 말라리아)

병태 & 증상

Plasmodium falciparum malaria

Anopheles mosquito: P. falciparum transmission

sporozoite: hepatocyte entry ➡ mature schizont 전환 (14일)

RNA Polymerase II ▶ antisense RNA 합성 ▶ p53 억제
▶ sporozoite DNA: malignant phenotype 전환
NOS gene: point mutation ▶ NO 생산 증가 ▶ peroxynitrite ($ONOO^-$) ↑
▶ sporozoite DNA: mutation
▶ T cell 면역 실패
estrogen Rc: 활성형 전환 ▶ sporozoite DNA 복제 증가
cholesterol ▶ sporozoite 영양분
hepatocyte TGF-β: 감소 ▶ TGF-β induced apoptosis 실패

bloodstream: mature schizont 출현

mature schizont: erythrocyte entry

P. falciparum: pfHRP1 (histidine-rich protein) ▶ erythrocyte 부착
erythrocyte membrane: anion exchange protein 1 (AE1)
▶ superoxide-mediated 활성화
▶ mature schizont 침투
erythrocyte: chloride channel family 활성화 ▶ 영양분 통로
P. falciparum 증식에 관여하는 효소
: cholesterol 합성효소 ▶ DOXP reductoisomerase
/ fatty acid 합성효소 ▶ FabI & FabZ
/ mitochondria dehydrogenase ▶ DHODH
erythrocyte: membrane bound PTK (protein tyrosine kinase) 증가
▶ P. falciparum 증식
erythrocyte VEGF Rc: VEGF influx ▶ P. falciparum 영양분

P. falciparum-infected erythrocyte (IRBCs): viscous fluid
➡ severe malaria

IRBCs splenic hematoma
IRBCs microvascular endothelium CD36 부착
▶ IRBCs antibody 출현
▶ IRBCs + antibody 복합체 형성
▶ neutrophil 유도
▶ neutrophil phagocytosis
▶ HClO 분비 via H2O2
▶ 혈관내피하 collagen 손상

▶ tissue factor 노출

▶ platelet independent thrombus formation

▶ thrombus 축적

▶ platelet thrombin Rc: thrombus 부착

▶ platelet-thrombin complex 형성

▶ platelet-thrombin complex 분리

▶ micro-emboli 작용

▶ tissue ischemia: lactatemia

▶ acute ranal failure: hyperphosphatemia
& noncardiogenic pulmonary edema

처방 목표 P. falciparum: antisense RNA 분해 / peroxynitrite ($ONOO^-$) 제거 / estrogen Rc: 활성형 억제 / hepatocyte: cholesterol 유입 억제 & 분해 촉진 / hepatocyte TGF-β: 전사 촉진 / bloodstream: mature schizont 제거 / P. falciparum: erythrocyte 부착 억제 / erythrocyte: superoxide 제거 / erythrocyte: chloride channel 차단 / DOXP reductoisomerase 억제 / FabI & FabZ 억제 / DHODH 억제 / erythrocyte: tyrosine kinase 차단 / erythrocyte VEGF Rc 차단 / splenic hematoma 제거 / HClO 분비 억제 / 혈관내피하 collagen 복구 / micro-emboli 제거 / lactatemia 교정 / hyperphosphatemia 교정 / noncardiogenic pulmonary edema 개선

처방 구성 鱉甲 十二分 (炙) / 烏扇 三分 (燒) / 黃芩 三分 / 柴胡 六分 / 鼠婦 三分 (熬) / 乾薑 三分 / 大黃 三分 / 芍藥 五分 / 桂枝 三分 / 葶藶 一分 (熬) / 石韋 三分 / 厚朴 三分 / 牡丹 五分 / 瞿麥 二分 / 紫葳 三分 / 半夏 一分 / 人參 一分 / 蟅蟲 五分 / 阿膠 三分 (炙) / 蜂窩 四分 (炙) / 赤硝 十二分 / 蜣螂 六分 (熬) / 桃仁 二分

처방 목표

시호 saikosaponin ➡ small interfering RNA (siRNA) (+) modulator
➡ P. falciparum: antisense RNA 분해

황금 baicalin ➡ peroxynitrite ($ONOO^-$) scavenger

도인 amygdalin
➡ 체내 활성 성분: thiocyanate (amygdalin metabolite)
➡ 4S estrogen receptor (ER) ▶ 5S estrogen receptor 전환 억제

(4S monomer: estrogen 저친화성, 5S dimer: estrogen 고친화성)

별갑 chitosan ➡ cholesterol absorption inhibitor

목단피 β-Sitosterol ➡ cholesterol ester hydrolase activator

인삼 panax ginsenoside
➡ Transforming growth factor β (TGF-β) (+) modulator

초석 Sodium Sulfate ➡ zwitterion (양쪽성 이온)
➡ 강한 산도: 음이온 흡착 / 약한 산도: 양이온 흡착
➡ blood: P. falciparum: pfHRP1 (histidine-rich protein) 흡착
봉와 (벌집): rosin ➡ Histidin binder ➡ P. falciparum: erythrocyte 부착 억제

작약 paeoniflorin ➡ superoxide scavenger

강랑 (쇠똥구리): ivermectin ➡ erythrocyte: chloride channel 차단
구맥 dianoside, 약리 추측 ➡ P. Falciparum: DOXP blocker

자위 (능소화) campenoside ➡ P. Falciparum: FabI blocker

오선 (범부채) iridin ➡ P. Falciparum: FabZ blocker

석위 fumaric acid ➡ P. Falciparum: DHODH blocker

대황 emodin ➡ tyrosine kinase blocker

후박 honokiol ➡ VEGF receptor blocker

자충 (흙바퀴) ESW extraction, 약리 추측
➡ erythrocyte C3b receptor (+) modulator
➡ 대식세포: hematoma 식균 촉진

아교 Glycine / Proline / Hydroxyproline / Alanine / 기타 아미노산
➡ collagen biosynthesis

건강 shogaol ➡ neutrophil H2O2 scavenger
➡ HClO 분비 억제

반하 triterpenoid (C30H48O7S)

➡ Rho GTPase family transcription promotor

➡ heparan sulfate 생성 촉진

➡ heparin 유사 작용

➡ micro-emboli 용해

계지 cinnamic acid ➡ lactate oxidizer

➡ Cori cycle: pyruvate 전환 촉진

서부 (쥐며느리) CaCO3 ➡ phosphate binder

➡ hyperphosphatemia 교정

정력자 helveticoside ➡ 강심배당체

➡ 심장 수축을 짧고 강하게 유도해서 확장기 길어짐

➡ 대정맥 유입 혈액량 증가

➡ 정맥 울혈 해소

➡ noncardiogenic pulmonary edema 개선

복령감초탕 (茯苓甘草湯)

원문 傷寒 汗出 而 渴 者, 五苓散 主 之; 不渴 者, 茯苓甘草湯 主之。

원문 해설 세포병변성 감염증으로 땀난 뒤 갈증이 있는 경우에는 오령산을 쓰고 갈증이 없는 경우에는 복령감초탕을 쓴다.

적응증 Streptococcal rheumatic myocarditis (연쇄구균 류마티스 심근염)

병태 & 증상

Streptococcal rheumatic myocarditis

➡ streptococcus infection

➡ streptococcus antigen & myocardium: cross reaction

➡ myocardium: IgG & IgM 부착

➡ complement 유도

➡ 심근 세포막: membrane attack complement 형성됨

➡ 심근 세포막: Na+/K+ pump 손상
➡ calcium 유입 ↑
➡ phospholipase A2 활성화
➡ arachidonic acid 생성
➡ superoxide ↑
➡ superoxide dismutase 작동: hydrogen peroxide ↑: 심근수축력 ↓
➡ superoxide dismutase2 고갈
➡ superoxide로 인해 Fe3+(ferric ions)가 Fe2+(ferrous ion)로 환원됨
➡ Ferrous ion-induced lipid peroxidation in mitochondria
➡ mitochondria membrane potential damage
➡ 세포질의 pyruvate가 mitochondria에 유입되지 못하고 lactate로 환원됨
➡ intracellular lactate ↑
➡ 수소이온 증가로 pH 감소
➡ 해당효소 glucose 6-phosphate와 phosphofructokinase 활성 감소됨
➡ ATP 생산 감소
➡ Na+/ K+ pump 손상 ↑
➡ myocarditis
➡ 좌심실 심첨부: thrombus formation

처방 목표 hydrogen peroxide 제거 / intracellular lactate 교정 / Na+/ K+ pump 활성화 / thrombus 억제

처방 구성 茯苓 二兩 / 桂枝 二兩 / 炙甘草 一兩 / 生薑 三兩

처방 약리

생강 gingerol ➡ hydrogen peroxide scavenger

계지 cinnamic acid ➡ lactate oxidizer
➡ pyruvate 전환 촉진

구감초 18β-24-Hydroxyglycyrrhetinic acid
➡ HSD11B2 inhibitor
➡ cortisol 분해 억제
➡ mineralocorticoid receptors 자극 지속
➡ Na+/ K+ pumps 전사 촉진

복령 pachymic acid ➡ glycoprotein IIb/IIIa (gpIIb/IIIa) (-) modulator
➡ thrombus formation 억제

복령계지감초대조탕 (茯苓桂枝甘草大棗湯)

원문 發汗 後, 其人 臍下 悸 者, 欲 作 奔豚, 茯苓桂枝甘草大棗湯 主之。

원문 해설 IL-1 매개 감염증 후 배꼽아래가 두근거리며 분돈증이 생기려고 하는 경우에는 복령계지감초대조탕을 쓴다.

적응증 Ventricular tachycardia (심실빈맥)

병태 & 증상

Ventricular tachycardia

➡ virus & bacteria infection
➡ 관상동맥경화증 진행
➡ myocardiocyte ischemia
➡ mitochondria: SOD2 감소
➡ ischemia-reperfusion: mitochondrial dysfunction
➡ intracellular lactate ↑
➡ ATP 감소
➡ Na+/ K+ pumps 손상
➡ myocardiocyte 손상
➡ ventricular tachycardia
➡ 좌심실 심첨부: thrombus formation

처방 목표 intracellular lactate 교정 / Na+/ K+ pumps 활성화 / 혈소판 1차, 2차 응집 억제

처방 구성 茯苓 半斤 / 桂枝 四兩 / 炙甘草 二兩 / 大棗 十五枚

처방 약리

계지 cinnamic acid ➡ lactate oxidizer
➡ pyruvate 전환 촉진
➡ intracellular lactate 교정

구감초 18β-24-Hydroxyglycyrrhetinic acid
➡ HSD11B2 inhibitor
➡ cortisol 분해 억제

➡ mineralocorticoid receptors 자극 지속
➡ Na+/ K+ pumps 전사 촉진

대조 c-AMP ➡ 혈소판, endoplasmic reticulum: inhibition of phosphorylation
➡ calcium blocking
➡ thromboxane 생성 억제
➡ 혈소판 1차 응집 억제

복령 pachymic acid ➡ glycoprotein IIb/IIIa (gpIIb/IIIa) (-) modulator
➡ 혈소판 2차 응집 억제

복령계지백출감초탕 (茯苓桂枝白朮甘草湯)

원문 傷寒 若 吐 若 下 後 , 心 下 逆滿 , 氣 上衝 胸 , 起 則 頭眩 , 脈 沉緊 , 發汗 則 動 經 , 身 為 振振搖 者, 茯苓桂枝白朮甘草湯 主之 。

원문 해설 세포병변성 감염병에서 최토법이나 사하법을 쓴 후 심장아래 부위가 빽근하고 호흡이 불편하면서 일어설 때 어지럽고, 맥이 가라앉으며 급하고, 땀이 난 뒤심방 전도가 불규칙해져서 몸이 벌벌 떨리며 흔들거리는 경우에는, 복령계지백출감초탕을 쓴다.

적응증 Atrial fibrilation (심방세동)

병태 & 증상

Atrial fibrilation

➡ 관상동맥 질환 / 류머티스성 판막 질환 / 갑상선 항진증 / 고혈압 / 기타 원인
➡ atrial myocardiocyte: ischemia
➡ myocardiocyte: lactate ↑
➡ myocardiocyte: Na+/ K+ pumps 손상
➡ 심방 전기 전도: 불규칙
➡ 심방 세동
➡ arrhythmia
➡ atrial endocardial endothelial cell: blood velocities ↓
➡ endocardial endothelial cell: nitric oxide 생성

➡ NADPH oxidase ↑
➡ oxidative stress
➡ VCAM-1 발현
➡ monocyte 부착
➡ endothelial cell: dysfunction
➡ platelet 응집
➡ thrombus formation
➡ silent cerebral infarction

처방 목표 lactate 교정 / Na+/ K+ pumps 활성화 / VCAM-1 차단 / thrombus 억제

처방 구성 茯苓 四兩 / 桂枝 三兩 / 白朮 二兩 / 炙甘草 二兩

처방 약리

계지 cinnamic acid ➡ lactate oxidizer
➡ pyruvate 전환 촉진
➡ intracellular lactate 교정

구감초 18β-24-Hydroxyglycyrrhetinic acid
➡ HSD11B2 inhibitor
➡ cortisol 분해 억제
➡ mineralocorticoid receptors 자극 지속
➡ Na+/ K+ pumps 전사 촉진

백출 atractylon ➡ vascular cell adhesion molecule-1 (VCAM-1) blocker

복령 pachymic acid ➡ glycoprotein IIb/IIIa (gpIIb/IIIa) (-) modulator
➡ thrombus formation 억제

복령사역탕 (茯苓四逆湯)

원문 發汗, 若 下之 , 病 仍 不解, 煩躁 者, 茯苓四逆湯 主之 。

원문 해설 IL-1 매개 감염증을 앓은 후 완전히 낫지 않고 괴롭고 초조한 경우에는 복령사역탕을 쓴다.

적응증 Viral myocarditis (바이러스성 심근염)

병태 & 증상

Viral myocarditis

➡ myocardiocyte: cardiotropic virus infection
: coxsackievirus / cytomegalovirus / enterovirus / rubellavirus. etc
➡ virus infected myocardiocyte: IL-12 분비
➡ natural killer cell 유도: IFN-γ 분비: sweating
➡ virus replication 억제
➡ IFN-γ: macrophage 유도
➡ macrophage: neutrophil chemotactic factor 분비
➡ neutrophil 유도
➡ neutrophil phagocytosis
➡ HClO 분비 via H2O2
➡ myocardiocyte: Na+/K+ pumps 손상
➡ myocarditis
➡ 심실 심첨부: thrombus formation

처방 목표 macrophage: neutrophil chemotactic factor 분비 억제 / HClO 분비 억제 / Na+/K+ pumps 활성화 / thrombus 억제 / myocardiocyte 증식 촉진

처방 구성 茯苓 四兩 / 人參 一兩 / 附子 一枚 / 炙甘草 二兩 / 乾薑 一兩

처방 약리

부자 hypaconitine
➡ 약리 추측: macrophage` Voltage-gated proton channels blocker
(식균작용에 의해 증가된 세포내 proton을 세포외로 방출시키는 채널)
➡ proton 방출 억제

➡ 세포내 pH ↓

➡ macrophage 대사 억제

➡ macrophage: neutrophil chemotactic factor 분비 억제

건강 shogaol ➡ neutrophil H2O2 scavenger

➡ HClO 분비 억제

구감초 18β-24-Hydroxyglycyrrhetinic acid

➡ HSD11B2 inhibitor

➡ cortisol 분해 억제

➡ mineralocorticoid receptors 자극 지속

➡ Na+/ K+ pumps 전사 촉진

복령 pachymic acid ➡ glycoprotein IIb/IIIa (gpIIb/IIIa) (-) modulator

➡ thrombus formation 억제

인삼 panax ginsenoside

➡ Transforming growth factor β (TGF-β) (+) modulator

➡ myocardiocyte proliferation 촉진

복령융염탕 (茯苓戎鹽湯)

원문 小便 不利，蒲灰散 主之 ； 滑石白魚散，茯苓戎鹽湯 并 主之 。

원문 해설 소변이 불편한 경우에는 포탄산, 활석백어산, 복령융염탕을 병용하여 쓴다.

적응증 Immune complexes-mediated Rapidly progressive glomerulonephritis (면역복합체 매개-급속진행성 사구체신염)

병태 & 증상

Immune complexes-mediated Rapidly progressive glomerulonephritis

➡ glomerulus: Immune complexes 침착

➡ glomerular capillary endothelium: VCAM-1 발현
➡ glomerular capillary endothelium: monocyte 부착
➡ monocyte ROS burst
➡ glomerular capillary injury: thrombus formation
➡ Rapidly progressive glomerulonephritis
➡ 보우만피막 파괴 / 세뇨관 위축
➡ 급성 신부전
➡ 핍뇨: 소변배설량 〈 30ml / 24hr
➡ 저나트륨혈증 / 저칼슘혈증
➡ 합병증: 울혈성심부전 / 폐부종 / 혼수

처방 목표 VCAM-1 발현 억제 / thrombus 제거 / 저나트륨혈증 / 저칼슘혈증 교정

처방 구성 茯苓 半斤 / 白朮 二兩 / 戎鹽 彈丸 大 一枚

처방 약리

백출 atractylon ➡ vascular cell adhesion molecule-1 (VCAM-1) blocker

복령 pachymic acid ➡ glycoprotein IIb/IIIa (gpIIb/IIIa) (-) modulator
➡ thrombus formation 억제

융염 (돌소금): NaCl, CaCO3 ➡ 저나트륨혈증 / 저칼슘혈증 교정

복령음 (茯苓飮)

원문 茯苓飮, 治 心胸 中 有 停痰 宿水 , 自 吐出 水 後 , 心胸 間 虛 , 氣滿 , 不 能 食 , 消 痰氣 , 令 能 食 。

원문 해설 복령음은 흉부의 조직부종을 치료하며 부종액이 토해진 후에, 흉부의 허탈감도 치료하며 신경순환이 원활하지 못해서 오는 식욕부진도 낫게 한다, 복령음으로 조직부종과 신경순환이 개선되면 음식을 먹을 수 있다.

적응증 Aortic aneurysm in Behcet's Disease (베체트 대동맥류)

병태 & 증상

Aortic aneurysm in Behcet's Disease

➡ streptococcus infection
➡ superantigen: CD4+ T cell activation
➡ aorta endothelium: HLA B51 발현
➡ aorta endothelium: CD4+ T cell 부착
➡ aorta endothelium: VCAM-1 발현
➡ aorta media & adventitia: CD4+ T cell 침윤
➡ CD4+ T cell: IFN-γ 분비
➡ macrophage 유도: matrix metalloproteinases (MMPs) 분비
➡ 혈관 media & adventitia: elastin degradation
➡ smooth muscle cell depletion
➡ aortic wall: weakness
➡ fibroblast: 섬유소 분비
➡ aorta media & adventitia: calcification
➡ aneurysm expansion
➡ 상대정맥 압박 (조직부종)
/ 미주신경 압박 ➡ myelin H_2O_2 ↑ ➡ myelitis ➡ myelin scar
➡ 폐신경얼기 (과호흡 유발) / 식도신경얼기 (구역 유발) / 위장 가지 (구토 유발) / 심장가지 (부정맥 유발)
➡ calcificated plaque: rupture
➡ thrombus frmation

처방 목표 VCAM-1 차단 / matrix metalloproteinases 차단 / calcification 억제 / myelin H_2O_2 제거 / myelin scar 제거 / thrombus 제거

처방 구성 茯苓 三兩 / 人參 三兩 / 白朮 三兩 / 枳實 二兩 / 橘皮 二兩半 / 生薑 四兩

처방 약리

백출 atractylon ➡ vascular cell adhesion molecule-1 (VCAM-1) blocker

지실 auraptene ➡ matrix metalloproteinases (MMPs) blocker

인삼 panax ginsenoside
➡ Transforming growth factor β (TGF-β) (+) modulator
➡ calcification 억제

생강 gingerol ➡ hydrogen peroxide scavenger

귤피 rutin ➡ proteolytic activator
➡ myelin scar 제거

복령 pachymic acid ➡ glycoprotein IIb/IIIa (gpIIb/IIIa) (-) modulator
➡ thrombus formation 억제

복령택사탕 (茯苓澤瀉湯)

원문 胃反, 吐 而 渴 欲 飮水 者, 茯苓澤瀉湯 主之。

원문 해설 속이 뒤집혀서 전부 토하고 갈증이 나서 계속 물을 마시려는 경우에는 복령택사탕을 쓴다.

적응증 Decompensated heart failure (보상기전 실패 심부전)

병태 & 증상

심부전 보상기전

➡ 콩팥: renin-angiotensin system ↑
➡ angiotensin II ↑
➡ 혈관평활근: 수축력 ↑
➡ 혈관평활근: lactate & hydrogen peroxide 축적
➡ 혈관평활근 손상
➡ vascular endothelium: VCAM-1 발현
➡ leukocyte 유도
➡ 혈관내피하 조직: leukocyte 이동
➡ 혈관내피 손상
➡ 혈소판 응집: thrombus formation
➡ 혈소판: 평활근 성장인자 분비
➡ 혈관평활근 증식
➡ vascular hypertropy
➡ 말초조직 허혈

➡ renin-angiotensin system ↑↑
➡ angiotensin II ↑↑
➡ 갈증 중추 자극
➡ 수분 섭취 ↑
➡ blood volume ↑
➡ 희석성 hyponatremia: vomitting

처방 목표 혈관평활근 lactate 교정 / 혈관평활근 hydrogen peroxide 제거 / VCAM-1 차단 / leukocyte 이동 억제 / 혈소판 응집 억제 / angiotensin II 차단

처방 구성 茯苓 半斤 / 澤瀉 四兩 / 甘草 二兩 / 桂枝 二兩 / 白朮 三兩 / 生薑 四兩

처방 약리

계지 cinnamic acid ➡ lactate oxidizer
➡ pyruvate 전환 촉진
➡ intracellular lactate 교정

생강 gingerol ➡ hydrogen peroxide scavenger

백출 atractylon ➡ vascular cell adhesion molecule-1 (VCAM-1) blocker

감초 glycyrrhetinic acid
➡ 11-beta-hydroxysteroid dehydrogenase1 (HSD11B1) inhibitor
➡ glucocorticoid 작용
➡ IκBα 생성
➡ NF-κB 억제
➡ leukocyte 대사 억제
➡ leukocyte 이동 억제됨

복령 pachymic acid ➡ glycoprotein IIb/IIIa (gpIIb/IIIa) (-) modulator
➡ thrombus formation 억제

택사 alisol ➡ angiotensin II receptor blocker

복령행인감초탕 (茯苓杏仁甘草湯)

원문 胸痹, 胸中氣塞, 短氣, 茯苓杏仁甘草湯 主之。

원문 해설 심장부위가 저리고 막히는 느낌이 있으면서 호흡이 짧아지는 경우에는 복령행인감초탕을 쓴다.

적응증 Rheumatic valvulitis (류마티스 판막염)

병태 & 증상

Rheumatic valvulitis

➡ valvular endothelium: MHC class II antigen expression
➡ CD4+ T cell 유도
➡ B cell 활성화
➡ antibody 생성
➡ CD8+ T cell 유도: TNF-α 분비
➡ valvular endothelium: 당대사 항진
➡ mitochondria 대사 ↑: hydroxyl radical ↑
➡ mitochondria dysfunction
➡ valvulitis
➡ 좌심실 심첨부: thrombus formation

처방 목표 antibody 생성 억제 / hydroxyl radical 제거 / thrombus 억제

처방 구성 茯苓 三兩 / 杏仁 五十個 / 甘草 一兩

처방 약리

감초 glycyrrhetinic acid ➡ HSD11B1 inhibitor
➡ cortisol 분해 억제
➡ glucocorticoid receptors 자극 지속
➡ IκBα 생성
➡ NF-κB 억제
➡ B cell 대사 억제
➡ 항체 형성 감소

행인 benzoic acid ➡ hydroxyl radical scavenger

복령 pachymic acid ➡ glycoprotein IIb/IIIa (gpIIb/IIIa) (-) modulator
➡ thrombus formation 억제

부자경미탕 (附子粳米湯)

원문 腹中 寒氣, 雷鳴 切痛, 胸 脅 逆滿, 嘔吐, 附子粳米湯 主之。

원문 해설 뱃속에 한기가 들고 장명이 심하면서 끊어질 듯 아프고 위장관과 쓸개관 부위에 역류가 있으면서 구토하면 부자경미탕을 쓴다.

적응증 Small intestine stenosis in Behcet's Disease (베체트 소장협착증)

병태 & 증상

Small intestine stenosis in Behcet's Disease

➡ streptococcus infection
➡ superantigen: CD4+ T cell activation
➡ small intestine mucosa: HLA B51 발현
➡ small intestine mucosa: CD4+ T cell 침윤
➡ CD4+ T cell: TNF-a, IL-8 분비
➡ TNF-a: chills
➡ IL-8: neutrophil 유도
➡ neutrophil cathepsin 분비
➡ mucosa cell: necrosis
➡ anion charge 소실
➡ small intestine stenosis
➡ obstruction: vomiting

처방 목표 CD4+ T cell 이동 억제 / neutrophil cathepsin 분비 억제 / mucosa cell 재생 및 상환 촉진

처방 구성 炮附子 一枚 / 半夏 半升 / 甘草 一兩 / 大棗 十枚 / 粳米 半升

처방 약리

감초 glycyrrhetinic acid

➡ 11-beta-hydroxysteroid dehydrogenase1 (HSD11B1) inhibitor
➡ glucocorticoid 작용과 동일
➡ Immune cell: IκBα 생성 증가
➡ NF-κB mediated transcription 억제됨
➡ CD4+ T cell 이동 & cytokine 생성 억제됨

포부자 aconitine

➡ 약리추측: neutrophil` Voltage-gated proton channels blocker
(식균작용에 의해 증가된 세포내 proton을 세포외로 방출시키는 채널)
➡ Voltage-gated proton channels 차단
➡ 호중구내 수소이온 축적
➡ neutrophil 대사 억제
➡ neutrophil cathepsin 분비 억제

경미 magnesium ➡ DNA replication cofactor

대조 c-AMP ➡ Protein kinase A avtivator
➡ ATP 합성 촉진
➡ cell cycle ↑

반하 triterpenoid (C30H48O7S)

➡ Rho GTPase family transcription promotor
➡ focal adhesion 생성 촉진
➡ 점막세포 이동 촉진

부자사심탕 (附子瀉心湯)

원문 心下痞 , 而 復 惡寒 汗出 者, 附子瀉心湯 主之 。

원문 해설 심장 아래쪽이 저리고 한기가 들며 땀 흘리는 경우에는 부자사심탕을 쓴다.

적응증 Cholecystitis (담낭염)

병태 & 증상

Cholecystitis

➡ cholesterol dietary
➡ cholesterol oversaturated bile prodicing
➡ gallbladder: cholesterol crystal formation
➡ plasma protein coated crystal: neutrophil 유도
➡ neutrophil: cathepsin 분비
➡ cholesterol crystal oxidation -> 음전하 ↑
➡ calcium cholesterol formation
➡ gallbladder: 상피세포 손상: heartburn
➡ adenomatous hyperplasia
➡ mucin overproduction (via EGFRc + TK domain)
➡ cholesterol gallstone formation
➡ gallstone: gallbladder neck 폐쇄
➡ bacteria 유입: 담낭 상피 -> IL-1 & IL-6 분비: sweating & chill
➡ fulminant Cholecystitis

처방 목표 neutrophil: cathepsin 분비 억제 / Tyrosine kinase 차단시킴 / 담낭에 유입된 bacteria를 살균시킴

처방 구성 大黃 二兩 / 黃連 一兩 / 黃芩 一兩 / 炮附子 一枚

처방 약리

포부자 aconitine
➡ 약리추측: neutrophil` Voltage-gated proton channels blocker
(식균작용에 의해 증가된 세포내 proton을 세포외로 방출시키는 채널)
➡ Voltage-gated proton channels 차단
➡ 호중구내 수소이온 축적
➡ neutrophil 대사 억제
➡ cathepsin 분비 억제

대황 emodin ➡ tyrosine kinase blocker
➡ gallbladder 상피세포: mucin overproduction 억제
➡ cholesterol gallstone 형성 억제됨

황련 berberine ➡ sortase inhibitor
➡ 담낭에 유입된 bacteria: peptidoglycan 합성 억제
➡ 삼투압 저항력이 감소되어 용균됨

황금 baicalin ➡ peroxynitrite ($ONOO^-$) scavenger
➡ peroxynitrite로 인한 담낭 손상을 억제시킴

부자탕 (附子湯)

원문 少陰病，身體痛，手足寒，骨節痛，脈 沉 者, 附子湯 主之。少陰病，得 之 一 二 日，口中和，其 背 惡寒 者，當 灸 之，附子湯 主之。

원문 해설 항체매개 감염병으로 몸 전체가 아프고 손발이 차며 관절통이 있으면서 맥이 가라앉아 있는 경우에는 부자탕을 쓴다. 항체매개 감염증에 걸린 후 1~2일째 입안이 건조하지 않고 갈증이 없으면서 등에 한기가 있는 경우에는 따뜻하게 해주어야 하며 부자탕을 쓴다.

적응증 p-ANCA associated vasculitis (핵주위 항호중구 세포질 항체-매개 혈관염), p-ANCA: protoplasmic-staining antineutrophil cytoplasmic antibodies

병태 & 증상

p-ANCA associated vasculitis

➡ small vessel: p-ANCA bind myeloperoxidase expressed neutrophil
➡ p-ANCA * neutrophil complex
➡ complement 유도
➡ vessel endothelial cell: superoxide mediated VCAM-1 발현
➡ neutrophil adhesion
➡ neutrophil elastase 분비
➡ small vessel vasculitis
➡ thrombus formation
➡ 침범 조직: Skin / Muscle / Joint / Nervous system
➡ 허혈 괴사: body ache, cold hands and feet, arthralgia

처방 목표 vascular endothelial cell 내 superoxide 제거 / vascular endothelial cell: VCAM-1 차단 / neutrophil: elastase 분비 억제 / thrombus 제거 / 괴사 조직 재생

처방 구성 炮附子 二枚 / 茯苓 三兩 / 人參 二兩 / 白朮 四兩 / 芍藥 三兩

처방 약리

작약 paeoniflorin ➡ superoxide scavenger

백출 atractylon ➡ vascular cell adhesion molecule-1 (VCAM-1) blocker

포부자 aconitine

➡ 약리추측: neutrophil` Voltage-gated proton channels blocker
(식균작용에 의해 증가된 세포내 proton을 세포외로 방출시키는 채널)

➡ Voltage-gated proton channels 차단

➡ 호중구내 수소이온 축적

➡ neutrophil 대사 억제

➡ elastase 분비 억제

복령 pachymic acid ➡ glycoprotein IIb/IIIa (gpIIb/IIIa) (-) modulator
➡ thrombus formation 억제

인삼 panax ginsenoside

➡ Transforming growth factor β (TGF-β) (+) modulator

➡ 괴사 조직 재생

분돈탕 (奔豚湯)

원문 病 有 奔豚 , 有 吐膿 , 有 驚怖 , 有 火邪 , 此 四 部 病 , 皆 從 驚 發 得 之 。奔豚病 , 從 少腹 起 , 上衝 咽喉 , 發作 欲 死 , 復 還 止 , 皆 從 驚恐 得 之 。奔豚氣 上衝 胸 , 腹痛 , 往來 寒熱 , 奔豚湯 主之 。

원문 해설 분돈증(새끼돼지가 이리저리 달리는 모습)과 농을 토하는 것, 놀라서 떠는 것 발열이 지속되는 것은 모두 놀라서 생기는 증상이다. 분돈병이 생기면 아랫배에서 인후

쪽으로 치밀어 오르는 상충감이 생기는 데, 죽을 지경까지 진행한 뒤에 멈추는 데, 공포감으로 인해 생기는 병이다. 분돈기는 심장으로 치밀어 오르는 상충감이 생기며, 복통이 있고 오한과 열이 반복되며 분돈탕을 쓴다.

적응증 Epinephrine-mediated encephalopathy (에피네프린-매개 뇌병증)

병태 & 증상

Epinephrine-mediated encephalopathy

➡ flight
➡ adrenal glands: epinephrine 분비 ▶ sputum secretion ↑
➡ 복강 지방세포 / 큰말초 지방세포 / 골격근 세포 / 간세포: Lipolysis
➡ 혈 중 유리 지방산
➡ 심근: 유리 지방산 산화 : cardiac toxicity
➡ brain microvessel: erythrocyte velocity ↓
➡ 적혈구 골격단백질 불안정화
➡ deformity erythrocyte 생성
➡ brain microvessel: deformity erythrocyte 부착
➡ brain microvessel: vwF 발현
➡ micro-emboli 형성
➡ brain microvessel endothelium: 허혈
➡ brain microvessel endothelium: superoxide 생성
➡ brain microvessel smooth muscle: α-adrenergic Rc Ca channel 자극
➡ brain microvessel spasm
➡ erythrocyte: s-nitrosothiol 분비
➡ superoxide + s-nitrosothiol: peroxynitrite 생성
➡ blood brain barrier: astrocyte 허혈
➡ 세포내 대사 ↓
➡ extracellular Ca2+ influx ↑
➡ hydrogen peroxide ↑
➡ NF-κB 활성화
➡ astrocyte inflammation
➡ synapse: glutamate 축적
➡ postsynaptic neuron NMDA Rc: glutamate 자극
➡ postsynaptic neuron: glutamate excitotoxicity
➡ 피질 손상

처방 목표 적혈구 골격단백질 유지 / micro-emboli 제거 / superoxide 제거 / α-adrenergic Rc 차단 / peroxynitrite 제거 / extracellular Ca2+ influx 억제 / hydrogen peroxide 제거 / NF-κB 억제 / postsynaptic neuron NMDA Rc 차단

처방 구성 甘草 二兩 / 芎藭 二兩 / 當歸 二兩 / 半夏 四兩 / 黃芩 二兩 / 生葛 五兩 / 芍藥 二兩 / 生薑 四兩 / 甘李根白皮 一升

처방 약리

당귀 decurcin ➡ erythrocyte protein kinase C inhibitor
➡ adducin-spectrin-actin complex 유지시킴

반하 triterpenoid (C30H48O7S)
➡ Rho GTPase family transcription promotor
➡ heparan sulfate 생성 촉진
➡ heparin 유사 작용
➡ micro-emboli 용해

작약 paeoniflorin ➡ superoxide scavenger

천궁 cnidilide ➡ α-adrenergic receptor blocker

황금 baicalin ➡ peroxynitrite ($ONOO^-$) scavenger

이근백피 potassium citrate ➡ extracellular Ca2+ influx inhibitor

생강 gingerol ➡ hydrogen peroxide scavenger

감초 glycyrrhetinic acid
➡ 11-beta-hydroxysteroid dehydrogenase1 (HSD11B1) inhibitor
➡ glucocorticoid 작용
➡ IκBα 생성
➡ NF-κB 억제

갈근 daidzein ➡ ionotropic glutamate receptor blocker

사심탕 (瀉心湯)

원문 心氣 不足 , 吐 血 `衄 血 , 瀉心湯 主之 。
,亦 治 霍 亂

원문 해설 부교감신경이 약해져서 (산화질소 분비가 감소하면 박테리아 독성이 증가되어) 토혈과 코피가 있는 경우에 사심탕을 쓴다. 사심탕은 갑자기 토하고 설사하는 것을 낫게 한다.

적응증 Helicobacter pylori-mediated stomach bleeding

병태 & 증상

Helicobacter pylori-mediated stomach bleeding

➡ Helicobacter pylori in Stomach body & antrum
➡ Helicobacter pylori: 병원성 균으로 형질전환
➡ Helicobacter pylori: Cag pathogenicity island (Cag PAI) 유전자 활동
➡ H. pylori peptidoglycan: type IV secretion system 형성
➡ CagA protein: epithelialium 주입
➡ tyrosine kinase: CagA 인산화
➡ epithelialium: cytoskeletal rearrangement
➡ epithelialium: scattering and elongation
➡ 위상피세포끼리의 단단한 결합력이 약해져서 상피세포끼리의 간격이 넓어짐
➡ peptidoglycan: macrophage 유도
➡ extracellular peroxynitrite ($ONOO^-$)
: 넓어진 상피세포사이의 틈을 통해 점막하조직까지 $ONOO^-$ 확산
➡ submucosa necrosis
➡ bleeding

처방 목표 H. pylori peptidoglycan 합성 억제 / tyrosine kinase 차단 / peroxynitrite ($ONOO^-$) 제거

처방 구성 大黃 二兩 / 黃連 一兩 / 黃芩 一兩

처방 약리

황련 berberine ➡ sortase inhibitor

➡ H. pylori peptidoglycan 합성 억제

대황 emodin ➡ tyrosine kinase blocker

황금 baicalin ➡ peroxynitrite ($ONOO^-$) scavenger

사역가인삼탕 (四逆加人參湯)

원문 惡寒 脈 微 而 復 利, 利 止 亡血 也, 四逆加人參湯 主之。

원문 해설 오한이 나고 맥은 약하며 설사를 반복하다가 멈추는 것은 탈수가 된 것으로 사역가 인삼탕을 쓴다.

적응증 Polymyositis-associated gastrointestinal myositis (다발성근염에 연관된 위장관근염)

병태 & 증상

Polymyositis associated gastrointestinal myositis

➡ virus antigen & muscle protein: molecular mimicry

➡ virus antigen: antidody

➡ muscle protein 공격

➡ antibody-dependent cell-mediated cytotoxicity (ADCC)

➡ macrophage 유도

➡ neutrophil chemotactic factor 분비

➡ neutrophil 유도

➡ neutrophil phagocytosis

➡ HClO 분비 via H2O2

➡ muscle cell: Na+/K+ pumps 손상

➡ 근육세포 부종

➡ myositis

➡ 침범부위: gastrointestinal smooth muscle cell

➡ severe diarrhea

처방 목표 macrophage: neutrophil chemotactic factor 분비 억제 / HClO 분비 억제 / muscle cell Na+/ K+ pumps 활성화 / 위장관 평활근 재생 촉진

처방 구성 炙甘草 二兩 / 附子 一枚 / 乾薑 一兩半 / 人參 一兩

처방 약리

부자 hypaconitine

➡ 약리 추측: macrophage` Voltage-gated proton channels blocker
(식균작용에 의해 증가된 세포내 proton을 세포외로 방출시키는 채널)

➡ proton 방출 억제

➡ 세포내 pH ↓

➡ macrophage 대사 억제

➡ neutrophil chemotactic factor 분비 억제

건강 shogaol ➡ neutrophil H2O2 scavenger

➡ HClO 분비 억제

구감초 18β-24-Hydroxyglycyrrhetinic acid

➡ HSD11B2 inhibitor

➡ cortisol 분해 억제

➡ mineralocorticoid receptors 자극 지속

➡ Na+/ K+ pumps 전사 촉진

인삼 panax ginsenoside

➡ Transforming growth factor β (TGF-β) (+) modulator

➡ cell proliferation 촉진

사역산 (四逆散)

원문 少陰病, 四逆, 其人 或 咳, 或 悸, 或 小便 不利 或 腹中痛, 或 泄利下重 者, 四逆散 主之。咳 者, 加 五味子 `乾薑 各 五分, 並 主 下利。悸 者, 加 桂枝 五分。小便 不利 者, 加 茯苓 五分。腹中痛 者, 加 炮附子 一枚。泄利下重 者, 先 以 水 五 升, 煮 薤白 三升。

원문 해설 항체매개 독성병으로 팔다리에 냉기가 있고 혹 기침하고, 혹 두근거리고 혹 소변이 불편하고, 혹 배가 아프고, 혹 흩어지는 설사가 있는 경우에는 사역산을 쓴다. 기침이 있을 때 오미자와 건강을 추가하면 설사도 잡힌다. 두근거리면 계지를 추가한다. 소변이 불편하면 복령을 추가한다. 배가 아프면 포부자를 추가한다. 흩어지는 설사가 있는 경우에는 총백을 추가한다.

적응증 Hashimoto's thyroiditis (하시모토 갑상선염)

병태 & 증상

Hashimoto's thyroiditis

➡ chronic hepatitis
➡ hepatis virus replication
➡ hepatis virus infected hepatocyte: IFN-a 분비
➡ thyrocyte receptor: IFN-a 부착
➡ proteasome 활성화
➡ thyrocyte receptor: degradation
➡ degradation debris
➡ antigen presenting cell: phagocytosis
➡ Th1 cell: antigen 전달
➡ macrophage 활성화
➡ matrix metalloproteinases 분비 ▶ 갑상선 연골 파괴
➡ Th1 cell: IFN-γ 분비
➡ IFN-γ: thyroid transcription factor-1 결합
➡ thyroid transcription factor-1: 억제됨
➡ thyroglobulin / thyroid peroxidase / TSH receptor: 발현 억제됨
➡ thyroid peroxidase ↓
➡ O2 (thyroid peroxidase 기질) 소모되지 못하고 산화
➡ superoxide 축적
➡ superoxide: thyrocyte Na+/ K+ pumps 손상
➡ thyroditis
➡ 대사기능 약해짐: 체온조절 / 심장박동 / 호흡기능 / 소화기능 / 배뇨기능

처방 목표 hepatis virus replication 억제 / matrix metalloproteinases 억제 / superoxide 제거 / Na+/ K+ pumps 활성화

처방 구성 炙甘草 / 枳實 (炙) / 柴胡 / 芍藥　各 十分

처방 약리

시호 saikosaponin, 약리추측

➡ small interfering RNA (siRNA) (+) modulator

➡ hepatitis virus RNA replication inhibition

지실 auraptene ➡ matrix metalloproteinases (MMPs) blocker

작약 paeoniflorin ➡ superoxide scavenger

구감초 18β-24-Hydroxyglycyrrhetinic acid

➡ HSD11B2 inhibitor

➡ cortisol 분해 억제

➡ mineralocorticoid receptors 자극 지속

➡ Na+/ K+ pumps 전사 촉진

사역탕 (四逆湯)

원문 少陰病，脈沉者，急溫之，宜四逆湯。少陰病，飮食入口則吐，心中溫溫欲吐，復不能吐，始得之，手足寒，脈弦遲者，此胸中實，不可下也，當吐之。若膈上有寒飮，乾嘔者，不可吐也，當溫之，宜四逆湯。吐利，汗出，發熱，惡寒，四肢拘急，手足厥冷者，四逆湯 主之。

원문 해설 항체매개 감염증에서 맥이 가라앉아 있으면 빨리 따뜻하게 해주어야 한다. 사역탕을 쓴다. 항체매개 감염증에서 음식을 먹으면 그대로 토하고 가슴부위가 더운 느낌이있어 더 토하고 싶은데, 토가 나오지 않으며 병이 시작될 때 손발이 차고 맥이 튕기는 듯하면서 느린 경우는 가슴부위가 막혀 있는 것이므로 내려 보낼 것이 아니라 토를 시켜야 한다. 만약 가슴부위에 허혈로 인한 정체감이 있어서 건구역이 있는 경우에는 토를 시키지 말고 따뜻하게 만들어 주어야 하며 사역탕을 쓴다. 토하고 설사하며 땀나고 열이 있으면서 오한이 나면서 팔다리가 땅기고 손발이 극도로 차가워지는 경우에는 사역탕을 쓴다.

적응증 Polymyositis (다발성근염)

병태 & 증상

Polymyositis

➡ virus antigen & muscle protein: molecular mimicry
➡ virus antigen: antidody
➡ muscle protein 공격
➡ antibody-dependent cell-mediated cytotoxicity (ADCC)
➡ macrophage 유도
➡ neutrophil chemotactic factor 분비
➡ neutrophil 유도
➡ neutrophil phagocytosis
➡ HClO 분비 via H2O2
➡ muscle cell: Na+/ K+ pumps 손상
➡ 근육세포 부종
➡ myositis
➡ 주로: 후두인두근 / 호흡근육 / 팔다리 근육
➡ 연하곤란 & 환기부족 & 근무력증

처방 목표 macrophage: neutrophil chemotactic factor 분비 억제 / HClO 분비 억제 / muscle cell Na+/ K+ pumps 활성화

처방 구성 炙甘草 二兩 / 乾薑 一兩半 / 附子 一枚

처방 약리

부자 hypaconitine
➡ 약리 추측: macrophage` Voltage-gated proton channels blocker
(식균작용에 의해 증가된 세포내 proton을 세포외로 방출시키는 채널)
➡ proton 방출 억제
➡ 세포내 pH ↓
➡ macrophage 대사 억제
➡ neutrophil chemotactic factor 분비 억제

건강 shogaol ➡ neutrophil H2O2 scavenger
➡ HClO 분비 억제

구감초 18β-24-Hydroxyglycyrrhetinic acid
➡ HSD11B2 inhibitor

➡ cortisol 분해 억제
➡ mineralocorticoid receptors 자극 지속
➡ Na+/ K+ pumps 전사 촉진

산조인탕 (酸棗仁湯)

원문 虛勞 虛煩 不得眠, 酸棗仁湯 主之。

원문 해설 과로로 인해 몸이 괴로우면서 불면증이 있는 경우에는 산조인탕을 쓴다.

적응증 basilar artery hemorrhage-mediated Insomnia (뇌저동맥 출혈에 의한 불면증)

병태 & 증상

basilar artery hemorrhage-mediated insomnia

➡ overwork
➡ cortisol ↑
➡ basilar artery (뇌바닥동맥) endothelium: endothelin-1 발현
➡ basilar artery endothelium: p-selectin 발현
➡ basilar artery endothelium: leukocyte 침윤
➡ leukocyte cytokine
➡ basilar artery: arteriovenous malformation
➡ basilar artery: hemorrhage
➡ thrombus 형성
➡ basilar artery: smaller branches ▶ ischemia
➡ smaller branches endothelium: superoxide 생성
➡ smaller branches: vascular smooth muscle ▶ α-adrenergic Rc Ca channel 자극
➡ smaller branches: vasospasm
➡ brain stem: ischemia & apoptosis
➡ locus coeruleus (청반핵) 손상 & raphe nucleus (솔기핵) 손상
➡ raphe nucleus: serotonin mediated NREM sleep 유도: 실패
& locus coeruleus: norepinephrine mediated REM sleep 유도: 실패
➡ 수면 생리작용 깨짐
➡ insomnia

처방 목표 leukocyte cytokine 억제 / thrombus 제거 / α-adrenergic Rc 차단 / locus coeruleus & raphe nucleus 다분화 촉진 / serotonin & norepinephrine 합성 촉진

처방 구성 酸棗仁 二升 / 甘草 一兩 / 知母 二兩 / 茯苓 二兩 / 芎藭 二兩

처방 약리

감초 glycyrrhetinic acid
➡ 11-beta-hydroxysteroid dehydrogenase1 (HSD11B1) inhibitor
➡ glucocorticoid 작용
➡ IκBα 생성
➡ NF-κB 억제
➡ cytokine 생성 억제

복령 pachymic acid ➡ glycoprotein IIb/IIIa (gpIIb/IIIa) (-) modulator
➡ thrombus formation 억제

천궁 cnidilide ➡ α-adrenergic receptor blocker

지모 timosaponin ➡ nestin (+) modulator
➡ multi-differentiation 세포에서 발현되는 단백질
➡ neural stem cell: locus coeruleus & raphe nucleus 다분화 촉진

산조인 jujuboside / sanjoinine
➡ serotonin (+) modulator / norepinephrine (+) modulator

삼물비급환 (三物備急丸)

원문 三物備急丸 方 : 主 心 腹 諸 卒暴 百病 , 若 中惡 客 忤 , 心 腹 脹滿, 卒 痛 如 錐 刺 , 氣急 口噤 , 停 尸 卒 死 者 。

원문 해설 삼물비급환은 흉부와 위장관이 막혀서 갑자기 죽을 것 같은 증상에 쓴다. 만약 어느 통로가 막혔는지 알아 차릴수 없이 흉부와 복부가 터질 것 같고, 송곳으로 찌르는 듯한 통증이 있으며, 호흡이 막혀서 입을 다물지 못하고, 그 자리에서 갑자기 주검이 되려고 하는 경우를 치료한다.

적응증 Esophageal adenocarcinoma (식도선암) & Small cell lung carcinoma (소세포폐암) & Gastrointestinal stromal tumor (위장관 간질세포암)

병태 & 증상

Esophageal adenocarcinoma & Small cell lung carcinoma
& Gastrointestinal stromal tumor

➡ Barrett`s esophagus & chronic bronchitis & Gastrointestinal stromal cell
➡ chronic inflammation
➡ cyclin D1 overexpression
➡ p53 inactiviation
➡ cell cycle 지속
➡ growth factor 전사 활성: autocrine, paracrine
➡ tyrosine kinase 활성화
➡ Esophageal adenocarcinoma & Small cell lung carcinoma
& Gastrointestinal stromal tumor
➡ IL-8 분비
➡ neutrophil 유도
➡ neutrophil phagocytosis
➡ HClO 분비 via H2O2
➡ tumor shedding (암세포 축적)
➡ lumen 좁아짐

처방 목표 p53 활성화 / tyrosine kinase Rc 차단 / HClO 분비 억제

처방 구성 大黃 一兩 / 乾薑 一兩 / 巴豆 一兩

처방 약리

파두 phorbol ester ➡ squamous cell: protein kinase C (PKC) activator
➡ p53 gene transcription 촉진
➡ cell cycle 정지

대황 emodin ➡ tyrosine kinase Rc blocker

건강 shogaol ➡ neutrophil H2O2 scavenger
➡ HClO 분비 억제

삼물황금탕 (三物黃芩湯)

원문 三物黃芩湯, 治 婦人 在 草蓐, 自發 露 得 風, 四肢 苦 煩熱, 頭痛 者 與 小柴胡湯, 頭 不痛 但 煩 者, 此湯 主之, 多 吐下 蟲 。

원문 해설 부인이 산 후 회복기에 찬바람을 쐬어 팔다리에 괴로운 열감이 있는 경우에는 삼물황금탕을 쓰며, 두통까지 있으면 소시호탕을 병용하고, 두통이 없이 단지 괴롭기만 한 경우는 삼물황금탕만 쓴다. 복용하면 충을 토하거나 배변하게 된다.

적응증 Amebic liver abscess (아메바성 간농양)

병태 & 증상

Amebic liver abscess

➡ 장내 정상 기생 원충: Entamoeba histolytica
➡ bacteriophage 감염
➡ amoeba transformation
➡ tyrosinase 생성
➡ 이동에 필요한 actin cytoskeleton 활성화
➡ 장간막 정맥 & 림프관을 통해 장외로 이동 (간/ 뇌/ 흉막/ 폐/ 비장/ 피부)
: colon epithelium ▶ IL-8 분비 ▶ fever
➡ portal entry
➡ kupffer cell: phagocytosis & respiratory burst
➡ extracellular: peroxynitrite ($ONOO^-$) ↑
➡ hepatocyte lysis: large necrotic area 형성
➡ amoeba trophozoites: erythrocyte 탐식
➡ anemia

처방 목표 Entamoeba histolytica tyrosinase 억제 / extracellular: peroxynitrite ($ONOO^-$) 제거 / anemia 교정

처방 구성 黃芩 一兩 / 苦參 二兩 / 乾地黃 四兩

처방 약리

고삼 trifolirhizin ➡ protozoa tyrosinase (-) modulator

황금 baicalin ➡ peroxynitrite ($ONOO^-$) scavenger

건지황 catalpol, 약리 추측 ➡ CD133+ CFU-GEMM (+) modulator
➡ hematopoietic stem cell 분화 촉진
➡ erythrocyte 생성 촉진

생강반하탕 (生薑半夏湯)

원문 病人 胸中 似 喘 不喘 , 似 嘔 不嘔 , 似 噦 不噦 , 徹 心 中 憒 憒 然 無 奈 者 , 生薑半夏湯 主之 。

원문 해설 가슴부위에 호흡곤란기와 구역기, 구토기가 있으며 심장에 괴로운 감이 있는데 특별히 악화되지 않고 넘어가는 경우에는 생강반하탕을 쓴다.

적응증 Herpesvirus vagus neuritis (헤르페스 미주신경염)

병태 & 증상

Herpesvirus vagus neuritis

➡ vagus nerve: herpesvirus activation
➡ cytopathic effects
➡ vagus neuritis
➡ vagus nerve palsy
➡ vagus nerve branches
➡ 폐신경얼기 (과호흡 유발) / 식도신경얼기 (구역 유발) / 위장 가지 (구토 유발) / 심장가지 (부정맥 유발)

처방 목표 신경세포 상환 촉진

처방 약리 半夏 半升 / 生薑汁 一升

처방 약리

반하 triterpenoid ($C_{30}H_{48}O_7S$)
➡ Rho GTPase family transcription promotor

➡ focal adhesion 생성
➡ 상피세포 이동 촉진

생강 gingerol ➡ hydrogen peroxide scavenger
➡ focal adhesion kinase 활성화
➡ 상피세포의 입체적 이동 촉진

생강사심탕 (生薑瀉心湯)

원문 傷寒, 汗出 , 解 之 後, 胃中 不和, 心下 痞硬, 乾噫 食臭, 脅 下 有 水氣, 腹中 雷鳴 , 下利 者, 生薑瀉心湯 主之 。

원문 해설 세포병변성 감염병이 발열하고 나은 후, 위장에 불편감이 있고, 명치 밑에 속 쓰림과 단단함 감이 있으며, 음식 냄새가 나는 트림을 하고 뱃속이 꼬르륵 거리며 설사하는 경우에는 생강사심탕을 쓴다.

적응증 Duodenal ulcer

병태 & 증상

Duodenal ulcer

➡ Chronic gastric ulcer
➡ gas ↑ : food smell burp
➡ 유문부 D cell 손상
➡ somatostatin ↓
➡ gastrin ↑ : 위산 분비 ↑
➡ 십이지장: 위산에 노출됨
➡ 십이지장 상피: 위산 & 펩신 자극
➡ 십이지장 상피세포의 위상피화
➡ 십이지장: Helicobacter pylori 정착
➡ Helicobacter pylori: 병원성 균으로 형질전환
➡ Helicobacter pylori: Cag pathogenicity island (Cag PAI) 유전자 활동
➡ H. pylori peptidoglycan: type IV secretion system 형성
➡ peptidoglycan: macrophage 유도

➡ extracellular peroxynitrite ($ONOO^-$)
➡ 상피세포 & 점막세포 손상
➡ mucin 분비 ↓ : heartburn
➡ Helicobacter pylori: CagE gene
➡ epithelial cell: IL-8 분비
➡ neutrophil 유도
➡ neutrophil phagocytosis
➡ HClO 분비 via H2O2
➡ 점막근층 손상
➡ duodenal epithelium 손상: secretin 분비 ↓
➡ 유문부에서 내려오는 내용물의 산도 조절 실패
➡ 유문 괄약근 수축: stiffness
➡ 췌장 소화액 & 중탄산염 분비 ↓
➡ 정상적인 소화작용 실패 & 이당류에서 gas 발생: stomach growling & diarrhea

처방 목표 H. pylori peptidoglycan 합성 억제: 병독성 감소됨 / extracellular $ONOO^-$ 제거 / 세포 상환 촉진 / 입체적 상환 촉진 / 상피 & 점막세포 증식 촉진 / HClO 분비 억제 / 위산 분비 억제시킴

처방 구성 生薑 四兩 / 炙甘草 三兩 / 人參 三兩 / 乾薑 一兩 / 黃芩 三兩 / 半夏 半升 / 黃連 一兩 / 大棗 十二枚

처방 약리

황련 berberine ➡ sortase inhibitor
➡ H. pylori peptidoglycan 합성 억제
➡ 병독성 감소됨

황금 baicalin ➡ peroxynitrite ($ONOO^-$) scavenger

반하 triterpenoid (C30H48O7S)
➡ Rho GTPase family transcription promotor
➡ focal adhesion 생성
➡ 상피세포 이동 촉진

생강 gingerol ➡ hydrogen peroxide scavenger
➡ focal adhesion kinase 활성화
➡ 상피세포의 입체적 이동 촉진

인삼 panax ginsenoside

➡ Transforming growth factor β (TGF-β) (+) modulator

➡ cell proliferation 촉진

대조 c-AMP ➡ protein kinase A avtivator

➡ ATP 합성 촉진

➡ cell cycle ↑

건강 shogaol ➡ neutrophil H2O2 scavenger

➡ HClO 분비 억제

구감초 18β-24-Hydroxyglycyrrhetinic acid

➡ 11-beta-hydroxysteroid dehydrogenase2 (HSD11B2) inhibitor

➡ aldosterone 생리작용과 동일

➡ H+ secretion

➡ 위산 분비 차단

서여환 (薯蕷丸)

원문 虛勞 諸 不足，風氣 百疾，薯蕷丸 主之。

원문 해설 영양부족으로 인한 백가지 질병에 서여탕을 쓴다.

적응증 Malnutrition-mediated disease (영양실조-매개 질병)

병태 & 증상

Malnutrition-mediated disease

@ protein breakdown ↑

➡ collagen 형성 ↓ / digestive enzymes ↓

@ macrophage: arachidonic acid metabolites ↑

➡ bacteria capsule 생성 촉진

➡ 병독성 증가

@ macrophage: IL-10 분비 ↓ ➡ NF-kB 활성화
➡ immune tolerance 깨짐
➡ intracellular pathogen 공격
➡ viral hepatitis & tuberculosis

@ endothelium: TNF-α ↓ ➡ commensal bacteria 활성화
➡ MyD88 억제 단백질 분비
➡ 내피세포 TLR signal 차단
➡ pathogen bacteria 전환

@ erythrocyte GLUT (glucose transpoter) ↓
➡ ATP ↓
➡ 적혈구 골격단백질 결함
➡ deformity erythrocyte 생성
➡ 산소포화도 감소
➡ 조직 허혈: superoxide 생성
➡ 혈관평활근: α-adrenergic Rc Ca channel 자극
➡ vasospasm
➡ tissue hypoxia
➡ lactatemia

@ neutrophil CD11b/CD18 ↓
➡ neutrophil exudation ↓
➡ neutrophil phagocytosis
➡ HClO 분비 via H2O2
➡ vascular endothelium: VCAM-1 발현
➡ leukocyte & monocyte adhesion
➡ 혈관내피하 공간: leukocyte & monocyte 이동
➡ 혈관내피 손상
➡ 혈소판 응집: thrombus formation

@ hemolysis ↑
➡ ferrous ion ↑
➡ neutrophil mediated H2O2
➡ hydroxyl radical 생성
-➡〉 tissue damage

처방 목표 protein 보충 / collagen 형성 촉진 / digestive enzymes 보충 / macrophage: arachidonic acid 대사 억제 / bacteria capsule 생성 억제 / macrophage: NF-kB 억제 / viral hepatitis 억제 / 내피세포 TLR signal 회복 / erythrocyte GLUT 발현 촉진 / 적혈구 골격단백질 유지 / superoxide 제거 / α-adrenergic Rc 차단 / lactatemia 교정 / HClO 분비 억제 / vascular endothelium: VCAM-1 차단 / thrombus 제거 / erythrocyte 생성 촉진 / hydroxyl radical 제거 / 손상된 조직: 세포 증식 촉진

처방 구성 薯蕷 三十分 / 當歸 十分 / 桂枝 十分 / 曲 十分 / 乾地黃 十分 / 豆黃卷 十分 / 甘草 二十八分 / 人參 七分 / 芎藭 六分 / 芍藥 六分 / 白朮 六分 / 麥門冬 六分 / 杏仁 六分 / 柴胡 五分 / 桔梗 五分 / 茯苓 五分 / 阿膠 七分 / 乾薑 三分 / 白斂 二分 / 防風 六分 / 大棗 百枚

처방 약리

두황 (콩가루) protein supplement

아교 glycine / proline / hydroxyproline / alanine ➡ collagen 주요 아미노산
➡ collagen 합성 촉진

곡 (누룩) α-amylase / protease / lipase ➡ digestive enzymes

방풍 deltoin ➡ cyclooxygenase-2 blocker
➡ arachidonic acid 대사 억제

백렴 gallotanin ➡ glucosyltransferase inhibitor
➡ bacteria capsule 생성 억제

감초 glycyrrhetinic acid
➡ 11-beta-hydroxysteroid dehydrogenase1 (HSD11B1) inhibitor
➡ glucocorticoid 작용
➡ IκBα 생성
➡ macrophage: NF-κB 억제

시호 saikosaponin, 약리 추측 ➡ small interfering RNA (siRNA) (+) modulator
➡ hepatitis virus RNA replication inhibition

맥문동 ophiopogonin, 약리 추측 ➡ M. tuberculosis` SigF transcription inhibitor

➡ M. tuberculosis growth 억제됨

길경 platycodin ➡ toll like receptor (+) modulator

서여 (산약) diosgenin ➡ erythrocyte GLUT (+) modulator
➡ glucose 유입 촉진
➡ ATP 증가

당귀 decurcin ➡ erythrocyte protein kinase C inhibitor
➡ adducin-spectrin-actin complex 유지시킴

작약 paeoniflorin ➡ superoxide scavenger

천궁 cnidilide ➡ α-adrenergic receptor blocker

계지 cinnamic acid ➡ lactate oxidizer
➡ Cori cycle: pyruvate 전환
➡ lactatemia 교정

건강 shogaol ➡ neutrophil H2O2 scavenger
➡ HClO 분비 억제

백출 atractylon ➡ vascular cell adhesion molecule-1 (VCAM-1) blocker

복령 pachymic acid ➡ glycoprotein IIb/IIIa (gpIIb/IIIa) (-) modulator
➡ thrombus formation 억제

건지황 catalpol, 약리 추측 ➡ CD133+ CFU-S (+) modulator
➡ hematopoietic stem cell 분화 촉진
➡ erythrocyte 생성 촉진

행인 benzoic acid ➡ hydroxyl radical scavenger

인삼 panax ginsenoside
➡ Transforming growth factor beta (TGF-β) (+) modulator
➡ 점막세포 증식 촉진

대조 c-AMP ➡ protein kinase A avtivator

➡ ATP 합성 촉진
➡ cell cycle

선복화탕 (旋覆花湯)

원문 肝 著, 其人 常 欲 蹈 其 胸 上, 先 未 苦 時, 但 欲 飮 熱, 旋覆花湯 主 之。

원문 해설 간문맥이 두꺼워지는 병에 걸리면 발을 동동거리고 가슴을 두드리게 된다. 아직 고통이 심하지는 않으며 오로지 뜨거운 것만 마시려고 하는 경우에는 선복화탕을 쓴다.

적응증 Portal vein thrombosis (간문맥 혈전증)

병태 & 증상

Portal vein thrombosis

➡ portal vein endothelium: cytomegalovirus infection
➡ cytomegalovirus replication: superoxide ↑
➡ portal vein endothelium: Cu2+ induced peroxidation
➡ portal vein endothelium: apoptosis
➡ tissue factor 분비
➡ thrombin formation
➡ fibrin formation
➡ fibrin 자극: smooth muscle cell 이동 & 증식
➡ vein wall: stiffness
➡ portal vein: outflow block

처방 목표 portal vein endothelium: Cu2+ induced peroxidation 억제 / thrombin formation 억제 / portal vein: smooth muscle cell 증식 억제
처방 구성 旋覆花 三兩 / 葱 十四莖 / 新絳 少許

처방 약리

선복화 teraxasterol ➡ Cu2+ induced lipid peroxidation inhibitor

총백 allicin ➡ factor VII, IX, X absorbent

➡ thrombin formation 억제

신강 (꼭두서니 뿌리) alizarin, 약리 추측

➡ vein smooth muscle cell: proliferation inhibitor

소건중탕 (小建中湯)

원문 傷寒 二 三 日，心中 悸 而 煩 者，小建中湯 主之。傷寒，陽脈 澀，陰脈 弦，法 當 腹中 急痛，先 與 小建中湯，不 差 者，與 小柴胡湯 主之。虛勞 裡急，悸 `衄，腹中痛，夢失精，四肢 痠疼, 手足 煩熱, 咽乾 口燥，小建中湯 主之。

원문 해설 세포병변성 감염병이 2~3일이 지난 후, 심장이 두근거리고 편하지 않은 경우에는 소건중탕을 쓴다. 세포병변성 감염병으로 양맥은 막혀 있고, 음맥은 팽팽하면, 배가 땅기면서 아플 것이다, 먼저 소건중탕을 쓰고, 낫지 않으면 소시호탕을 쓴다. 과로하여 신체가 땅기고, 두근거림과 코피 및 복통이 있고, 과도한 성교에 의해 팔다리가 저리고 쑤시며, 손과 발에 불편한 열감이 있고, 목구멍이 건조하고 입이 마르면 소건중탕을 쓴다.

적응증 Picornavirus infection / Hypoglycemia (저혈당)

병태 & 증상

Picornavirus infection

➡ small intestine epithelium: maltose receptor

▶ picornavirus (coxsackievirus & hepatitis A virus) binding

➡ small intestine epithelium: coxsackievirus & hepatitis A virus

▶ first replication

➡ viremia

➡ coxsackievirus: cardiomyocyte 이동 ▶ cardiomyositis

& hepatitis A virus: hepatocyte 이동 ▶ hepatitis

처방 목표 small intestine epithelium: maltose receptor 차단 / picornavirus replication 억제

처방 구성 桂枝 三兩 / 芍藥 六兩 / 生薑 三兩 / 炙甘草 二兩 / 大棗 十二枚 / 膠飴 一升

처방 약리

교이 maltose ➡ small intestine epithelium: maltose receptor 부착
➡ picornavirus 부착 차단

계지탕 heat shock protein 생산 ➡ viral replication 억제

소반하가복령탕 (小半夏加茯苓湯)

원문 卒 嘔 吐 , 心 下 痞 , 膈 間 有 水 , 眩 悸 者 , 小半夏加茯苓湯 主之 。

원문 해설 죽을 것 같은 구토를 하고 심장이 저리며 흉부에 수분이 축적되고 어지럼증이 있는 경우에는 소반하가복령탕을 쓴다.

적응증 Superior vena cava thrombosis in Behcet's Disease (베체트 상대정맥 혈전증)

병태 & 증상

Superior vena cava thrombosis in Behcet's Disease

➡ streptococcus infection
➡ streptococcus surface protein & 상대정맥 epithelium: molecular mimicry
➡ streptococcus surface protein: antibody 생성
➡ 상대정맥 epithelium: antibody 부착
➡ antibody-dependent cell-mediated cytotoxicity: macrophage 유도
➡ 상대정맥 epithelium: vasculitis
➡ thrombus formation
➡ superior vena cava syndrome: vomiting, chest pain, swelling, dizziness

처방 목표 상대정맥 내피세포 상환 촉진 / thrombus 제거

처방 구성 半夏 一升 / 生薑 半斤 / 茯苓 三兩 一法 四兩 。

처방 약리

반하 triterpenoid (C30H48O7S)

➡ Rho GTPase family transcription promotor
➡ focal adhesion 생성
➡ 상피세포 이동 촉진

생강 gingerol ➡ hydrogen peroxide scavenger
➡ focal adhesion kinase 활성화
➡ 상피세포의 입체적 이동 촉진

복령 pachymic acid ➡ glycoprotein IIb/IIIa (gpIIb/IIIa) (-) modulator
➡ thrombus formation 억제

소반하탕 (小半夏湯)

원문 嘔家本渴, 渴者為欲解, 今反不渴, 心下有支飮故也, 小半夏湯主之。

원문 해설 구역이 있으면 본래 갈증이 생기는데 (기저막 콜라겐 재생 시에 물 소모), 갈증이 있는 것은 병이 나으려고 하는 것이다.(기저막 재생) 지금 반대로 갈증이 없는 것은 식도부위에 혈관내피 부종이 있고 기저막은 손상되지 않은 것이다. 소반하탕을 쓴다.

적응증 Esophagitis in Behcet's Disease (베체트 식도염)

병태 & 증상

Esophagitis in Behcet's Disease

➡ streptococcus infection
➡ streptococcus surface protein & 식도세동맥 pericyte desmin: molecular mimicry
➡ streptococcus surface protein: antibody 생성
➡ pericyte desmin: antibody 부착
➡ antibody-dependent cell-mediated cytotoxicity: macrophage 유도
➡ pericyte 손상
➡ 혈관내피 부종
➡ 식도 상피세포: 허혈 손상
➡ esophagitis

처방 목표 식도 상피세포 상환 촉진

처방 구성 半夏 一升 / 生薑 半斤

처방 약리

반하 triterpenoid (C30H48O7S)

➡ Rho GTPase family transcription promotor

➡ focal adhesion 생성

➡ 상피세포 이동 촉진

생강 gingerol ➡ hydrogen peroxide scavenger

➡ focal adhesion kinase 활성화

➡ 상피세포의 입체적 이동 촉진

소승기탕 (小承氣湯)

원문 下利 譫語 者， 有 燥屎 也，小承氣湯 主之。

원문 해설 설사하고 헛소리를 하며 변이 딱딱한 경우에는 소승기탕을 쓴다.

적응증 Diffuse large B cell lymphoma of gastric MALT
(위장 점막림프조직의 미만성 B세포 림프종)

병태 & 증상

Diffuse large B cell lymphoma of gastric MALT

➡ gastric MALT lymphoma

➡ VEGF autocrine

➡ diffuse large B cell lymphoma 형성

➡ diffuse large B cell lymphoma: growth factor autocrine

➡ tyrosine kinase Rc: diffuse large B cell lymphoma 성장

➡ diffuse large B cell: matrix metalloproteinases (MMP) 분비

➡ lymph node: destruction

➡ diffuse large B cell: dissemination

➡ 주로 small intestine & brain
▶diffuse large B cell lymphoma 침투
▶ diarrhea, clouded consciousness, hard stool

처방 목표 VEGF Rc 차단 ➡ B cell transformation 억제 / tyrosine kinase Rc 차단 / matrix metalloproteinases (MMP) 차단

처방 구성 大黃 四兩 / 厚朴 二兩 / 枳實 大者 三枚

처방 약리

대황 emodin ➡ tyrosine kinase Rc blocker
➡ diffuse large B cell lymphoma 성장 억제

후박 honokiol ➡ VEGF receptor blocker
➡ B cell lymphoma transformation 억제

지실 auraptene ➡ matrix metalloproteinases (MMPs) blocker
➡ diffuse large B cell 전이 억제

소시호탕 (小柴胡湯)

원문 少陽 之 為 病，口苦，咽乾，目眩 也。傷寒，脈 弦 細，頭痛 發熱 者，屬 少陽。少陽 不可 發汗，發汗 則 譫語，此 屬 胃，胃 和 則 愈，胃 不和，煩 而 悸。傷寒 五 六 日，中風，往來 寒熱，胸脅 苦滿，嘿嘿 不 欲 飮食，心煩 喜 嘔, 或 胸 中 煩 而 不 嘔，或 渴，或 腹 中 痛，或 脅 下 痞 硬，或 心 下 悸 ˋ小便不利，或 不 渴 ˋ身 有 微熱，或 咳 者，小柴胡湯 主之。

원문 해설 간 세망내피계 감염병은 입이 쓰며 목이 건조해지고 눈 어지럼증이 생긴다. 세포병변성 감염병으로 맥이 울리면서 가늘고 두통과 발열이 있는 경우는 간 세망내피계에 병이 생긴 것이다. 간 세망내피계 감염병은 계지탕류를 쓰지 않는다, 계지탕류로 발한을 유도하면 대식세포가 활성화되어 간염이 더 심해져서 간성혼수가 올 수 있다. 이 병은 소장에서 1차 증식하는 장바이러스 질병으로 여기서 바이러스가 억제되면 낫고, 그렇지 않으면 심근으로 이동될 수 있다. 세포병변성 감염병이 5~6일이 지나 IL-1 매개증상이 생겨, 추위와 더위가 번갈아 있고, 가슴 옆 부위에 불쾌한 팽만감이 있으며, 매사가 귀찮고 식욕이 없으며 마음이 괴롭고 구역이 생긴 경우,

혹 괴롭기는 하나 구역은 없으며, 혹 갈증이 있고, 혹 배가 아프고, 혹 갈빗대 아래로 아리고 딱딱한 감이 있고, 혹 가슴이 두근거리고, 소변이 불편하고, 혹 갈증 없이 미열이 있고, 혹 기침이 있는 경우에는 소시호탕을 쓴다.

若 胸 中 煩 而 不 嘔 者, 去 半夏 `人參, 加 栝蔞實 一枚。若 渴 者, 去 半夏, 加 人參 合 前 成 四兩半, 栝蔞根 四兩。若 腹 中 痛 者, 去 黃芩, 加 芍藥 三兩。若 脅 下 痞 硬, 去 大棗, 加 牡蠣 四兩。若 心 下 悸 `小便 不利 者, 去 黃芩, 加 茯苓 四兩。若 不 渴 `外 有 微熱 者, 去 人參, 加 桂枝 三兩, 溫 覆 微 汗 癒。若 咳 者, 去 人參 `大棗 `生薑, 加 五味子 半升, 乾薑 二兩。

원문 해설 만약 구역이 없으면 간세포 재생은 없는 것이므로 반하와 인삼을 빼고 간성상세포가 근섬유모세포로 표현형이 변하지 않도록 과루실을 추가한다. 갈증이 있는 경우에는 간섬유화가 진행되고 있는 것이므로 반하는 빼고 섬유소용해에 필요한 TGF-β를 발현하도록 인삼을 추가하고, 섬유소 생산을 억제하도록 과루근도 추가한다. 만약 배가 아프면 간염바이러스의 증식에 의한 superoxide 배출증가가 원인이므로 황금은 빼고 작약을 추가한다. 갈빗대 밑에 단단한 감이 있는 것은 간경변 증상으로 알부민이 감소하여 저나트륨혈증이 생길 수 있으므로 대조를 빼고 모려를 추가한다. 간염이 있으면서 두근거림과 소변이 불편한 증상이 있는 것은 간기능이 저하되어 혈액응고인자가 감소해서 생기는 것이므로 황금을 빼고 복령을 추가한다.
갈증이 끝난 것은 간경변이 있는 것으로 TGF-β에 의해 용해가 되지 않으므로 인삼은 빼고, 간문맥 내피세포와 간세포의 허혈이 있으므로 계지를 추가한다. 간염이 있으면서 기침이 있는 것은 만성간염에서 바이러스항원에 대한 항체에 폐간질이 자가면역반응을 일으켜 collagen vascular disease가 생긴 것으로 alveolitis에 의한 기침이 발생되며 인삼/대조/생강은 빼고 오미자와 건강을 추가한다.

傷寒, 陽脈 濇, 陰脈 弦, 法 當 腹 中 急 痛, 先 與 小建中湯, 不 差 者, 與 小柴胡湯 主之。傷寒 中風, 有 柴胡證, 但 見 一 證 便 是, 不 必 悉 具。凡 柴胡湯 病證 而 下 之, 若 柴胡證 不 罷 者, 復 與 柴胡湯, 必 蒸 蒸 而 振, 卻 復 發熱 汗出 而 解。陽明病, 發 潮 熱, 大便 溏, 小便 自 可, 胸脅滿 不去 者, 與 小柴胡湯。陽明病, 脅下 硬滿, 不 大便, 而 嘔, 舌上 白胎 者, 可 與 小柴胡湯, 上焦 得 通, 津液 得 下, 胃氣 因 和, 身 濈 然 汗出 而 解。

원문 해설 세포병변성 감염병으로 양맥은 막히는 느낌이 있고, 음맥은 울리는 것 같으면 당연히 배가 아플 것이다, 먼저 소건중탕을 쓰고 낫지 않으면 소시호탕을 쓴다. 세포병변성 감염병과 IL-1매개 감염병에서 모든 증상이 구비되지 않더라도 한가지 증상이

라도 있으면 시호를 쓸 수 있다. 시호탕 병증을 치료했는데도 여전히 증상이 계속되면 다시 시호탕을 쓰며 이후에는 반드시 찌는 듯이 열이 나고 몸이 떨리게 되며, 다시 발열하고 땀이 나면서 낫게 된다. 위장관 점막림프절 감염병으로 조수가 반복되는 듯한 열이 있고, 대변이 묽고, 갈빗대옆 쪽으로 팽만감이 가시지 않으면 소시호탕을 쓴다. 위장관 점막림프절 감염병으로 갈빗대 옆쪽으로 딱딱한 팽만감이 있으면서 대변이 힘들고 구역이 있으면서 백태가 보이는 경우에 소시호탕을 쓰면, 간경변에 의한 저나트륨혈증이 교정되어 뇌독성이 치료되며, 알부민 생성도 촉진되고, 간세포 허혈도 개선되어 소화기능도 회복되고, 땀을 흥건히 흘리고 낫게 된다.

적응증 Viral hepatitis (type A, B) (바이러스성 간염)

병태 & 증상

Type A hepatitis

contaminated water & food: digestion

intestinal endothelium : hepatitis A virus (HAV) infection

➡ HAV virion 성숙

➡ intestinal lumen: 방출

➡ portal vein endothelium: 침투

➡ HAV infected endothelium: collagenase 분비

➡ 문맥기저막 분해 후 간실질로 침투

➡ Kupffer cells: HAV infection

➡ phagocytosis & respiratory burst

➡ extracellular: peroxynitrite ($ONOO^-$) ↑

➡ hepatitis

&

➡ hepatocyte: HAV infection

➡ RNA polymerase

➡ virus replicon RNAs

➡ hepatocyte: viral antigen 발현

➡ cytotoxic T cell 유도

➡ hepatitis

* Type B hepatitis

➡ blood & body fluid: transmission

➡ Kupffer cells: HBV infection

➡ phagocytosis & respiratory burst
➡ extracellular: peroxynitrite ($ONOO^-$) ↑
➡ hepatitis
&
➡ hepatocyte: hepatitis B virus (HBV) infection
➡ RNA Polymerase II
➡ virus replicon RNAs
➡ hepatocyte: viral antigen 발현
➡ cytotoxic T cell 유도
➡ hepatitis
&
➡ HBV infected hepatocyte: NOS2 gene expression ↑
➡ nitric oxide + superoxide
➡ peroxynitrite ($ONOO^-$) ↑
➡ HBV DNA: mutation
➡ hepatocyte: viral antigen 발현 실패
➡ chronic hepatitis

처방 목표 peroxynitrite ($ONOO^-$) 제거 / virus replicon RNAs 제거 / hepatocyte 재생 / 재생된 hepatocyte 이동 & 대사 촉진

처방 구성 柴胡 半斤 / 黃芩 三兩 / 人參 三兩 / 半夏 半升 / 炙甘草 三兩 / 生薑 三兩 / 大棗 十二枚

처방 약리

황금 baicalin ➡ peroxynitrite ($ONOO^-$) scavenger

시호 saikosaponin, 약리추측 ➡ small interfering RNA (siRNA) (+) modulator
➡ hepatitis virus RNA replication inhibition

인삼 panax ginsenoside
➡ Transforming growth factor β (TGF-β) (+) modulator
➡ hepatocyte proliferation 촉진

반하 triterpenoid (C30H48O7S)
➡ Rho GTPase family transcription promotor
➡ focal adhesion 생성
➡ 상피세포 이동 촉진

생강 gingerol ➡ hydrogen peroxide scavenger
➡ focal adhesion kinase 활성화
➡ 상피세포의 입체적 이동 촉진

대조 c-AMP ➡ Protein kinase A avtivator
➡ ATP 합성 촉진
➡ cell cycle ↑

구감초 18β-24-Hydroxyglycyrrhetinic acid
➡ HSD11B2 inhibitor
➡ cortisol 분해 억제
➡ mineralocorticoid receptors 자극 지속
➡ 재생된 hepatocyte Na+/ K+ pumps 활성화

소청룡탕 (小青龍湯)

원문 傷寒, 表不解, 心下 有 水氣, 乾嘔, 發熱 而 咳, 或 渴 , 或 利 , 或 噎 , 或 小便 不利 , 少腹滿 , 或 喘 者, 小青龍湯 主之 。

원문 해설 세포병변성 감염병에서(숙주세포에서 바이러스 증식 후 세포 파괴) 발열과 오한이 해소되지 않으며, 폐포 간질에 수분이 축적되고, 구역이 있으며 열나면서 기침하고, 혹 갈증, 설사, 기도 이물감, 소변불리, 아랫배 팽만감, 호흡곤란이 있는 경우에는 소청룡탕을 쓴다.

적응증 Viral pneumonia (바이러스성 폐렴)

병태 & 증상

Viral pneumonia

➡ main cause: influenza virus
➡ bronchial cell infection
➡ CC chemokine 분비
➡ eosinophil 유도
➡ eosinophil degranulation: neusea, feeling of irritation, fever

➡ bronchitis: cough, wheezing
➡ alveolar epithelial cell infection
➡ IL-8 분비
➡ neutrophil 유도
➡ neutrophil phagocytosis
➡ HClO 분비 via H2O2
➡ alveolar-capillary barrier 손상
➡ 폐포 간질: erythrocyte 유입 & 수분 축적: thirsty
➡ Met hemoglobin 형성
➡ alveolar epithelium: ischemia
➡ alveolitis
➡ hypoxemia
➡ tissue hypoxia: superoxide ↑ & lactate ↑ & Na+/ K+ pumps 약화
➡ urine retention, abdominal distension, diarrhea

처방 목표 eosinophil degranulation 억제 / HClO 분비 억제 / Met hemoglobin 환원 / 폐포 세포 상환 촉진 / tissue hypoxia: superoxide 제거 / tissue hypoxia: lactate 교정 / tissue hypoxia: Na+/ K+ pumps 활성화 / 폐환기량 증가: 횡격막근 수축 강화

처방 구성 麻黃 / 芍藥 / 細辛 / 乾薑 / 炙甘草 / 桂枝　各 三兩 / 五味子 半升 / 半夏 半升

처방 약리

마황 ephedrine ➡ Epinephrine receptors agonist
➡ adenylate cyclase 활성화
➡ cAMP ↑
➡ eosinophil degranulation 억제

건강 shogaol ➡ neutrophil H2O2 scavenger
➡ HClO 분비 억제

세신 eugenol ➡ MetHb reducer

반하 triterpenoid (C30H48O7S)
➡ Rho GTPase family transcription promotor

➡ focal adhesion 생성
➡ 폐포 상피세포 이동 촉진

작약 paeoniflorin ➡ superoxide scavenger

계지 cinnamic acid ➡ lactate oxidizer
➡ pyruvate 전환

구감초 18β-24-Hydroxyglycyrrhetinic acid
➡ HSD11B2 inhibitor
➡ cortisol 분해 억제
➡ mineralocorticoid receptors 자극 지속
➡ Na+/ K+ pumps 전사 활성화

오미자 schizandrin ➡ acetylcholinesterase inhibitor
➡ 횡격막근 수축 강화

소함흉탕 (小陷胸湯)

원문 小結胸 病 , 正 在 心下 , 按 之 則 痛 , 脈 浮 滑 者, 小陷胸湯 主之 。

원문 해설 위장에 침습성궤양이 생기는 병으로, 명치 밑 중앙부위에 병소가 있고, 누르면 통증이 있으며, 맥이 뜨면서 매끈한 경우에는 소함흉탕을 쓴다.

적응증 Gastric adenocarcinoma (위암)

병태 & 증상

Gastric adenocarcinoma

➡ Stomach body & antrum: Helicobacter pylori 감염
➡ Helicobacter pylori: 병원성 균으로 형질전환
➡ H. pylori peptidoglycan: type IV secretion system 형성
➡ mucosal cell: CagA protein 주입
➡ mucosal cell: cytoskeleton 붕괴

➡ gastric ulcer 반복
➡ gastric mucosal cells: metaplasia (intestine epithelium)
➡ chronic atrophic gastritis
➡ gastric mucosal cells: syndecan 소실
➡ gastric mucosal cells: phenotypic transition
➡ fibroblast-like cell 전환
➡ fibroblast-like cell: collagenase 분비
➡ invasion & metastasis

처방 목표 H. pylori peptidoglycan 합성 억제 / gastric mucosal cells: syndecan 형성 촉진 / fibroblast-like cell 전환 억제

처방 구성 黃連 一兩 / 半夏 半升 / 栝蔞實 大者 一枚

처방 약리

황련 berberine ➡ sortase inhibitor
➡ H. pylori peptidoglycan 합성 억제

반하 triterpenoid (C30H48O7S)
➡ Rho GTPase family transcription promotor
➡ syndecan 생성 촉진

과루실 cucurbitacin
➡ endothelium의 fibroblast 분화에 필요한 actin cytoskeleton 붕괴시킴
➡ gastric mucosal cells ▶ fibroblast-like cell 전환 억제

속명탕 (續命湯)

원문 續命湯, 治 中風痱 , 身體 不能 自收持 , 口 不能 言 , 冒 昧 不 知 痛 處 , 或 拘 急 不 得 轉 側 。

원문 해설 속명탕은 반신불수를 낫게 하며, 스스로 움직이지 못하는 것과 언어장애와 아픈 곳을 느끼지 못하면서 몸이 땅겨서 움직이지 못하는 것을 치료한다.

적응증 Intracerebral hemorrhage (뇌출혈)

병태 & 증상

Intracerebral hemorrhage

➡ blood pressure ↑
➡ intracerebral hemorrhage
➡ 흔한 발생 부위: lateral lenticulo-striate artery (선조체동맥 외측지)
➡ 손상부위와 증상: 피각부 ▶ 반신마비, 언어장애, 시상부 ▶ 반대측 사지저림, 피질하 ▶ 계산불능, 좌우인지 불능, 실서증, 뇌교 ▶ 사지마비, 호흡장애, 의식장애, 소뇌 ▶ 어지럼증, 구토, 진전
➡ 뇌실질: erythrocyte 유출
➡ 적혈구 골격단백질 손상
➡ complement 부착
➡ complement cascade: membrane attack complement (MAC) 생성
➡ MAC mediated erythrocyte lysis
➡ hematoma 생성
➡ ferrous ion: neutrophil 유도
➡ neutrophil phagocytosis
➡ HClO 분비 via H2O2
➡ HClO + ferrous ion ▶ hydroxyl radical 생성
➡ hydroxyl radical ▶ basilar artery α-adrenergic Rc 자극
➡ vasospasm
➡ 허혈 ↑ ▶ 세포질 lactate ↑ ▶ 세포내 산증 ▶ ATP 고갈
▶ ion pump 손상 ▶ 세포외액 유입 ▶ 뇌세포부종
➡ hematoma: microglia 유도
➡ microglia secretion: IL-1, TNF-α
➡ blood-brain barrier: leakage
➡ T cell 유입
➡ B cell 유도: myelin autoantibody 생성
➡ demyelination

처방 목표 적혈구 골격단백질 유지 / HClO 분비 억제 / hydroxyl radical 제거 / α-adrenergic Rc 차단 / 세포질 lactate 교정 / microglia secretion 억제 / T cell apoptosis 유도 / myelin autoantibody 생성 억제 / neuron & oligodendrocyte 재생

처방 구성 麻黃 / 桂枝 / 當歸 / 人參 / 石膏 / 乾薑 / 甘草 各 三兩 / 芎藭 一兩 / 杏

仁 四十枚

처방 약리

당귀 decurcin ➡ erythrocyte protein kinase C inhibitor
➡ adducin-spectrin-actin complex 유지시킴

건강 shogaol ➡ neutrophil H_2O_2 scavenger
➡ HClO 분비 억제

행인 benzoic acid ➡ hydroxyl radical scavenger

천궁 cnidilide ➡ α-adrenergic receptor blocker

계지 cinnamic acid ➡ lactate oxidizer
➡ pyruvate 전환

마황 ephedrine ➡ Epinephrine receptors agonist
➡ adenylate cyclase 활성화
➡ cAMP ↑
➡ microglia secretion 억제

석고 $CaSO_4$ ➡ calcium mediated T-cell apoptosis 유도

감초 glycyrrhetinic acid
➡ 11-beta-hydroxysteroid dehydrogenase1 (HSD11B1) inhibitor
➡ glucocorticoid 작용
➡ IκBα 생성
➡ NF-κB 억제
➡ 항체 생성 억제

인삼 panax ginsenoside
➡ Transforming growth factor β (TGF-β) (+) modulator
➡ SVZ neuronal progenitors: TGF-β (+) modulation
➡ neuron & oligodendrocyte: proliferation 촉진

승마별갑탕 (升麻鱉甲湯)

원문 陽毒 之 為 病，面 赤 斑 斑 如 錦 紋，咽喉痛，唾 膿 血, 五日 可 治, 七日 不可 治，升麻鱉甲湯 主之。陰毒 之 為 病，面目 青，身痛 如 被杖，咽喉痛。五日 可 治，七日 不可 治, 升麻鱉甲湯 去 雄黃 `蜀椒 主之。

원문 해설 세포 외 톡소플라스마증이 생기면 얼굴에 비단결 같은 붉은 반진이 생기고 인후통과 토혈이 있게 되는데, 5일 안으로는 치료가 가능하고, 7일이 지나면 치료가 안 된다. 승마별갑탕을 쓴다. 대식세포내에서 톡소플라스마증이 생기면 안면과 눈이 파래지고 몽둥이로 맞은 것처럼 몸이 아프며, 인후통이 생긴다. 5일안으로는 치료가 가능하고 7일이 지나면 치료가 안 된다. 승마별갑탕에서 웅황을 빼고 촉초를 가하여 쓴다.

적응증 Toxoplasmosis (톡소플라즈마증)

병태 & 증상

Toxoplasmosis

➡ cyst 섭취: toxoplasma gondii infection

➡ tachyzoites: erythrocyte 침입

➡ erythrocyte: calcium influx ↑ ▶ protein kinase C 활성화
▶ mitochondria respiration ↑
▶ tachyzoites multiplication

➡ tachyzoites 방출

➡ toxoplasma antibody & complement

➡ vasculitis: flat rash, sore throat, hemoptysis

➡ tissue 이동

➡ tissue macrophage: tachyzoites infection

➡ intracellular macrophage
: tubulovesicular membrane ▶ cholesterol 유입 ▶ 세포내 소기관 합성

➡ tachyzoites: microneme protein (EGF-like) 분비

➡ intracellular macrophage: Inositol trisphosphate 활성화
▶ mitogen-activated protein kinase 활성화
▶ gene transcription ↑

➡ microneme protein (EGF-like): p53 phoshorylation 억제
▶ cell cycle 지속

➡ intracellular macrophage: parasitophorous vacuole membrane

▶ IκB 인산화 ▶ NF-κB 활성화

▶ antiapoptosis gene 전사 촉진

➡ tachyzoites infected macrophage: potassium channel ▶ K+ 유출

➡ membrane permeabilization ↑

➡ toxoplasma gondii: 세포외 방출

➡ macrophage lysis: swollen lymph nodes ▶ sore throat, body ache

➡ tissue dissemination

: dermal infiltration / eye infiltration

/ encephalitis / myocarditis / pneumonia / hepatitis

➡ severe toxoplasmosis: death

처방 목표 erythrocyte: protein kinase C 억제 / toxoplasma gondii: pyruvate kinase 억제 / tubulovesicular membrane ▶ cholesterol 유입 억제 / p53 phoshorylation 촉진 / IκB 생성 촉진 / macrophage: potassium channel 차단

처방 구성 升麻 二兩 / 當歸 一兩 / 甘草 二兩 / 雄黃 半兩 / 鱉甲 手指 大 一片 (炙) / 蜀椒 一兩

처방 약리

당귀 decurcin ➡ erythrocyte protein kinase C inhibitor

웅황 arsenic ➡ toxoplasma gondii: pyruvate kinase 억제

➡ mitochondria respiration 억제

별갑 chitosan ➡ cholesterol absorption inhibitor

승마 cimigenol, 약리 추측 ➡ p53 phoshorylation activator

감초 glycyrrhetinic acid

➡ 11-beta-hydroxysteroid dehydrogenase1 (HSD11B1) inhibitor

➡ glucocorticoid 작용

➡ IκBα 생성

➡ NF-κB 억제

촉초 sanshool ➡ potassium channel blocker

시호가망초탕 (柴胡加芒硝湯)

원문 傷寒 十 三 日 不解，胸脅 滿 而 嘔，日晡 所 發 潮熱，已 而 微 利。此 本 柴胡 證，下 之 以 不 得 利，今 反 利 者，知 醫 以 丸藥 下 之，此 非 其 治 也。潮熱 者，實 也。 先 宜 服 小柴胡湯 以 解 外，後 以 柴胡加芒硝湯 主之。

원문 해설 세포병변성 감염병이 13일이 지나도 낫지 않고 갈빗대 옆이 그득해지고 구역이 나며, 해가 질 무렵에 조수가 반복되는 듯한 열이 있고, 열이가시면 약하게 설사를 하게 된다. 이는 본래 시호증이므로 시호제를 쓰면 설사 없이 나아야 되는데, 반대로 설사를 하는 것은 의사가 시호제를 쓰지 않고 사하제만 쓴 탓이다. 조수가 반복되는 듯한 열이 있는 것은 바이러스 증식이 활발한 상태이므로 먼저 소시호탕을 써서 열을 없애고 이후에 시호가망초탕을 써서 완치시킨다.

적응증 Type C hepatitis (C형 간염)

병태 & 증상

Type C hepatitis

➡ blood: transmission
➡ intestinal endothelium : hepatitis C virus (HCV) infection
➡ HCV: lipo-viro-particles 생산 --> HCV 복제에 필요한 지단백입자
➡ intestinal endothelium lysis: 방출
➡ portal vein endothelium: 침투
➡ HCV infected endothelium: collagenase 분비
➡ 문맥기저막 분해 후 간실질로 침투
➡ Kupffer cells: HCV infection
➡ phagocytosis & respiratory burst
➡ extracellular: peroxynitrite ($ONOO^-$) ↑
➡ hepatitis
&
➡ hepatocyte: hepatitis C virus (HCV) infection
➡ RNA-dependent RNA polymerase
➡ virus replicon RNAs
➡ hepatocyte: viral antigen 발현
➡ cytotoxic T cell 유도
➡ hepatitis

&

➡ HCV infected hepatocyte: NOS2 gene expression ↑

➡ nitric oxide + superoxide

➡ peroxynitrite ($ONOO^-$) ↑

➡ HCV RNA: mutation

➡ hepatocyte: viral antigen 발현 실패

➡ chronic hepatitis

처방 목표 Intraluminal distention pressure 상승시켜서 lipo-viro-particles 제거 / peroxynitrite ($ONOO^-$) 제거 / virus replicon RNAs 제거 / hepatocyte 재생

처방 구성 柴胡 二兩 十六銖 / 黃芩 一兩 / 人參 一兩 / 炙甘草 一兩 / 生薑 一兩 / 半夏 二十銖 / 大棗 四枚 / 芒硝 二兩

처방 약리

망초 Sodium Sulfate ➡ Intraluminal distention pressure 상승시킴
➡ lipo-viro-particles 제거

황금 baicalin ➡ peroxynitrite ($ONOO^-$) scavenger

시호 saikosaponin, 약리추측 ➡ small interfering RNA (siRNA) (+) modulator
➡ hepatitis virus RNA replication inhibition

인삼 panax ginsenoside
➡ Transforming growth factor β (TGF-β) (+) modulator
➡ hepatocyte proliferation 촉진

반하 triterpenoid (C30H48O7S)
➡ Rho GTPase family transcription promotor
➡ focal adhesion 생성
➡ hepatocyte 이동 촉진

생강 gingerol ➡ hydrogen peroxide scavenger
➡ focal adhesion kinase 활성화
➡ 상피세포의 입체적 이동 촉진

대조 c-AMP ➡ Protein kinase A avtivator
➡ ATP 합성 촉진
➡ cell cycle

구감초 18β-24-Hydroxyglycyrrhetinic acid
➡ HSD11B2 inhibitor
➡ cortisol 분해 억제
➡ mineralocorticoid receptors 자극 지속
➡ 재생된 hepatocyte Na+/ K+ pumps 활성화

시호가용골모려탕 (柴胡加龍骨牡蠣湯)

원문 傷寒 八 九 日 , 下 之 , 胸 滿 煩 驚 , 小便 不利 , 譫 語, 一 身 盡 重 , 不 可 轉 側 者, 柴胡加龍骨牡蠣湯 主之 。

원문 해설 세포병변성 감염증이 8~9일이 지나 심장이 빠근하고 괴로우며 신경이 예민해지고, 소변이 불편하고 헛소리를 하며 몸이 무거워 돌아눕기도 힘든 경우에는 시호가용골모려탕을 쓴다.

적응증 Viral fulminant hepatitis (바이러스 전격성간염)

병태 & 증상

Viral fulminant hepatitis

➡ 선행질환: 주로, EBV 감염
➡ EBV infected B cell: cytokine 분비
➡ T cell proliferation ↑
➡ Tc lymphoproliferative disease
➡ hepatitis virus infection
➡ Kupffer cells: hepatitis virus infection
➡ phagocytosis & respiratory burst
➡ extracellular: peroxynitrite ($ONOO^-$) ↓
➡ hepatitis
➡ virus replicon RNAs

➡ hepatocyte: viral antigen 발현
➡ cytotoxic T cell 유도
➡ 과잉 증식된 cytotoxic T cell: cytokine storm
➡ fulminant hepatitis
➡ 간부전
➡ albumin 생산 감소 ▶ rapid hyponatremia: 뇌세포 부종
lactate 대사 감소 ▶ lactic acidosis
detoxication 감소 ▶ 친자성 이온 증가 (Mn/Cu/Fe): 뇌세포 축적
혈액응고인자 감소 ▶ 출혈 증가: thrombus 형성

처방 목표 Tc lymphoproliferative disease 억제 / peroxynitrite ($ONOO^-$) 제거 / virus replicon RNAs 제거 / rapid hyponatremia 교정 / lactic acidosis 교정 / 친자성 이온 증가 (Mn/Cu/Fe) 제거 / thrombus 제거 / hepatocyte 재생

처방 구성 柴胡 四兩 / 龍骨 / 黃芩 / 生薑 / 鉛丹 / 人參 / 桂枝 / 茯苓 各 一兩半 / 半夏 二合半 / 大黃 二兩 / 牡蠣 一兩半 / 大棗 六枚

처방 약리

대황 emodin tyrosine kinase blocker
➡ cytotoxic T cell 성장 억제

황금 baicalin ➡ peroxynitrite ($ONOO^-$) scavenger

시호 saikosaponin, 약리추측 ➡ small interfering RNA (siRNA) (+) modulator
➡ hepatitis virus RNA replication inhibition

모려 NaCl ➡ hyponatremia & hypernatremia 교정

용골 $CaCO_3$ ➡ $NaHCO_3$ 공급원 ➡ 산증 교정

계지 cinnamic acid ➡ lactate oxidizer
➡ Cori cycle: pyruvate 전환 촉진
➡ lactatemia 교정

연단 사산화삼납 (Pb_3O_4), 약리추측
➡ 3개의 산소음전하가 친자성이온을 킬레이션 시킴

복령 pachymic acid ➡ glycoprotein IIb/IIIa (gpIIb/IIIa) (-) modulator

➡ thrombus formation 억제

인삼 panax ginsenoside

➡ Transforming growth factor β (TGF-β) (+) modulator

➡ hepatocyte proliferation 촉진

반하 triterpenoid ($C_{30}H_{48}O_7S$)

➡ Rho GTPase family transcription promotor

➡ focal adhesion 생성

➡ 상피세포 이동 촉진

생강 gingerol ➡ hydrogen peroxide scavenger

➡ focal adhesion kinase 활성화

➡ 상피세포의 입체적 이동 촉진

대조 c-AMP ➡ Protein kinase A avtivator

➡ ATP 합성 촉진

➡ cell cycle ↑

시호계지건강탕 (柴胡桂枝乾薑湯)

원문 傷寒 五 六 日 , 已 發 汗 而 復 下 之 , 胸脅 滿 微 結 , 小便 不利, 渴 而 不嘔 , 但 頭汗出 , 往來寒熱 , 心煩 者 , 此 為 未 解 也, 柴胡桂枝乾薑湯 主之 。

원문 해설 세포병변성 감염병이 5~6일째 IL-1매개 면역반응을 유도해서 낫게했는데, 갈빗대 옆이 뭉치는 느낌이 들고 소변이 불편하며, 구역은 없고 갈증이 나며, 머리에서만 땀이 흐르고, 추웠다 더웠다 하며, 마음이 괴로운 경우에는 병이 진행 중이므로 시호계지건강탕을 쓴다.

적응증 Liver cirrhosis (간경변)

병태 & 증상

Liver cirrhosis

➡ chronic hepatitis

➡ HBV & HCV replication

➡ hepatocyte: viral antigen 발현
➡ cytotoxic T cell 유도
➡ hepatitis 반복
➡ hepatocyte necrotic body
➡ Kupffer cells: 식균 ▶ cytokine 분비
➡ hepatic stellate cell 활성화
➡ hepatic stellate cell ▶ myofibroblast 분화
➡ collagen mRNA 생성 ↑
➡ collagen 분비
➡ collagen polymerization: 비수용성 섬유
➡ 간세포: 허혈 ▶ lactate 축적 & Na+/ K+ pumps 약화: hepatitis
➡ 재관류
➡ Kupffer cells: peroxynitrite ($ONOO^-$) ↑ : hepatitis
&
➡ 간문맥동 내피세포: 허혈
➡ 간문맥동 내피세포: selectin 발현
➡ neutrophil 유도
➡ neutrophil ▶ phagocytosis
➡ HClO 분비 via H2O2
➡ hepatitis
➡ 간기능 장애
➡ 저알부민혈증
➡ 혈관 삼투압이 낮아져서 Na이 혈관밖으로 빠져나감
➡ hyponatremia
➡ 뇌세포외액 ▶ 뇌척수액으로 이동: head sweating
➡ 뇌세포외액 용적 감소되어 저나트륨혈증이 교정됨

처방 목표 HBV & HCV replication 억제 / collagen mRNA 번역 차단 / lactate 교정 / Na+/ K+ pumps 활성화 / peroxynitrite ($ONOO^-$) 제거 / HClO 분비 억제 / hyponatremia 교정

처방 구성 柴胡 半斤 / 桂枝 三兩 / 乾薑 二兩 / 栝蔞根 四兩 / 黃芩 三兩 / 牡蠣 二兩 / 炙甘草 二兩

처방 약리

시호 saikosaponin, 약리추측 ➡ small interfering RNA (siRNA) (+) modulator
➡ hepatitis virus RNA replication inhibition

괄루근 trichosanthin ➡ ribosome inactivating protein
➡ collagen 합성 억제

계지 cinnamic acid ➡ lactate oxidizer
➡ pyruvate 전환 촉진

구감초 18β-24-Hydroxyglycyrrhetinic acid
➡ HSD11B2 inhibitor
➡ cortisol 분해 억제
➡ mineralocorticoid receptors 자극 지속
➡ 재생된 hepatocyte Na+/ K+ pumps 활성화

황금 baicalin ➡ peroxynitrite ($ONOO^-$) scavenger

건강 shogaol ➡ neutrophil H2O2 scavenger
➡ HClO 분비 억제

모려 NaCl ➡ hyponatremia & hypernatremia 교정

시호계지탕 (柴胡桂枝湯)

원문 傷寒 六 七 日，發熱，微 惡寒，支節 煩疼，微嘔，心下 結，外 證 未 去 者, 柴胡桂枝湯 主之。

원문 해설 세포병변성 감염병이 6~7일이 된 후 발열하고 약간 한기가 들며 관절부위가 괴롭게 쑤시고 심장부위가 뭉친 것 같은 표증이 계속되면 시호계지탕을 쓴다.

적응증 Type B hepatitis-mediated immune complex disease

병태 & 증상

Type B hepatitis-mediated immune complex disease

➡ acute hepatitis B virus infection
➡ blood & body fluid: transmission

➡ Kupffer cells: HBV infection
➡ phagocytosis & respiratory burst
➡ extracellular: peroxynitrite ($ONOO^-$) ↑
➡ hepatitis
&
➡ hepatocyte: hepatitis B virus (HBV) infection
➡ RNA Polymerase II
➡ virus replicon RNAs
➡ hepatocyte: viral antigen 발현
➡ cytotoxic T cell 유도
➡ hepatitis
&
➡ circulatory HBsAg 출현
➡ anti-HBsAg & HBsAg: immune complex 형성
➡ synovium (활액막): 침착
➡ complement 유도
➡ synovium: membrane attack complement (MAC) 결합
➡ Ca influx ↑
➡ mitochondria respiration ↑
➡ superoxide ↑
➡ mitochondria membrane potential damage
➡ lactate 축적
➡ ATP 생산 감소
➡ 세포부종
➡ synovitis: IL-6 분비 ▶ fever, chills
➡ immune complex: angioedema ▶ rapid heart rate

처방 목표 peroxynitrite ($ONOO^-$) 제거 / virus replicon RNAs 제거 / hepatocyte 재생 / synovium superoxide 제거 / synovium lactate 교정

처방 구성 桂枝 一兩半 / 黃芩 一兩半 / 芍藥 一兩半 / 人參一兩半 / 炙甘草 一兩 / 半夏 二合半 / 大棗 六枚 / 生薑 一兩半 / 柴胡 四兩

처방 약리

황금 baicalin ➡ peroxynitrite ($ONOO^-$) scavenger

시호 saikosaponin, 약리추측 ➡ small interfering RNA (siRNA) (+) modulator

➡ hepatitis virus RNA replication inhibition

인삼 panax ginsenoside
➡ Transforming growth factor β (TGF-β) (+) modulator
➡ hepatocyte proliferation 촉진

반하 triterpenoid (C30H48O7S)
➡ Rho GTPase family transcription promotor
➡ focal adhesion 생성
➡ hepatocyte 이동 촉진

생강 gingerol ➡ hydrogen peroxide scavenger
➡ focal adhesion kinase 활성화
➡ 상피세포의 입체적 이동 촉진

대조 c-AMP ➡ Protein kinase A avtivator
➡ ATP 합성 촉진
➡ cell cycle ↑

구감초 18β-24-Hydroxyglycyrrhetinic acid
➡ HSD11B2 inhibitor
➡ cortisol 분해 억제
➡ mineralocorticoid receptors 자극 지속
➡ 재생된 hepatocyte Na+/ K+ pumps 활성화

작약 paeoniflorin ➡ superoxide scavenger

계지 cinnamic acid ➡ lactate oxidizer
➡ pyruvate 전환 촉진

오두계지탕 (烏頭桂枝湯)

원문 寒疝 腹中痛 , 逆冷 , 手足 不仁 , 若 身 疼痛 , 灸 刺 諸藥 不能 治, 抵 當 烏頭 桂枝湯 主之 。

원문 해설 오한이 들면서 배가 아픈데, 손발이 차갑고 저려오며, 몸이 쑤시고 통증이 있으며, 뜸이나 침과 다른 약이 모두 효과가 없는 경우에는 오두계지탕을 쓴다.

적응증 Mesenteritis-mediated volvulus (장간막염-매개 장꼬임증)

병태 & 증상

Mesenteritis-mediated volvulus

➡ Peyer's patch: macrophage
➡ enterovirus infection
➡ enterovirus infected macrophage: mesentery lymph node 이동
➡ enterovirus replication
➡ macrophage lysis
➡ mesenteritis
➡ mesentery & bowel: adhesion
➡ volvulus
➡ bowel obstruction: TNF-α ▶ cold hands and feet

처방 목표 enterovirus infected macrophage: mesentery lymph node 이동 억제 / enterovirus replication 억제 / mesentery & retroperitoneum: adhesion 억제

처방 구성 烏頭 五枚 / 蜜 二斤 / 桂枝湯 五合

처방 약리

오두 hypaconitine
➡ 약리 추측: macrophage` Voltage-gated proton channels blocker
➡ Voltage-gated proton channels 차단
➡ 조직 대식세포내 수소이온 축적
➡ tissue macrophage 대사 억제
➡ mesentery lymph node 이동 억제

계지탕 heat shock protein 생산 ➡ viral replication 억제

밀 (꿀) xylose & galactose ➡ heparan sulfate 구성 단당류
➡ 장간막 & 후복막 유착 억제

오두적석지환 (烏頭赤石脂丸)

원문 心 痛 徹 背, 背 痛 徹 心, 烏頭赤石脂丸 主之。

원문 해설 가슴에서 등쪽으로 뚫고 나가는 듯한 통증이 있거나,
등에서 가슴쪽으로 뚫고 들어오는 듯한 통증이 있는 경우에는
오두적석지환을 쓴다.

적응증 Liver clonorchiasis (간흡충증)

병태 & 증상

Liver clonorchiasis

➡ intrahepatic bile duct: adult liver fluke 감염
➡ adult liver fluke: excreting secretory product 분비
➡ bile duct endothelium 손상
➡ IL-8 분비
➡ neutrophil 유도
➡ neutrophil phagocytosis & degranulation
➡ HClO 분비 via H2O2 & elastase 분비
➡ 담도 손상
➡ dead neutrophil: protein-rich fluid
➡ pus 생성: 농양
➡ adult liver fluke: ATP-sensitive K+ channels ▶ 영양분 통로
➡ egg 방출
➡ egg antigen: CD4+ T cell 유도
➡ CD4+ T cell: cytokine
➡ liver macrophage 유도: egg 식균
➡ liver macrophage: TNF-α 분비
➡ eosinophil, B cell, T cell 유도
➡ granuloma formation
➡ hepatomegaly: radiating pain

처방 목표 HClO 분비 억제 / neutrophil: elastase 분비 / pus 제거 / adult liver fluke: ATP-sensitive K+ channels 차단 / liver macrophage: TNF-α 분비 억제

처방 구성 蜀椒 一兩 / 炮烏頭 一分 / 炮附子 半兩 / 乾薑 一兩 / 赤石脂 一兩

처방 약리

포부자 aconitine

➡ 약리추측: neutrophil` Voltage-gated proton channels blocker
(식균작용에 의해 증가된 세포내 proton을 세포외로 방출시키는 채널)
➡ Voltage-gated proton channels 차단
➡ 호중구내 수소이온 축적
➡ neutrophil 대사 억제
➡ elastase 분비 억제

건강 shogaol ➡ neutrophil H2O2 scavenger
➡ HClO 분비 억제

적석지 Al2O3, 2SiO2·4H2O ➡ Cation absorbent
➡ pus 주성분: 양이온 단백
➡ pus 흡착-제거

촉초 sanshool ➡ potassium channel blocker

오두 hypaconitine
➡ 약리 추측: macrophage` Voltage-gated proton channels blocker
➡ Voltage-gated proton channels 차단
➡ 조직 대식세포내 수소이온 축적
➡ tissue macrophage 대사 억제
➡ mesentery lymph node 이동 억제
➡ liver macrophage: TNF-α 분비 억제

오두탕 (烏頭湯)

원문 病 歷節 不 可 屈伸，疼痛，烏頭湯 主之。

원문 해설 퇴행성관절염으로 관절움직임이 불가능해지고, 쑤시고 아픈 경우에는 오두탕을 쓴다.

적응증 Osteoarthritis (퇴행성 관절염)

병태 & 증상

Osteoarthritis

➡ aging: blood acidity ↑
➡ synovial membranes: fibronectin
➡ fibronectin: advanced glycation end products (AGEs) 생성
▶ proteoglycan 탈락
▶ synoviocyte: tissue factor 발현
▶ fibrin 생성
➡ synovial macrophage: fibrin 청소
➡ synovial macrophage: IL-1, TNF-α, IGF-1 분비
➡ fibroblast like synoviocyte (FLS): hyperplasia
➡ hyaluronate: advanced glycation end products (AGEs) 생성
➡ FLS AGEs Rc: advanced glycation end products 부착
➡ FLS: superoxide ↑
➡ FLS: DNA 손상 ▶ 형질전환
➡ 침습성 획득
➡ FLS: cartilage 침투
➡ cartilage destruction & bone erosion
➡ osteoarthritis
➡ synovial fluid: hyaluronate
➡ aging
➡ hyaluronate: advanced glycation end products (AGEs) 생성
➡ type II collagen 산화: browning
➡ type II collagen: IgG 생성
➡ synovial mast cell FcR γ: IgG binding
➡ synovial mast cell: histamine degranulation
➡ vasodilation: body fluid influx
➡ synovial tissue: swelling

처방 목표 blood acidity 교정 / fibrin 제거 / synovial macrophage: IL-1, TNF-α, IGF-1 분비 억제 / FLS: superoxide 제거 / synovial mast cell: histamine degranulation 억제 / hyaluronate & glucosaminoglycan & chondroitin: 합성 촉진

처방 구성 麻黃 三兩 / 芍藥 三兩 / 黃耆 三兩 / 炙甘草 三兩 / 川烏 五枚 / 蜜 二升

처방 약리

구감초 18β-24-Hydroxyglycyrrhetinic acid

➡ 11-beta-hydroxysteroid dehydrogenase2 (HSD11B2) inhibitor

➡ aldosterone 생리작용과 동일

➡ H+ secretion

➡ acidity 교정

황기 astragaloside ➡ Tissue plasminogen activator (+) modulator

➡ fibrin 용해

천오 (오두) hypaconitine

➡ 약리 추측: macrophage` Voltage-gated proton channels blocker

➡ Voltage-gated proton channels 차단

➡ 조직 대식세포내 수소이온 축적

➡ tissue macrophage 대사 억제

➡ synovial macrophage: IL-1, TNF-α, IGF-1 분비 억제

작약 paeoniflorin ➡ superoxide scavenger

마황 ephedrine ➡ Epinephrine receptors agonist

➡ adenylate cyclase 활성화

➡ cAMP ↑

➡ mast cell: degranulation 억제

밀(꿀) xylose & galactose ➡ heparan sulfate 구성 단당류

오령산 (五苓散)

원문 太陽病, 發汗 後, 大汗出, 胃中 乾, 煩躁 不得 眠, 欲 得 飮水 者, 少少 與 飮之, 令 胃氣 和 則 愈。若 脈 浮, 小便 不利, 微熱 消渴 者, 五苓散 主 之。中風 發熱, 六 七 日 不解 而 煩, 有 表裡 證, 渴 欲 飮水, 水入 則 吐 者, 名曰 水逆, 五苓散 主 之。本 以 下 之, 故 心下痞, 與 瀉心湯。, 痞 不 解, 其人 渴 而 口燥 煩, 小便 不利 者, 五苓散 主 之。

원문 해설 IL-1 매개 림프절 감염병에서 땀이 크게 난 후 위장이 마르고 마음이 편치 않으며 잠 못 자고 갈증이 있어 조금씩 물을 마시는데 위장이 편하면 낫고, 맥이 뜨면서 소변이 불편하고 미열이 있으면서 갈증이 있는 경우에는 오령산을 쓴다. 시상하부 발열점이 상승된 감염병에서 발열하며 6~7일이 지나도 낫지 않고, 괴로우면서 체표와 내과증상이 모두 있고 갈증이 나서 물을 마시는데 마시자마자 토하는 경우를 수역이라고 부르며 오령산을 쓴다. 원래 위장관 점막림프절을 배출한 뒤 명치 밑이 쓰릴 때는 사심탕을 쓰는데, 그래도 낫지 않고 갈증이 나며 입안이 마르면서 괴롭고 소변이 불편할 때는 오령산을 쓴다.

적응증 Immune complex-mediated glomerulonephritis (면역복합체-매개 사구체신염)

병태 & 증상

Immune complex-mediated glomerulonephritis

➡ glomerulus 혈관: Immune complex 침착
➡ mesangial cell: phagocytosis
➡ mesangial cell: IL-1 분비
➡ glomerulus vessel: VCAM-1 발현
➡ monocyte 유도
➡ monocyte: 사구체 혈관 부착
➡ monocyte ROS burst
➡ 사구체 혈관 손상: thrombus formation
➡ 수출소동맥 저산소증
➡ 수출소동맥 수축
➡ 사구체내 압력 ↑
➡ 사구체 모세혈관 손상: glomerulonephritis
➡ glomerular filtration rate ▶ 수분배설 감소: vomiting
➡ podocyte contraction
➡ podocyte: intracellular lactate ↑
➡ podocyte apoptosis
➡ monocyte: mesangial cell growth factor 분비
➡ mesangial cell proliferation

처방 목표 glomerulus endothelial cell: VCAM-1 발현 억제 / thrombus formation 억제 / 수출소동맥 수축 억제 / podocyte: intracellular lactate 제거 / mesangial cell: proliferation 억제

처방 구성 豬苓 十八銖 / 澤瀉 一兩 六銖 / 白朮 十八銖 / 茯苓 十八銖 / 桂枝 半兩

처방 약리

백출 atractylon ➡ vascular cell adhesion molecule-1 (VCAM-1) blocker

복령 pachymic acid ➡ glycoprotein IIb/IIIa (gpIIb/IIIa) (-) modulator
➡ thrombus formation 억제

택사 alisol ➡ angiotensin II receptor blocker
➡ 수출소동맥 수축 억제

계지 cinnamic acid ➡ lactate oxidizer
➡ pyruvate 전환 촉진

저령 ergosterol ➡ mesangial cell proliferation inhibitor

오수유탕 (吳茱萸湯)

원문 食穀 欲 嘔, 屬 陽明 也, 吳茱萸湯 主 之 ; 得 湯 反 劇 者, 屬 上焦 也。少陰病, 吐利, 手足逆冷, 煩燥 欲 死 者, 吳茱萸湯 主之。乾嘔, 吐涎沫, 頭痛 者, 吳茱萸湯 主之。

원문 해설 식사 중에 구토하고 싶어지는 것은 담도내 증식성질환, 즉 담석 때문으로 오수유탕을 쓴다. 복용 후 구토가 더 심해지면 식도질환을 의심해야 된다. 항체매개 감염병에서 토하고 설사하면서 손발이 차갑고 죽을 정도로 괴로우면 오수유탕을 쓴다. 구역기가 있으면서 멀건물을 토하고 두통이 있는 경우에는 오수유탕을 쓴다.

적응증 Pancreatitis

병태 & 증상

Pancreatitis

➡ gallstone / autoimmune pancreatitis / virus infection
➡ 췌장 선방세포의 직접적 손상 또는 췌관 손상
➡ 췌장 선방세포내 산성화
➡ low-affinity Cholecystokinine (CCK) receptor 자극

➡ phospholipase C 활성화
➡ diacylglycerol 생성
➡ hydrogen peroxide: Ca+2 / calmodulin ↑
➡ protein kinase C 활성화
➡ 선방세포 vacuole내 pro-enzyme 활성화
➡ 산성화 조건: 췌장 선방세포내 공포 깨짐
➡ pro-enzyme: 세포질로 방출
➡ 선방세포 자가분해됨
➡ pancreatitis

처방 목표 low-affinity CCK receptor 차단 / hydrogen peroxide 제거 / 선방세포 증식 촉진

처방 구성 吳茱萸 一升 / 人參 三兩 / 生薑 六兩 / 大棗 十二枚

처방 약리

오수유 evodiamine ➡ low-affinity CCK receptor blocker
➡ vacuole: pro-enzyme 활성화 억제

생강 gingerol ➡ hydrogen peroxide scavenger
➡ 선방세포 protein kinase C 억제됨

인삼 panax ginsenoside
➡ Transforming growth factor β (TGF-β) (+) modulator
➡ cell proliferation 촉진

대조 c-AMP ➡ protein kinase A avtivator
➡ ATP 합성 촉진
➡ cell cycle ↑

온경탕 (溫經湯)

원문 婦人 年 五十 所，病 下利 數 十日 不止，暮 即 發熱，少腹 裡急，腹滿，手掌 煩熱，唇口 乾燥，何 也 師 曰 :此 病 屬 帶下，何 以 故 ? 曾 經 半產, 瘀血

在 少腹 不去。何 以 知 之 ? 其 證 唇口 乾燥, 故 知 之。當 以 溫經湯 主 之。亦 主 婦人 少腹 寒, 久 不 受胎 ; 兼 取 崩中 去 血, 或 月 水 來 過多, 及 至 期 不 來。

원문 해설 부인이 50세가 되어 질분비물이 잦으며 그치지 않고, 해가 질 무렵에 발열하며, 아래 뱃속이 땅기고 팽만감이 있으며, 손바닥에 불편한 열감이 있고, 입술이 건조한 것은 왜입니까? 이 병은 대하병에 속하며, 반복된 유산으로 인한 굳은 피 때문에 발병된다. 입술이 건조한 것으로 대하병을 판단할 수 있으며, 온경탕을 쓴다. 또한, 부인의 아랫배가 차가워서 오랫동안 착상이 안 되거나, 자궁이 헐어서 출혈이 생기거나, 생리량이 너무 많거나, 무월경일 때에도 온경탕을 쓴다.

적응증 Tuberculous endometritis (결핵성 자궁내막염)

병태 & 증상

Tuberculous endometritis (결핵성 자궁내막염)

➡ endometrium macrophage: latent tuberculosis infection
➡ starvation & low oxygen pressure
➡ M. tuberculosis: thehalose dimycolate 합성
➡ macrophage: focal adhesion kinase 활성화
➡ macrophage fusion 형성
➡ blood macrophage 유도됨
➡ macrophage fusion 증가
➡ granuloma formation
➡ M. tuberculosis: SigF overexpression
➡ M. tuberculosis: intracellular growth
➡ M. tuberculosis: hydrolytic enzyme 분비
➡ macrophage necrosis
➡ cavity formation & stromal breakdown
: uterine bleeding, vaginal dischage, menopause endometritis
➡ cavity formation ▶ capillary pressing ▶ deformity erythrocyte 생성
& capillary leakage ▶ hematoma 형성
▶ artery α-adrenergic Rc 자극 ▶ vasospasm
➡ deformity erythrocyte + vasospasm
➡ myometrium ischemia & reperfusion: intracelluar lactate ↑, superoxide ↑
➡ manganese superoxide dismutase & glutathione peroxidase 고갈
➡ myometrium necrosis
➡ myometritis

처방 목표 granuloma formation 억제 / M. tuberculosis: SigF 전사 억제 / endometrium cell 상환 촉진 / endometrium cell 재생 / deformity erythrocyte 교정 / artery α-adrenergic Rc 차단 / myometrium: intracelluar lactate ↑, superoxide ↑ 교정 / manganese superoxide dismutase & glutathione peroxidase 전사 촉진 / myometrium 재생 / myometrium 수축 억제

처방 구성 吳茱萸 三兩 / 當歸 二兩 / 芎藭 二兩 / 芍藥 二兩 / 人參 二兩 / 桂枝 二兩 / 阿膠 二兩 / 生薑 二兩 / 牧丹皮 二兩 / 甘草 二兩 / 半夏 半升 / 麥門冬 一升

처방 약리

감초 glycyrrhetinic acid ➡ HSD11B1 inhibitor
➡ cortisol 분해 억제
➡ glucocorticoid receptors 자극 지속
➡ IκBα 생성
➡ NF-κB 억제
➡ macrophage 대사 & 이동에 필요한 cytokine 생성 억제
➡ granuloma formation 억제

맥문동 ophiopogonin, 약리 추측 ➡ M. tuberculosis' SigF transcription inhibitor
➡ M. tuberculosis growth 억제됨

반하 triterpenoid (C30H48O7S)
➡ Rho GTPase family transcription promotor
➡ focal adhesion 생성
➡ endometrium cell 이동 촉진

인삼 panax ginsenoside
➡ Transforming growth factor β (TGF-β) (+) modulator
➡ endometrium cell proliferation 촉진

당귀 decurcin ➡ erythrocyte protein kinase C inhibitor
➡ adducin-spectrin-actin complex 유지시킴

천궁 cnidilide ➡ α-adrenergic receptor blocker

계지 cinnamic acid ➡ lactate oxidizer
➡ pyruvate 전환

작약 paeoniflorin ➡ superoxide scavenger

목단피 β-Sitosterol
➡ manganese superoxide dismutase & glutathione peroxidase (+) modulator
➡ myometrium necrosis 억제

아교 Glycine / Proline / Hydroxyproline / Alanine
➡ collagen 주요 아미노산
➡ myometrium 합성 촉진

오수유 evodiamine ➡ low-affinity CCK receptor blocker
➡ myometrium CCK receptor blocking
➡ myometrium relaxation

생강 gingerol ➡ hydrogen peroxide scavenger
➡ myometrium relaxation

왕불류행산 (王不留行散)

원문 病 金 瘡，王不留行散 主之，小瘡 即 粉 之，大瘡 但 服 之，產後 亦 可 服。

원문 해설 쇠붙이에 베어 상처가 난 경우에는 왕불류행산을 쓴다. 조금 베인 경우는 가루를 내어 붙이고, 크게 베인 경우에는 복용한다. 출산 후에도 복용할 수 있다.

적응증 Tetanus (파상풍)

병태 & 증상

Tetanus

➡ rusty metal: wound
➡ Clostridium tetani infection

➡ lymphatic system & blood 재배치
➡ Clostridium tetani: tetanospasmin 분비

➡ peripheral motor neurons: tetanospasmin infection
▶ motor neuron membrane disialoganglioside: tetanospasmin B chain 부착
▶ phospholipase C & D 활성화: endocytosis
➡ retro-axonal transport
➡ spinal cord interneuron: infection
▶ interneuron membrane disialoganglioside: tetanospasmin B chain 부착
▶ phospholipase C & D 활성화: endocytosis
▶ tetanospasmin A chain: proteolytic activity
▶ synaptobrevin degrading
▶ GABA & glycine 분비 차단
▶ inhibitory impulse 중단
▶ neuromuscler junction: acethycholine 지속
▶ muscle cell: potassium channel open ▶ K 배출
▶ 근수축 지속
▶ spastic paralysis
➡ circulating tetanospasmin: blood-brain barrier (BBB) 부착
➡ BBB endothelium: cytokine
➡ BBB endothelium: neutrophil 이동
➡ neutrophil phagocytosis
➡ HClO 분비 via H2O2
➡ BBB endothelium: GDP-> GTP 전환
➡ BBB endothelium : NF-κB 활성화 ▶ VEGF gene expression
➡ BBB endothelium : VEGF 분비
➡ BBB endothelium VEGF Rc: VEGF 부착
➡ BBB endothelium: permeability ↑
➡ tetanospasmin 유입
➡ tetanospasmin IgG 출현
➡ microglia: tetanospasmin phagocytosis
➡ extracellular peroxynitrite ($ONOO^-$) ↑
➡ neuron damage

처방 목표 Clostridium tetani 살균 / phospholipase C & D 억제 / tetanospasmin A chain: proteolytic activity 억제 / muscle cell: potassium channel 차단 / muscle cell: capsaicin-sensitive channel 차단 / HClO 분비 억제 / BBB endothelium: GDP➡

GTP 전환 억제 / BBB endothelium : NF-κB 억제 / BBB endothelium: VEGF Rc 차단 / extracellular peroxynitrite (ONOO⁻) 제거

처방 구성 王不留行 十分 (八月 八日 採) / 蒴藋 細葉 十分 (七月 七日 採) / 桑東南根 白皮 十分 (三月 三日 採) / 甘草 十八分 / 黃芩 二分 / 川椒 三分 (除目 及 閉口 , 去 汗) / 乾薑 二分 / 厚朴 二分 / 芍藥 二分

처방 약리

왕불류행 vaccaroside, 약리 추측 ➡ Clostridium tetani 살균

삭조 (말오줌나무잎): cyanidin-3-xylosylglucoside, 약리 추측
➡ phospholipase C & D inhibitor
➡ tetanospasmin endocytosis 억제
& metal ion chelator
➡ tetanospasmin A chain: zinc 제거
➡ synaptobrevin degrading 억제

천초 sanshool ➡ potassium channel blocker

상백피 α-amyrin, 약리 추측: capsaicin-sensitive channel blocker
➡ 근육세포에서 척수로의 구심성신호 차단됨

건강 shogaol ➡ neutrophil H2O2 scavenger
➡ HClO 분비 억제

작약 paeoniflorin ➡ superoxide scavenger
➡ BBB endothelium: GDP ▶ GTP 전환 억제

감초 glycyrrhetinic acid
➡ 11-beta-hydroxysteroid dehydrogenase1 (HSD11B1) inhibitor
➡ glucocorticoid 작용
➡ IκBα 생성
➡ NF-κB 억제

후박 honokiol ➡ VEGF receptor blocker
황금 baicalin ➡ peroxynitrite (ONOO⁻) scavenger

월비가반하탕 (越婢加半夏湯)

원문 咳 而 上氣 , 此 為 肺脹 , 其 人 喘 , 目 如 脫 狀 , 脈 浮 大 者, 越婢加半夏湯 主之 。

원문 해설 기침을 하는데 그치지 않고 계속하는 것은 폐포에 병이 있는 것으로 호흡이 곤란해지고 눈점막이 탈락될 것 같으며 맥이 뜨고 큰 경우에는 월비가반하탕을 쓴다.

적응증 Hypersensitivity pneumonitis (과민성 폐렴)

병태 & 증상

Hypersensitivity pneumonitis

➡ pulmonary alveoli: allergen inhalation 반복
➡ B cell allergen specific IgE Rc: allergen binding
➡ CD4+ Th cell: CD4+ Rc ▶ allergen binding
➡ CD4+ Th cell: IL-4 분비
➡ B cell: memory cell & plasma cell 분화
➡ B cell: allergen specific IgE 생산 ↑
➡ mast cell FcR γ: IgE binding
➡ mast cell FcR γ: high affinity IgE Rc ▶ allergen: mutiple binding
➡ Phospholipase C activation
➡ diacylglycerol & Inositol trisphosphate 생성
➡ Inositol trisphosphate -> endoplasmic reticulum: calcium 분비
➡ 세포질: granule-bound adenylate cyclase 활성화
➡ cAMP ↑
➡ cAMP-dependent protein kinase 활성화
➡ cAMP ↓
➡ 세포질 granule-membrane protein: phospholylation
➡ 세포질 granule swelling
➡ mast cell FcR γ: high affinity IgE Rc ▶ allergen: mutiple binding
➡ mast cell: Fyn/Gab2/RhoA-signaling pathway 활성화
➡ microtubule polymerization via hydrogen peroxide
➡ 세포질 granule: translocation
➡ plasma membrane: granule fusion
➡ vasoactive amines degranulation

: histamine / serine proteases / serotonin / heparin

➡ lipid mediator: prostaglandin D2 / leukotrienes

➡ alveolitis: cough, dyspnea

처방 목표 CD4+ Th cell apoptosis 유도 / B cell: allergen specific IgE 생산 억제 / 세포질 cAMP 농도 지속 ➡ 세포질 granule-membrane protein: phospholylation 억제 / hydrogen peroxide 제거 / degranulation 억제 / 폐포상피 상환 촉진

처방 구성 麻黃 六兩 / 石膏 半斤 / 生薑 三兩 / 甘草 二兩 / 大棗 十五枚 / 半夏 半升

처방 약리

석고 CaSO4 ➡ Calcium Mediated T-Cell Apoptosis 유도

감초 glycyrrhetinic acid

➡ 11-beta-hydroxysteroid dehydrogenase1 (HSD11B1) inhibitor

➡ glucocorticoid 작용

➡ B cell: IκBα 생성

➡ NF-κB 억제

➡ 항체 생성 억제

대조 cAMP ➡ inhibition of granular organelles phosphorylation

➡ granule swelling 억제

생강 gingerol ➡ hydrogen peroxide scavenger

➡ 세포질 granule: translocation 억제

마황 ephedrine ➡ Epinephrine receptors agonist

➡ adenylate cyclase 활성화

➡ cAMP ↑

➡ degranulation 억제

반하 triterpenoid (C30H48O7S)

➡ Rho GTPase family transcription promotor

➡ focal adhesion 생성

➡ 상피세포 이동 촉진

월비가부자탕 (越婢加附子湯)

원문 風水 惡風，一身 悉 腫, 脈 浮 不渴，續 自汗出，無 大熱，惡風 者, 越婢加附子湯 主之。

원문 해설 피하 부종이 있고 추위를 타며 몸 전체가 붓고 맥은 떠 있으며 갈증은 없고 땀이 저절로 흐르면서 큰 열은 없고 추위를 많이 타는 경우에는 월비가부자탕을 쓴다.

적응증 Type I hypersensitive reaction: neutrophil mediated late phase reaction

병태 & 증상

Type I hypersensitive reaction: late phase reaction

➡ allergen 침입
➡ B cell allergen specific IgE Rc: allergen binding
➡ CD4+ Th cell: CD4+ Rc ▶ allergen binding
➡ CD4+ Th cell: IL-4 분비
➡ B cell: memory cell & plasma cell 분화
➡ B cell: allergen specific IgE 생산 ↑
➡ mast cell FcR γ: IgE binding
➡ mast cell FcR γ: high affinity IgE Rc ▶ allergen: mutiple binding
➡ Phospholipase C activation
➡ diacylglycerol & Inositol trisphosphate 생성
➡ Inositol trisphosphate ➡ endoplasmic reticulum: calcium 분비
➡ 세포질: granule-bound adenylate cyclase 활성화
➡ cAMP ↓
➡ cAMP-dependent protein kinase 활성화
➡ cAMP ↓
➡ 세포질 granule-membrane protein: phospholylation
➡ 세포질 granule swelling
➡ mast cell FcR γ: high affinity IgE Rc ▶ allergen: mutiple binding
➡ mast cell: Fyn/Gab2/RhoA-signaling pathway 활성화
➡ microtubule polymerization via hydrogen peroxide
➡ 세포질 granule: translocation
➡ plasma membrane: granule fusion
➡ vasoactive amines degranulation

: histamine / serine proteases / serotonin / heparin

➡ vasodilation: coldness

➡ body fluid influx: body swelling

➡ lipid mediator: prostaglandin D2 / leukotrienes: sweating

➡ mast cell: IL-8 분비

➡ intravascular neutrophil 유도

➡ neutrophil: extravation ▶ coldness ↑

➡ neutrophil elastase 분비

➡ tissue damage

처방 목표 CD4+ Th cell apoptosis 유도 / B cell: allergen specific IgE 생산 억제 / 세포질 cAMP 농도 지속 ➡ 세포질 granule-membrane protein: phospholylation 억제 / hydrogen peroxide 제거 / mast cell degranulation 억제 / neutrophil elastase 분비

처방 구성 麻黄 六兩 / 石膏 半斤 / 生薑 三兩 / 甘草 二兩 / 大棗 十五枚 / 炮附子 一枚

처방 약리

석고 CaSO4 ➡ Calcium Mediated T-Cell Apoptosis 유도

감초 glycyrrhetinic acid

➡ 11-beta-hydroxysteroid dehydrogenase1 (HSD11B1) inhibitor

➡ glucocorticoid 작용

➡ B cell: IκBα 생성

➡ NF-κB 억제

➡ 항체 생성 억제

대조 cAMP ➡ inhibition of granular organelles phosphorylation

➡ granule swelling 억제

생강 gingerol ➡ hydrogen peroxide scavenger

➡ 세포질 granule: translocation 억제

마황 ephedrine ➡ Epinephrine receptors agonist

➡ adenylate cyclase 활성화

➡ cAMP ↑

➡ degranulation 억제

포부자 aconitine

➡ 약리추측: neutrophil` Voltage-gated proton channels blocker
(식균작용에 의해 증가된 세포내 proton을 세포외로 방출시키는 채널)
➡ Voltage-gated proton channels 차단
➡ 호중구내 수소이온 축적
➡ neutrophil 대사 억제
➡ elastase 분비 억제

월비가출탕 (越婢加朮湯)

원문 風水 惡風, 一身 悉 腫, 脈 浮 不渴, 續 自汗出, 無 大熱, 風水 者, 越婢加朮湯 主之。

원문 해설 피하 부종이 있고 추위를 타며 몸 전체가 붓고 맥은 떠 있으며 갈증은 없고 땀이 저절로 흐르면서 큰 열은 없으며 피하부종이 심한 경우에는 월비가출탕을 쓴다.

적응증 Type I hypersensitive reaction: eosinophil-mediated late phase reaction

병태 & 증상

Type I hypersensitive reaction: eosinophil-mediated late phase reaction

➡ allergen 침입
➡ B cell allergen specific IgE Rc: allergen binding
➡ CD4+ Th cell: CD4+ Rc ▶ allergen binding
➡ CD4+ Th cell: IL-4 분비
➡ B cell: memory cell & plasma cell 분화
➡ B cell: allergen specific IgE 생산 ↑
➡ mast cell FcR γ: IgE binding
➡ mast cell FcR γ: high affinity IgE Rc ▶ allergen: mutiple binding
➡ Phospholipase C activation
➡ diacylglycerol & Inositol trisphosphate 생성
➡ Inositol trisphosphate -> endoplasmic reticulum: calcium 분비
➡ 세포질: granule-bound adenylate cyclase 활성화
➡ cAMP ↑

➡ cAMP-dependent protein kinase 활성화
➡ cAMP ↓
➡ 세포질 granule-membrane protein: phospholylation
➡ 세포질 granule swelling
➡ mast cell FcR γ: high affinity IgE Rc - -> allergen: mutiple binding
➡ mast cell: Fyn/ Gab2/ RhoA-signaling pathway 활성화
➡ microtubule polymerization via hydrogen peroxide
➡ 세포질 granule: translocation
➡ plasma membrane: granule fusion
➡ vasoactive amines degranulation
: histamine / serine proteases / serotonin / heparin
➡ vasodilation: coldness
➡ body fluid influx: body swelling
➡ lipid mediator: prostaglandin D2 / leukotrienes: sweating
➡ mast cell: IL-1 & TNF-α 분비
➡ vascular endithelium: VCAM-1 발현
➡ eosinophil 유도
➡ eosinophil: vasoactive amines degranulation ↑
➡ vasodilation
➡ body fluid influx: body swelling ↑

처방 목표 CD4+ Th cell apoptosis 유도 / B cell: allergen specific IgE 생산 억제 / 세포질 cAMP 농도 지속 ➡ 세포질 granule-membrane protein: phospholylation 억제 / hydrogen peroxide 제거 / mast cell degranulation 억제 / VCAM-1 발현 억제

처방 구성 麻黃 六兩 / 石膏 半斤 / 生薑 三兩 / 甘草 二兩 / 大棗 十五枚 / 白朮 四兩

처방 약리

석고 CaSO4 ➡ Calcium Mediated T-Cell Apoptosis 유도

감초 glycyrrhetinic acid
➡ 11-beta-hydroxysteroid dehydrogenase1 (HSD11B1) inhibitor
➡ glucocorticoid 작용
➡ B cell: IκBα 생성
➡ NF-κB 억제
➡ 항체 생성 억제

대조 cAMP ➡ inhibition of granular organelles phosphorylation
➡ granule swelling 억제

생강 gingerol ➡ hydrogen peroxide scavenger
➡ 세포질 granule: translocation 억제

마황 ephedrine ➡ Epinephrine receptors agonist
➡ adenylate cyclase 활성화
➡ cAMP ↑
➡ degranulation 억제

백출 atractylon ➡ vascular cell adhesion molecule-1 (VCAM-1) blocker

월비탕 (越婢湯)

원문 風水 惡風，一身 悉 腫，脈 浮 不渴，續 自汗出，無 大熱，越婢湯 主之。

원문 해설 피하 부종이 있고 추위를 타며 몸 전체가 붓고 맥은 떠 있으며 갈증은 없고 땀이 저절로 흐르면서 큰 열이 없는 경우에는 월비탕을 쓴다.

적응증 Type I hypersensitive reaction: second sensitization

병태 & 증상

Type I hypersensitive reaction: second sensitization

➡ allergen 침입
➡ B cell allergen specific IgE Rc: allergen binding
➡ CD4+ Th cell: CD4+ Rc ▶ allergen binding
➡ CD4+ Th cell: IL-4 분비
➡ B cell: memory cell & plasma cell 분화
➡ B cell: allergen specific IgE 생산 ↑
➡ mast cell FcR γ: IgE binding
➡ mast cell FcR γ: high affinity IgE Rc --> allergen: mutiple binding
➡ Phospholipase C activation

➡ diacylglycerol & Inositol trisphosphate 생성
➡ Inositol trisphosphate -> endoplasmic reticulum: calcium 분비
➡ 세포질: granule-bound adenylate cyclase 활성화
➡ cAMP ↑
➡ cAMP-dependent protein kinase 활성화
➡ cAMP ↓
➡ 세포질 granule-membrane protein: phospholylation
➡ 세포질 granule swelling
➡ mast cell FcR γ: high affinity IgE Rc ▶ allergen: mutiple binding
➡ mast cell: Fyn/Gab2/RhoA-signaling pathway 활성화
➡ microtubule polymerization via hydrogen peroxide
➡ 세포질 granule: translocation
➡ plasma membrane: granule fusion
➡ vasoactive amines degranulation
: histamine / serine proteases / serotonin / heparin
➡ vasodilation: coldness
➡ body fluid influx: body swelling
➡ lipid mediator: prostaglandin D2 / leukotrienes: sweating

처방 목표 CD4+ Th cell apoptosis 유도 / B cell: allergen specific IgE 생산 억제 / 세포질 cAMP 농도 지속 ➡ 세포질 granule-membrane protein: phospholylation 억제 / hydrogen peroxide 제거 / degranulation 억제

처방 구성 麻黃 六兩 / 石膏 半斤 / 生薑 三兩 / 甘草 二兩 / 大棗 十五枚

처방 약리

석고 $CaSO_4$ ➡ Calcium Mediated T-Cell Apoptosis 유도

감초 glycyrrhetinic acid
➡ 11-beta-hydroxysteroid dehydrogenase1 (HSD11B1) inhibitor
➡ glucocorticoid 작용
➡ B cell: IκBα 생성
➡ NF-κB 억제
➡ 항체 생성 억제

대조 cAMP ➡ inhibition of granular organelles phosphorylation

➡ granule swelling 억제

생강 gingerol ➡ hydrogen peroxide scavenger
➡ 세포질 granule: translocation 억제

마황 ephedrine ➡ Epinephrine receptors agonist
➡ adenylate cyclase 활성화
➡ cAMP ↑
➡ degranulation 억제

육물황금탕 (六物黃芩湯)

원문 六物黃芩湯, 治 乾嘔 下利 。

원문 해설 육물황금탕은 마른 구역과 설사를 치료한다.

적응증 Pathogenic E. coli infection

병태 & 증상

Pathogenic E. coli infection

➡ intestine epithelial microvilli: pathogenic E. coli 부착
➡ epithelial microvilli: protein kinase C 활성화
▶ calmodulin 활성화
▶ actin bundle 형성
▶ pathogenic E. coli 정착
➡ pathogenic E. coli LPS: macrophage 유도
▶ phagocytosis & respiratory burst
▶ extracellular: peroxynitrite ($ONOO^-$) ↑
▶ enteritis
➡ pathogenic E. coli antigen: neutrophil 유도
➡ neutrophil phagocytosis
➡ HClO 분비 via H2O2
➡ pathogenic E. coli: CD9 strain ▶ neutrophil granule 저항

➡ neutrophil granule: pathogenic E. coli 활성화

▶ verotoxin 생산

➡ epithelial microvilli: verotoxin 부착

➡ attachment elongation mechanism

➡ epithelial microvilli: necrosis ▶ diarrhea, vommiting

➡ verotoxin: blood 유입

➡ fascia (근막) 정착: 근막 대사 증가 ▶ intracellular lactate ↑

▶ necrotizing fasciitis

처방 목표 epithelial microvilli: calmodulin 억제 / extracellular: peroxynitrite ($ONOO^-$) 제거 / HClO 분비 억제 / epithelial microvilli 재생 & 상환 / 근막 intracellular lactate 교정

처방 구성 黃芩 三兩 / 人參 三兩 / 乾薑 三兩 / 桂枝 一兩 / 大棗 十二枚 / 半夏 半斤

처방 약리

대조 cAMP ➡ inhibition of granular organelles phosphorylation

➡ endoplasmic reticulum: calcium 분비 억제

➡ calmodulin 억제

황금 baicalin ➡ peroxynitrite ($ONOO^-$) scavenger

건강 shogaol ➡ neutrophil H2O2 scavenger

➡ HClO 분비 억제

인삼 panax ginsenoside

➡ Transforming growth factor β (TGF-β) (+) modulator

➡ epithelial microvilli proliferation 촉진

반하 triterpenoid (C30H48O7S)

➡ Rho GTPase family transcription promotor

➡ focal adhesion 생성

➡ epithelial microvilli 이동 촉진

계지 cinnamic acid ➡ lactate oxidizer

➡ pyruvate 전환

REFERENCE

Helen Nazareth,1,2,3 Stacy A. Genagon,1,3 and Thomas A. Russo1,2,3,4*, Extraintestinal Pathogenic *Escherichia coli* Survives within Neutrophils. Infection and Immunity, June 2007, p. 2776-2785, Vol. 75, No. 6

의이부자산 (薏苡附子散)

원문 胸痺 緩急 者 , 薏苡附子散 主之 。

원문 해설 흉부가 저리는데, 증상에 완급이 있는 경우에는 의이부자산을 쓴다.

적응증 Postherpetic neuralgia (대상포진 후 신경통)

병태 & 증상

Postherpetic neuralgia

➡ reactivation of varicella zoster virus
➡ VZV antibody 출현
➡ thorax intercostal nerve: HLA class I (MHC class I allele) 발현
➡ molecular mimic response
➡ HLA class I: VZV antibody 부착
➡ antibody-dependent cellular cytotoxicity
➡ neutrophil 유도
➡ neutrophil cathepsin 분비
➡ intercostal nerve: neuritis ▶ neuralgia

처방 목표 thorax intercostal nerve: HLA class I (MHC class I allele) 발현 억제 / neutrophil cathepsin 분비 억제

처방 구성 薏苡仁 十五兩 / 炮大附子 十枚

처방 약리

의이인 stigmasterol, 약리 추측 ➡ MHC class I molecule (-) modulator

포부자 aconitine

➡ 약리추측: neutrophil` Voltage-gated proton channels blocker
(식균작용에 의해 증가된 세포내 proton을 세포외로 방출시키는 채널)

➡ Voltage-gated proton channels 차단

➡ 호중구내 수소이온 축적

➡ 대사 억제

➡ cathepsin 분비 억제

의이부자패장산 (薏苡附子敗醬散)

원문 腸癰 之 為 病，其 身 甲錯，腹 皮 急，按 之 濡，如 腫狀，腹 無 積聚, 身 無 熱，脈 數，此 為 腹 內 有 癰膿，薏苡附子敗醬散 主之。

원문 해설 장 부속기에 병이 생기면 피부가 거칠어지고, 배가 땅기며, 누르면 물에 젖은 듯하고, 종기가 있는 것처럼 보이나, 뱃속에 큰 덩어리는 없어 보이고, 발열 없이 맥이 빠른 것은, 장 부속기(충수)에 농이 생긴 것으로 의이부자패장산을 쓴다.

적응증 Appendicitis (충수염)

병태 & 증상

Appendicitis

➡ bacterial infection

➡ Yersinia spp / Campylobacter spp / Salmonella spp / etc

➡ bacteria antibody 출현

➡ appendix endothelium: HLA-B27 (MHC class I allele) 발현

➡ molecular mimic response

➡ HLA-B27: bacteria antibody 부착

➡ antibody-dependent cellular cytotoxicity

➡ macrophage 유도: phagocytosis

➡ TNF-α 분비

➡ appendix endothelium: TNF Rc 부착

➡ 세포막 대사 증가 & 미토콘드리아 대사 증가

➡ reactive oxygen species ↑

➡ NF-κB ↑
➡ p53 활성화
➡ appendix endothelium: apoptosis

처방 목표 appendix endothelium: HLA-B27 (MHC class I allele) 발현 억제 / macrophage TNF-α 분비 억제 / p53 활성화 억제

처방 구성 薏苡仁 十分 / 附子 二分 / 敗醬 五分

처방 약리

의이인 stigmasterol, 약리 추측 ➡ MHC class I molecule (-) modulator

부자 hypaconitine
➡ 약리 추측: macrophage` Voltage-gated proton channels blocker
(식균작용에 의해 증가된 세포내 proton을 세포외로 방출시키는 채널)
➡ voltage-gated proton channels 차단
➡ 수소이온 축적
➡ 대사 억제
➡ TNF-α 분비 억제

패장 (마타리) oleanolic acid
➡ PPAR (peroxisome proliferator-activated receptors) activator
➡ p53 억제

이중환 (理中丸)

원문 霍亂 頭痛, 發熱 身疼痛, 熱多 欲 飲水 者, 五苓散 主之, 寒多 不 用 水 者, 理中丸 主之。

원문 해설 식중독으로 구토하고 설사하는데, 발열하고 몸이 쑤시고 아프며, 열이 많으면서 물을 마시려하면 오령산을 쓰고, 오한이 많으면서 물을 마시지 않으면 이 중환을 쓴다.

적응증 Clostridial necrotic enteritis (클로스트리디움균 괴사성장염)

병태 & 증상

Clostridial necrotic enteritis

➡ food poisoning
➡ small intestine mucosa: Clostridium perfringens 감염
➡ Clostridium perfringens: β-toxin 생산
➡ proteolytic enzymes: β-toxin 분해
➡ β-toxin: monocyte 유도
➡ monocyte: IL-6 / IL-1 / TNF-α 분비: chills , fever, headache
➡ C. perfringens capsule: phagocytosis 회피
➡ monocyte: IL-8 분비
➡ microvascular endothelium: VCAM-1 발현
➡ neutrophil 부착
➡ mucosal lamina propria: neutrophil infiltration
➡ C. perfringens capsule: phagocytosis 회피
➡ neutrophil phagocytosis
➡ HClO 분비 via H2O2
➡ mucosal endothelium: necrosis ▶ vomitting, diarrhea

처방 목표 microvascular endothelium: VCAM-1 차단 / HClO 분비 억제 / mucosal endothelium 재생

처방 구성 人參 / 乾薑 / 炙甘草 / 白朮 各 三兩

처방 약리

백출 atractylon ➡ vascular cell adhesion molecule-1 (VCAM-1) blocker

건강 shogaol ➡ neutrophil H2O2 scavenger
➡ HClO 분비 억제

인삼 panax ginsenoside
➡ Transforming growth factor β (TGF-β) (+) modulator
➡ small intestine mucosa 재생 촉진

구감초 18β-24-Hydroxyglycyrrhetinic acid
➡ HSD11B2 inhibitor
➡ cortisol 분해 억제

➡ mineralocorticoid receptors 자극 지속
➡ small intestine mucosa: Na+/ K+ pumps 전사 촉진

인삼탕 (人參湯)

원문 胸痹 心 中 痞 , 留氣 結 在 胸 , 胸滿 , 脅下 逆 搶 心, 枳實薤白桂枝湯 主之 ; 人參湯 亦 主之 。

원문 해설 가슴부위에 마비감이 있고 심장이 저리며 심박동이 불안정하면서 그득해지고, 저리는 기운이 겨드랑이까지 뻗치는 경우에는 지실해백계지탕을 쓰며, 인삼탕도 쓸 수 있다.

적응증 Unstable angina-mediated coronary calcification
(불안정형 협심증-매개 관상동맥 석회화)

병태 & 증상

Unstable angina-mediated coronary calcification

➡ coronary artery: unstable fibrous cap
➡ fibrous cap 내부: 신생혈관 출혈
➡ smooth muscle cell 괴사
➡ smooth muscle cell 내부: lipid 유출
➡ fibrous cap 내부: lipid ↑
➡ fibrous cap 내부: 압력 증가
➡ fibrous cap: expansion
➡ coronary artery: 내강 좁아짐
➡ coronary endothelium: ischemia
➡ coronary endothelium: VCAM-1 발현
➡ neutrophil 부착 & 내피하 이동
➡ neutrophil phagocytosis
➡ HClO 분비 via H2O2
➡ coronary collagen: hydrolysis
➡ coronary smooth muscle cell: NF-κB 활성화
➡ smooth muscle cell: phenotypic transition

➡ osteoblastic differentiation

➡ coronary calcification

처방 목표 coronary endothelium: VCAM-1 차단 / HClO 분비 억제 / coronary smooth muscle cell: NF-κB 억제 / coronary calcification 억제

처방 구성 人參 / 甘草 / 乾薑 / 白朮 各 三兩

처방 약리

백출 atractylon ➡ vascular cell adhesion molecule-1 (VCAM-1) blocker

건강 shogaol ➡ neutrophil H2O2 scavenger

➡ HClO 분비 억제

감초 glycyrrhetinic acid

➡ 11-beta-hydroxysteroid dehydrogenase1 (HSD11B1) inhibitor

➡ glucocorticoid 작용

➡ IκBα 생성

➡ NF-κB 억제

인삼 panax ginsenoside

➡ Transforming growth factor β (TGF-β) (+) modulator

➡ coronary calcification 억제

인진오령산 (茵陳五苓散)

원문 黃疸病，茵陳五苓散 主之。

원문 해설 황달병에는 인진오령산을 쓴다.

적응증 Free bile acids-mediated glomerulonephritis (자유담즙산-매개 사구체신염)

병태 & 증상

Free bile acids-mediated glomerulonephritis

➡ cholestasis
➡ bile 역류: jaundice
➡ serum bile acids ↑
➡ bile acids: plasma proteins 부착
➡ serum bile acids plasma proteins
➡ free bile acids 생성
➡ free bile acids: uncharged hydrophilic group
➡ glomerular filtration
➡ mesangial cell: phagocytosis
➡ mesangial cell: IL-1 분비
➡ glomerulus vessel: VCAM-1 발현
➡ monocyte 유도
➡ monocyte: 사구체 혈관 부착
➡ monocyte ROS burst
➡ 사구체 혈관 손상: thrombus formation
➡ 수출소동맥 저산소증
➡ 수출소동맥 수축
➡ 사구체내 압력 ↑
➡ 사구체 모세혈관 손상: glomerulonephritis
➡ glomerular filtration rate ↓ ▶ 수분배설 감소: vomiting
➡ podocyte contraction
➡ podocyte: intracellular lactate ↑
➡ podocyte apoptosis
➡ monocyte: mesangial cell growth factor 분비
➡ mesangial cell proliferation

처방 목표 free bile acids: uncharged hydrophilic group 감소 / glomerulus endothelial cell: VCAM-1 발현 억제 / thrombus formation 억제 / 수출소동맥 수축 억제 / podocyte: intracellular lactate 제거 / mesangial cell: proliferation 억제

처방 구성 茵陳蒿 末 十分 / 五苓散 五分

처방 약리

인진호 capillarisin ➡ CDCA hydrophilic group: detoxicant
➡ glomerular filtration 억제

➡ tubular secretion 유도

백출 atractylon ➡ vascular cell adhesion molecule-1 (VCAM-1) blocker

복령 pachymic acid ➡ glycoprotein IIb/IIIa (gpIIb/IIIa) (-) modulator
➡ thrombus formation 억제

택사 alisol ➡ angiotensin II receptor blocker
➡ 수출소동맥 수축 억제

계지 cinnamic acid ➡ lactate oxidizer
➡ pyruvate 전환 촉진

저령 ergosterol ➡ mesangial cell proliferation inhibitor

인진호탕 (茵陳蒿湯)

원문 陽明病 / 發熱 汗出 者 , 此 為 熱 越 , 不 能 發黃 也;但 頭汗出 , 身 無汗, 劑 頸 而 還 , 小便 不利 , 渴 引 水 漿 者 此 為 瘀熱 在裡 , 身 必 發黃 。傷寒 七 八 日 , 身黃 如 橘子色 , 小便 不利 , 腹 微滿 者, 茵陳蒿湯 主之。

원문 해설 위장관 점막림프절 감염증에서 열나고 땀나는 것은 열이 빠져나가는 것으므로 황달이 생기지 않는다. 단지 머리에서만 땀나고 목 부위 밑으로는 땀이 없으면서 소변이 불편하고 갈증이 나서 물을 찾는 것은 속열이 있는 있기 때문이며 반드시 황달이 생긴다. 세포병변성 감염증이 7~8일 후 몸이 귤 알맹이처럼 누래지고 소변이 불편하며 복부팽만감이 있는 경우에는 인진호탕으로 치료한다.

적응증 Intrahepatic cholangiocarcinoma (간내담도암)

병태 & 증상

Intrahepatic cholangiocarcinoma

➡ HBV, HCV: chronic cholangiocyte infection
➡ intrahepatic cholangitis

➡ cholangiocyte: adenomatous hyperplasia
➡ chlangiocarcinoma
➡ intrahepatic bile duct: obstruction
➡ hepatocyte: chenodeoxycholic acid (CDCA) 축적
➡ CDCA: hydrophilic group 독성
➡ ROS 발생
➡ GSH 고갈
➡ mitochondria dysfunction
➡ hepatocyte apoptosis
➡ conjugated bilirubin 역류
➡ 혈 중: conjugated bilirubin ↑
➡ jaundice

처방 목표 chlangiocarcinoma 성장 억제 / CDCA: hydrophilic group 감소 (CDCA의 소수성 그룹이 hepatocyte의 mitochondria dysfunction 원인) / conjugated bilirubin ➡ 산화 촉진

처방 구성 茵陳蒿 六兩 / 梔子 十四枚 / 大黃 二兩

처방 약리

대황 emodin ➡ tyrosine kinase blocker
➡ chlangiocarcinoma 성장 억제

인진호 capillarisin ➡ CDCA hydrophilic group: detoxicant

치자 crocin ➡ conjugated bilirubin oxidation
➡ bilirubin degradation

일물과체탕 (一物瓜蒂湯)

원문 太陽 中暍 , 身熱 疼 重 , 而 脈 微 弱 , 此 以 夏月 傷 冷水, 水行 皮中 所 致 也 , 一物瓜蒂湯 主之 。

원문 해설 온열 중추 과흥분으로 갈증이 있고, 몸에 열이 나며, 쑤시고 무거우며, 맥이 가늘고 약한 것은 여름철에 냉수를 많이 먹은 것으로서, 찬물이 체내에서 병을 일으킨 것이다, 일물과체산을 쓴다.

적응증 hyperthermia (악성고열증)

병태 & 증상

hyperthermia

➡ heat stroke & sun stroke
➡ hypothalamic or spinal: thermal stimulation
➡ smooth muscle cell: heat producing 자극
➡ hyperthermia

처방 목표 smooth muscle cell: F-actin 분해

처방 구성 瓜蔕 二十個

처방 약리

과체 cucurbitacin ➡ smooth muscle cell: F-actin aggregation inhibitor
➡ smooth muscle cell: contraction 억제
➡ heat producing 차단

작약감초부자탕 (芍藥甘草附子湯)

원문 發汗 , 病 不解 , 反 惡寒 者 , 虛 故 也, 芍藥甘草附子湯 主之 。

원문 해설 땀을 낸 뒤에 병이 풀리지 않고 오히려 오한이 나는 경우는 몸이 약하기 때문이며 작약감초부자탕을 쓴다.

적응증 Human T-Lymphotropic Virus (HTLV) infection

병태 & 증상

HTLV infection

➡ HTLV replication
➡ endoplasmic reticulum (ER): HTLV protein 조립 반복
➡ endoplasmic reticulum: superoxide 축적
➡ endoplasmic reticulum: SOD 고갈
➡ ER stress
➡ Na+/ K+ pumps ↓
➡ HTLV infected cell: apoptosis
➡ IL-6 분비: chills
➡ neutrophil 유도
➡ neutrophil elastase 분비
➡ 조직 손상

처방 목표 superoxide 제거 / Na+/ K+ pumps 전사 촉진 / neutrophil elastase 분비 억제

처방 구성 芍藥 三兩 / 炙甘草 三兩 / 炮附子 一枚

처방 약리

작약 paeoniflorin ➡ superoxide scavenger

구감초 18β-24-Hydroxyglycyrrhetinic acid ➡ HSD11B2 inhibitor
➡ cortisol 분해 억제
➡ mineralocorticoid receptors 자극 지속
➡ Na+/ K+ pumps 전사 촉진

포부자 aconitine
➡ 약리추측: neutrophil` Voltage-gated proton channels blocker
(식균작용에 의해 증가된 세포내 proton을 세포외로 방출시키는 채널)
➡ Voltage-gated proton channels 차단
➡ 호중구내 수소이온 축적
➡ neutrophil 대사 억제
➡ elastase 분비 억제

작약감초탕 (芍藥甘草湯)

원문 傷寒 脈浮，自汗出，小便 數，心煩，微 惡寒，脚 攣急，反 與 桂枝，欲 攻 其 表，此 誤 也。 得之 便 厥，咽中 乾，煩躁 吐逆 者，作 甘草乾薑湯 與 之, 以 復 其 陽 ; 若 厥愈 ` 足 溫 者, 更 作 芍藥甘草湯 與 之.

원문 해설 세포병변성 감염증으로 맥이 뜨고 땀나고 소변이 잦으며 마음이 괴롭고 약간 오한이 들며 다리가 땅기어 오므라드는 경우에 계지탕을 쓰면 안 된다. 병의 초기에 곧바로 수족냉증이 나타나고 목구멍이 건조하며 괴롭고 구토하는 경우에는 감초건강탕을 써서 양(면역기능)을 회복해야 하며 수족냉증이 해소되고 발이 따뜻해지는 경우에는 이어서 작약감초탕을 쓴다.

적응증 Inclusion body myositis (봉입체 근염)

병태 & 증상

Inclusion body myositis

➡ muscle fiber: endogenous retrovirus 활성화
➡ endoplasmic reticulum (ER): retrovirus protein 조립 반복
➡ endoplasmic reticulum: superoxide 축적
➡ endoplasmic reticulum: SOD 고갈
➡ ER stress: retrovirus protein misfolding ↑ ➡ 봉입체
➡ Na+/ K+ pumps ↓
➡ 근육세포 부종
➡ 근력 약화

처방 목표 superoxide 제거 / Na+/ K+ pumps 전사 촉진

처방 구성 芍藥 四兩 / 炙甘草 四兩

처방 약리

작약 paeoniflorin ➡ superoxide scavenger

구감초 18β-24-Hydroxyglycyrrhetinic acid
➡ HSD11B2 inhibitor

➡ cortisol 분해 억제
➡ mineralocorticoid receptors 자극 지속
➡ Na+/ K+ pumps 전사 촉진

저고발전 (豬膏髮煎)

원문 諸 黃, 豬膏髮煎 主之, 病 從 小便 出。

원문 해설 모든 황달병에 저고발전을 쓴다. 소변을 통해 병소가 배출된다.

적응증 Free conjugated bilirubin-mediated renal failure
(유리형 결합빌리루빈-매개 신부전)

병태 & 증상

Free conjugated bilirubin-mediated renal failure

➡ obstructive jaundice & hepatitis
➡ hyperbilirubinemia: conjugated bilirubin
➡ albumin: conjugated bilirubin 부착
▶ biliprotein 형성 ▶ liver & kidney 이동 안됨
▶ albumin 붕괴와 더불어 bilirubin 소실
➡ albumin 〈 conjugated bilirubin
➡ free conjugated bilirubin 출현
➡ renal tubular epithelium: endocytosis
➡ tubular epithelium: lysosome pH
➡ tubular epithelium: necrosis
➡ renal failure

처방 목표 renal tubular epithelium: conjugated bilirubin endocytosis 억제 / conjugated bilirubin: urine 배설 촉진

처방 구성 豬膏 半斤 / 亂髮 如 雞子大 三枚

처방 약리

저고 (돼지기름) fatty acid ➡ albumin bounded fatty acid
➡ renal tubular epithelium: endocytosis
➡ free conjugated bilirubin 유입 억제

난발 (머리털) keratin ➡ metal & organic-amines chelator
➡ free conjugated bilirubin: chelation
➡ urine 배설 촉진

저당탕 (抵當湯)

원문 太陽病，六 七 日 表證 仍 在，脈 微 而 沉，反 不 結胸, 其人 發狂 者, 以 熱 在 下焦，少腹 當 硬滿，小便 自利 者,下血 乃 愈. 所 以 然 者，以 太陽 隨 經，瘀熱 在 裡 故 也, 抵當湯 主 之。婦 人 經 水 不 利 下， 抵 當 湯 主 之 。

원문 해설 림프절 감염병이 6~7일이 지난 후 표증이 계속 있고 맥이 가늘고 가라앉아 있는데 결흉증은 보이지 않으면서 미친 것처럼 보이면 아랫배에 종괴가 있는 것으로 빈뇨를 보이면 하혈시키면 낫는다. 이는 림프절을 따라 자궁내막 기질세포가 이동하여 종괴를 만든 것이므로 저당탕을 쓴다. 부인이 생리가 잘 나오지 않거나 하혈이 반복되면 저당탕을 쓴다.

적응증 Endometrioma in uterine serosa & ovary
(자궁장막 & 난소에 발생된 자궁내막종)

병태 & 증상

Endometrioma (자궁내막종)

➡ endometrial stroma cell: 자궁장막 & 난소 이동
➡ endometrial stroma cell: estrogen receptor
➡ estrogen signal: growth factor 생산
➡ growth factor: autocrine
➡ tyrosine kinase 활성화
➡ endometrial stroma cell: proliferation

➡ endometrioma: urinary frequency, ovulation disorder
➡ mense without heparin
➡ 탈락
➡ thrombi-fibrin formation
➡ fibrin clot

처방 목표 estrogen receptor 차단 / tyrosine kinase 차단 / fibrin clot 용해

처방 구성 水蛭 三十個 / 䗪蟲 各 三十個 / 桃仁 二十個 / 大黃 三兩

처방 약리

도인 amygdalin
➡ 체내 활성 성분: thiocyanate (amygdalin metabolite)
➡ 4S estrogen receptor (ER) ▶ 5S estrogen receptor 전환 억제
(4S monomer: estrogen 저친화성, 5S dimer: estrogen 고친화성)

대황 emodin ➡ tyrosine kinase blocker

수질 hirudin ➡ thrombolytic activator
➡ hirudin C-terminus: thrombin 부착
➡ thrombolysis
➡ thrombi-fibrin formation 용해

맹충 anophelin ➡ thrombin esterase blocker
➡ antithrombin activation

저당환 (抵當丸)

원문 傷寒 有熱, 少腹 滿, 應 小便 不利, 今 反 利 者, 為 有 血 也. 當 下 之, 不可 餘藥, 宜 抵當丸。服 之, 晬 時 當 下 血, 若 不 下 者, 更 服。

원문 해설 세포병변성 감염병에서 열이 있으면서 아랫배가 그득하면 당연히 소변이 불편해 지는데, 반대로 빈뇨가 있다면 혈괴가 있는 것이므로 빼내야 되며 다른 약으로는 안 되고 저당환을 쓴다. 복용하면 당연히 하혈하게 되는데, 하혈이 없는 경우에는 다시 복용한다.

적응증 Endometrial adenocarcinoma (자궁내막선종)

병태 & 증상

Endometrial adenocarcinoma

➡ endometrial gland cell: 자궁근육속으로 이동
➡ endometrial gland cell: estrogen receptor
➡ estrogen signal: growth factor 생산
➡ growth factor: autocrine
➡ tyrosine kinase 활성화
➡ endometrial gland cell: proliferation
➡ endometrial adenocarcinoma: urinary frequency
➡ mense without heparin
➡ 탈락
➡ thrombi-fibrin formation
➡ fibrin clot

처방 목표 estrogen receptor 차단 / tyrosine kinase 차단 / fibrin clot 용해

처방 구성 水蛭 二十個 / 蝱蟲 二十個 / 桃仁 二十五個 / 大黃 三兩

처방 약리

도인 amygdalin
- ➡ 체내 활성 성분: thiocyanate (amygdalin metabolite)
- ➡ 4S estrogen receptor (ER) ▶ 5S estrogen receptor 전환 억제
  (4S monomer: estrogen 저친화성, 5S dimer: estrogen 고친화성)

대황 emodin ➡ tyrosine kinase blocker

수질 hirudin ➡ thrombolytic activator
➡ hirudin C-terminus: thrombin 부착
➡ thrombolysis
➡ thrombi-fibrin formation 용해

맹충 anophelin ➡ thrombin esterase blocker
➡ antithrombin activation

저령산 (豬苓散)

원문 嘔吐 而 病 在 膈 上, 後 思 水 者, 解, 急 與 之。 思 水 者, 豬苓散 主之。

원문 해설 구토가 있는 경우에 소화기계통에 원인이 있지 않다면, 수분축적에 의한 것으로 생각해야 하며, 저령산을 쓴다.

적응증 IgA nephropathy (IgA 신병증)

병태 & 증상

IgA nephropathy

➡ glomerulus 모세혈관: IgA 침착
➡ mesangial cell: phagocytosis
➡ mesangial cell: IL-1 분비
➡ glomerulus capillary: VCAM-1 발현
➡ monocyte 유도
➡ monocyte: 사구체 모세혈관 부착
➡ monocyte ROS burst
➡ 사구체 모세혈관 손상: thrombus formation
➡ glomerular filtration rate ↓ ▶ uremia: vomiting
➡ monocyte: mesangial cell growth factor 분비
➡ mesangial cell proliferation

처방 목표 glomerulus capillary: VCAM-1 차단 / 사구체 모세혈관: thrombus formation 제거 / mesangial cell proliferation 억제

처방 구성 豬苓 / 茯苓 / 白朮 各 等分

처방 약리

백출 atractylon ➡ vascular cell adhesion molecule-1 (VCAM-1) blocker

복령 pachymic acid ➡ glycoprotein IIb/IIIa (gpIIb/IIIa) (-) modulator
➡ thrombus formation 억제

저령 ergosterol ➡ mesangial cell proliferation inhibitor

저령탕 (豬苓湯)

원문 脈 浮 發熱 , 渴 欲 飮水 , 小便 不利 者 。, 少陰病, 下利六七日, 咳而嘔渴, 心煩 不得眠者 。

원문 해설 맥이 뜨고 발열하며 갈증이 나서 물을 마시려 하는 경우, 항체매개독성증에서 6~7 일간 설사하고 기침하며 구역과 갈증이 있고 흉부가 괴롭고 잠들지 못하는 경우

적응증 Goodpasture's syndrome ➡ Anti-GBM glomerulonephritis (항-기저막 사구체신염) , GBM: glomerular basement membrane, Goodpasture's syndrome: type IV collagen autoantibodies mediated disease
➡ glomerulonephritis & lung hemorrhage & gastrointestinal bleeding 일으킴

병태 & 증상

anti-GBM glomerulonephritis

➡ glomerular basement membrane: IgG autoantibodies
➡ complement 유도
➡ GBM injury
➡ mesangial cell: GBM에서 이탈
➡ mesangial cell proliferation
➡ mesangial cell: proteinase 분비
➡ elastic laminin 손상
➡ crescent formation
➡ 사구체 모세혈관 손상: thrombus formation
➡ Bowman's capsule: 단백질 & 당 유출 ▶ thirst
➡ 수출소동맥 저산소증
➡ 수출소동맥 수축
➡ 사구체내 압력 ↑
➡ 사구체 손상 ↑

처방 목표 mesangial cell proliferation 억제 / elastic laminin 합성 촉진 / thrombus formation / Bowman's capsule: 단백질 유출 / 수출소동맥 수축 억제시킴

처방 구성 豬苓 / 茯苓 / 澤瀉 / 阿膠 / 滑石 各 一兩

처방 약리

저령 ergosterol ➡ mesangial cell proliferation inhibitor

아교 Glycine / Proline / Hydroxyproline / Alanine
➡ collagen의 주요 아미노산
➡ elastic laminin biosynthesis 촉진

복령 pachymic acid ➡ 약리추측: glycoprotein IIb/IIIa (gpIIb/IIIa) (-) modulator
➡ thrombus formation inhibition

활석 Mg3(Si4O10)(OH)2 ➡ ammonia & Nucleic acid absorbent
➡ 단백질 유출 억제

택사 alisol ➡ angiotensin II receptor blocker
➡ 수출소동맥 수축 억제됨

적두당귀산 (赤豆當歸散)

원문 病 者 脈 數 , 無熱 , 微 煩, 默默 但 欲 臥, 汗出 , 初得 之 三 `四日, 目 赤 如 鳩 眼 ; 七 `八 日, 目 四 眥 黑 。若 能 食 者 , 膿 已 成 也 , 赤豆當歸散 主之 。

원문 해설 환자의 맥이 빠르고 열은 없으며, 약간 괴롭고, 말없이 눕고만 싶어하며 땀이 나는데, 병이 시작된 지 3~4일 후 비둘기 눈처럼 눈이 벌겋게 되고 7~8일 후 눈꼬리가 검게 된다. 만약 식사를 하면 농이 나오게 된다. 적소당귀산을 쓴다.

적응증 Polyclonal IgM cold agglutinins - mediated hemolytic anemia
(다클론IgM 한냉응집소-매개 용혈성빈혈)

병태 & 증상

Polyclonal IgM cold agglutinins - mediated hemolytic anemia

➡ Mycoplasma pneumoniae & infectious mononucleosis (전염성 단핵구증)
& other infections
➡ 병원성 IgM 자가항체 생성

➡ erythrocyte membrane: cross reaction
➡ 손발 저온말초순환: erythrocyte membrane ▶ IgM 부착
➡ IgM Fc region: complement 부착
➡ 보체연쇄반응: C3b 생성
➡ erythrocyte CR1: C3b 부착
➡ C3b coated erythrocyte 생성
➡ liver reticuloendothelial system 접촉
➡ macrophage CR1: C3b coated erythrocyte 부착
➡ macrophage: protease 분비
➡ erythrocyte: protein kinase C 활성화
➡ adducin phosphorylation
➡ adducin-spectrin-actin complex: 분리됨
➡ erythrocyte membrane: 불안정해짐
➡ spherocyte 생성
➡ spleen: hemolysis
➡ anemia
➡ polycythemia (적혈구 증다증)
➡ hypertension / conjunctival haemorrhage / capillary haemorrhage / oropharynx haemorrhage

처방 목표 IgM Fc region: complement 부착 억제 / erythrocyte: protein kinase C 억제

처방 구성 赤小豆 三升 / 當歸 十兩

처방 약리

적소두 (팥) albumin, 약리추측 ➡ immunoglobulin Fc region binder
➡ IgM Fc region: complement 부착 억제

당귀 decurcin ➡ erythrocyte protein kinase C inhibitor
➡ adducin-spectrin-actin complex 유지시킴
➡ spherocyte 생성 억제

적석지우여량탕 (赤石脂禹餘糧湯)

원문 傷寒 服 湯藥，下利 不止，心下 痞硬。服 瀉心湯 已，復 以 他藥 下之，利 不止。醫 以 理中 與 之，利 益 甚。理 中 者，理 中 焦，此 利 在 下焦，赤石脂禹餘糧湯 主之。復 不止 者，當 利 其 小便。

원문 해설 세포병변성 감염증에서 약을 복용해도 설사가 멈추지 않고 속 쓰림과 복부경직이 있으면 사심탕을 쓴다. 그래도 설사가 계속 되면 보통 이중탕을 쓰는데, 복용 후 설사가 오히려 심해지면 이 설사는 소장병이 아니고 대장병이므로 적석지우여량탕을 쓴다. 만약 적석지우여량탕으로도 설사가 멈추지 않으면 콩팥에 병이 있는 것이다.

적응증 Cytomegalovirus inclusion colitis (사이토메가로바이러스 봉입체대장염)

병태 & 증상

Cytomegalovirus inclusion colitis

➡ colon mucosa: capillary endothelial cells
➡ cytomegalovirus (CMV) replication
➡ inclusion body 형성
➡ capillary endothelial cells: giant cell
➡ 모세혈관 내강 좁아져서 점막상피에 혈류량 감소됨
➡ mucosa cell: necrosis
➡ dead mucosa cell: protein-rich fluid
➡ pus 생성
➡ 수분 흡수 불량: diarrhea

처방 목표 inclusion body cell: apoptosis 유도 / pus 제거

처방 구성 赤石脂 一斤 / 太 一 禹餘糧 一斤

처방 약리

우여량 Fe_2O_3 ➡ 체내 활성 성분은 위액에 분해된 $FeCl_2$
➡ 소장에서 흡수되지 않고 대장으로 이동
➡ 저산소 상태의 점막하 모세혈관 내피: $FeCl_2$ 흡수 증가됨
➡ 모세혈관 내피 세포막 침착

➡ Fe^{2+}: Haber-Weiss 반응
➡ hydroxyl radicals (•OH) 생성
➡ 세포막 지질 과산화
➡ 봉입체 형성한 대장 모세혈관 내피세포: apoptosis
➡ 점막상피 허혈 개선

적석지 Al_2O_3, $2SiO_2 \cdot 4H_2O$ ➡ Cation absorbent

적환 (赤丸)

원문 寒 氣 厥 逆 , 赤丸 主之 。

원문 해설 조직 허혈이 있고 손발이 심하게 차가워 지는 경우에는 적환을 쓴다.

적응증 Complement-mediated vasculitis (보체-매개 혈관염)

병태 & 증상

Complement-mediated vasculitis

➡ blood: Ag-Ab complex, microorganism
➡ complement activation
➡ C3b ↑
➡ marginated neutrophil C3b Rc: C3b 부착
➡ marginated neutrophil 활성화
➡ superoxide 배출: vascular endothelium 자극
➡ vascular endothelium: vwF 분비
➡ vwF + thrombin: 1차 응집
➡ platelet 활성화
➡ platelet GP IIb/IIIa + fibrinogen: 2차 응집
➡ thrombus 형성: tissue ischemia
➡ superoxide
➡ hemoglobin ferrous ion ▶ ferric ion
➡ methemoglobin 형성: cold hands and feet

처방 목표 marginated neutrophil 활성화 억제 / vwF + thrombin: 1차 응집 억제 / thrombus 제거 / methemoglobin 환원

처방 구성 茯苓 四兩 / 炮烏頭 二兩 / 半夏 四兩 / 細辛 一兩

처방 약리

포오두 aconitine, 약리추측

➡ marginated neutrophil` Voltage-gated proton channels blocker
(식균작용에 의해 증가된 세포내 proton을 세포외로 방출시키는 채널)

➡ Voltage-gated proton channels 차단

➡ 호중구내 수소이온 축적

➡ marginated neutrophil 대사 억제

반하 triterpenoid (C30H48O7S)

➡ Rho GTPase family transcription promotor

➡ heparan sulfate 생성 촉진

➡ heparin 유사 작용

➡ thrombin 용해

복령 pachymic acid ➡ glycoprotein IIb/IIIa (gpIIb/IIIa) (-) modulator
➡ thrombus formation 억제

세신 eugenol ➡ Met-hemoglobin reducer

정력대조사폐탕 (葶藶大棗瀉肺湯)

원문 肺癰 , 喘 不 得 臥, 葶藶大棗瀉肺湯 主之 。

원문 해설 폐농양으로 호흡이 곤란하며, 눕지 못하는 경우에는 정력대조사폐탕을 쓴다.

적응증 Lung abscess (폐농양)

병태 & 증상

Lung abscess

➡ pneumonia compliation

➡ lung abcess

➡ bronchial dilation: purulent sputum excretion
➡ bronchial dilation: pulmonary vein 확장
➡ myocardial sleeve 자극
➡ atrial arrhythmia

처방 목표 bronchial dilation 지속 / atrial arrhythmia 억제

처방 구성 葶藶 熬 令 黃色，搗 丸 如 彈子大 / 大棗 十二枚

처방 약리

대조 cAMP ➡ airway smooth muscle: β2-receptors 활성 지속
➡ bronchial dilation

정력자 helveticoside ➡ cardiac glycoside
➡ 심방세동 억제

조위승기탕 (調胃承氣湯)

원문 太陽病 三日，發汗 不解，蒸蒸 發熱 者，屬 胃 也，調胃承氣湯 主之。傷寒 吐 後，腹脹滿 者，與 調胃承氣湯。陽明病，不吐 不下，心煩 者，可 與 調胃承氣湯。

원문 해설 림프절감염증이 3일이 되어, 땀을 흘리고도 낫지 않고, 찌는 듯이 열이 나는 것은 위점막림프절에 병이 생긴 것이고 조위승기탕을 쓴다. 세포병변성 감염증으로 토한 뒤에 복부팽만감이 있는 경우에는 조위승기탕을 쓴다. 위점막림프절 감염병으로 토해지지도 않고 설사도 없으면서, 흉부가 괴로운 경우에는 조위승기탕을 쓴다.

적응증 Small intestine MALT lymphoma (소장 점막림프조직 림프종)

병태 & 증상

Small intestine MALT lymphoma

➡ 주로 ileum: pathogenic microorganisms: persistent infection
➡ B cell infiltration

➡ Peyer`s patch: B cell clones formation
➡ pathogenic microorganisms: persistent antigenic stimulation
➡ B cell: genetic alteration
➡ B cell: neoplastic transformation

처방 목표 B cell infiltration 억제 / Peyer`s patch: microorganisms & B cell clones 장외로 배출 / neoplastic B cell: apoptosis 시킴

처방 구성 甘草 二兩 / 芒硝 半升 / 大黃 四兩

처방 약리

감초 glycyrrhetinic acid
➡ 11-beta-hydroxysteroid dehydrogenase1 (HSD11B1) inhibitor
➡ glucocorticoid 작용
➡ IκBα 생성
➡ NF-κB 억제
➡ B cell 이동 억제

망초 Sodium Sulfate ➡ Intraluminal distention pressure 상승시킴
➡ submucosa: leacking
➡ Peyer`s patch: microorganisms & B cell clones 배출

대황 emodin ➡ tyrosine kinase Rc blocker
➡ neoplastic B cell 성장 정지

조협환 (皂莢丸)

원문 咳 逆 上氣，時 時 吐 濁，但 坐 不 得 眠，皂莢丸 主之。

원문 해설 얼굴이 붉어질 정도의 심한 기침을 하고, 때때로 탁한 가래가 나오며, 앉아 있으려고 하고 누워서 자기 힘든 경우에는 조협환을 쓴다.

적응증 Bronchiectasis (기관지 확장증)

병태 & 증상

Bronchiectasis

➡ bronchitis / emphysema / cystic fibrosis
➡ bronchial tree: irreversible dilation
➡ mucopurulent sputum production 축적: cough, sputum

처방 목표 기도 확장

처방 구성 皂莢 八兩

처방 약리

조협 triacanthin ➡ Phosphodiesterase (PDE) blocker
➡ 기관지 평활근 이완
➡ 기도 확장

주마탕 (走馬湯)

원문 走馬湯 :治 中惡 心痛 腹脹 , 大便 不通 。

원문 해설 주마탕은 통로에 병이 생긴 것과 흉통이 있는 것,
복부팽만과 대변이 막힌 것을 치료한다.

적응증 Squamous cell carcinoma (편평세포암)

병태 & 증상

Squamous cell carcinoma

➡ 종류: head and neck cancer / esophageal squamous cell carcinoma / squamous cell lung carcinoma / anal cancer
➡ squamous cell: chronic inflammation
➡ cyclin D1 overexpression
➡ p53 inactiviation
➡ cell cycle 지속

➡ squamous cell carcinoma

처방 목표 p53 활성화 / squamous cell carcinoma: apoptosis 유도

처방 구성 杏仁 二枚 / 巴豆 二枚

처방 약리

파두 phorbol ester ➡ squamous cell: protein kinase C (PKC) activator
➡ p53 gene transcription 촉진
➡ cell cycle 정지

행인 cyanide ➡ squamous cell carcinoma: apoptosis 유도
(중층편평상피세포: rhodanese 부족
, cyanide ▶ thiocyanate 무독화되지 않고 축적됨)

죽엽석고탕 (竹葉石膏湯)

원문 傷寒 解 後, 虛 羸 少 氣, 氣逆 欲 吐, 竹葉石膏湯 主之。

원문 해설 세포병변성 감염증이 나은 후 몸이 야위고 호흡이 짧아지며 넘어갈 것 같은 기침과 구토가 있는 경우 죽엽석고탕을 쓴다.

적응증 Secondary tuberculosis (이차성 결핵)

병태 & 증상

Secondary tuberculosis

➡ pulmonary: cavitation
➡ M. tuberculosis: reactivation
➡ systemic spread
➡ pulmonary upper lobe / peripheral lymph node / brain / heart / pancreas / kidney / thyroid / skeletal muscle / bone
➡ M. tuberculosis infected cell: MHC class II 발현
➡ cytotoxic T cell 유도

➡ perforin & granulysin 분비
➡ M. tuberculosis infected cell: Na+/ K+ pump 손상
➡ M. tuberculosis infected cell: necrosis
➡ tissue destruction
➡ amyloidosis
➡ amyloid fibrosis

처방 목표 cavitation 복구시킴 / M. tuberculosis reactivation 억제시킴 / cytotoxic T cell apoptosis 시킴 / M. tuberculosis infected cell: Na+/ K+ pump 활성화시킴 / amyloidosis 억제시킴

처방 구성 竹葉 二把 / 石膏 一斤 / 半夏 半升 / 麥門冬 一升 / 人參 二兩 / 炙甘草 二兩 / 粳米 半升

처방 약리

인삼 panax ginsenoside
➡ Transforming growth factor β (TGF-β) (+) modulator
➡ cell proliferation 촉진

반하 triterpenoid (C30H48O7S)
➡ Rho GTPase family transcription promotor
➡ focal adhesion 생성
➡ 상피세포 이동 촉진

경미 magnesium ➡ DNA replication cofactor

맥문동 ophiopogonin ➡ M. tuberculosis` SigF transcription inhibitor
➡ M. tuberculosis growth 억제됨

석고 CaSO4 ➡ calcium mediated T-cell apoptosis 유도

구감초 18β-24-Hydroxyglycyrrhetinic acid
➡ HSD11B2 inhibitor
➡ cortisol 분해 억제
➡ mineralocorticoid receptors 자극 지속
➡ Na+/ K+ pumps 전사 촉진

죽엽 arundoin ➡ 약리 추측: β-Amyloid gene expression (-) modulator
➡ β-Amyloid 생성 억제시킴

죽엽탕 (竹葉湯)

원문 産後 中風 `發熱 正面 赤 `喘 而 頭痛 , 竹葉湯 主之 。, 頸 項 強 , 用 大 附 子 一 枚 。 嘔 者 加 半夏 半升 。

원문 해설 산 후 중풍으로 발열하며 얼굴이 붉고 호흡이 곤란하며 두통이 있는 경우에는 죽엽탕을 쓴다. 목 앞뒤로 강직감이 있으면 부자를 추가한다. 구역이 있으면 반하를 추가한다.

적응증 Postpartum mononucleosis (산 후 단핵구증)

병태 & 증상

Postpartum mononucleosis

➡ postpartum
➡ Th1 cell activation
➡ macrophage activation
➡ macrophage & chronic inactivated EBV infected astrocyte: 상호작용 깨짐
➡ Epstein-Barr virus (EBV) activation: IL-1 ↑ ▶ fever
➡ EBV specific antibody 생성
➡ antibody-dependent cell-mediated cytotoxicity (ADCC)
➡ neutrophil 유도
➡ neutrophil: leukotriene B4 합성
➡ neutrophil: receptor 변화 ▶ phagocytosis ↑
➡ EBV infected astrocyte: necrosis
➡ astrocyte loss: glutamate uptake ↓
➡ synaptic space: glutamate ↑
➡ postneuron NMDA Rc: glutamate excessive binding
➡ postneuron exciting: intracellular lactate ↑
➡ postneuron 방어기전 작동
➡ postneuron: amyloid-β gene transcription ↑

➡ amyloid-β 분비: axon으로의 전기신호 감소됨
➡ amyloid-β 분비 ↑: axon 전체에 amyloid-β fibril 침착
➡ 뇌신경 전도 감소: 중풍 유사 증상
➡ 침범신경: 후각신경 / 시신경 / 동안신경 / 삼차신경 / 활차신경 / 외전신경 / 안면신경 / 청 신경 / 설인신경 / 미주신경 / 부신경 / 설하신경

처방 목표 macrophage activation 억제 / EBV specific antibody 생성 억제 / leukotriene B4 합성 억제 / neutrophil phagocytosis 억제 / astrocyte 재생 / NMDA Rc 차단 / intracellular lactate 교정 / amyloid-β gene transcription 억제 / amyloid-β fibril 제거

처방 구성 竹葉 一把 / 葛根 三兩 / 防風 一兩 / 桔梗 一兩 / 桂枝 一兩 / 人參 一兩 / 甘草 一兩 / 炮附子 一枚 / 大棗 十五枚 / 生薑 五兩 / 頸 項 強, 用 大 附 子 一 枚。 嘔 者 加 半夏 半升。

처방 약리

부자 hypaconitine
➡ 약리 추측: macrophage` Voltage-gated proton channels blocker
(식균작용에 의해 증가된 세포내 proton을 세포외로 방출시키는 채널)
➡ 세포내 pH ↓
➡ macrophage 대사 억제
➡ macrophage activation

감초 glycyrrhetinic acid -> HSD11B1 inhibitor
➡ cortisol 분해 억제
➡ glucocorticoid receptors 자극 지속
➡ IκBα 생성
➡ NF-κB 억제
➡ B cell 대사 억제
➡ 항체형성 감소

포부자 aconitine
➡ 약리추측: neutrophil` Voltage-gated proton channels blocker
(식균작용에 의해 증가된 세포내 proton을 세포외로 방출시키는 채널)
➡ Voltage-gated proton channels 차단
➡ 호중구내 수소이온 축적

➡ neutrophil 대사 억제
➡ phagocytosis 억제

방풍 deltoin ➡ cyclooxygenase-2 blocker

인삼 panax ginsenoside
➡ Transforming growth factor β (TGF-β) (+) modulator
➡ cell proliferation 촉진

대조 c-AMP ➡ protein kinase A avtivator: cell cycle

반하 triterpenoid (C30H48O7S)
➡ Rho GTPase family transcription promotor
➡ focal adhesion 생성
➡ 상피세포 이동 촉진

생강 gingerol ➡ hydrogen peroxide scavenger
➡ focal adhesion kinase 활성화
➡ 상피세포의 입체적 이동 촉진

죽엽 arundoin, 약리 추측 ➡ β-Amyloid gene expression (-) modulator

길경 platycodin ➡ toll like receptor (TLR) activator
➡ Microglia TLR ↑
➡ amyloid-β fibril 식균력 향상

죽피대환 (竹皮大丸)

원문 婦人 乳 中 虛, 煩 亂 嘔逆, 安 中 益 氣, 竹皮大丸 主之。

원문 해설 부인 출산 도중에 근력이 떨어지고 괴로운 상태가 되며 구역이 있는 경우에는 자궁 운동력과 호흡력을 증진시켜야 되므로 죽피대환을 쓴다.

적응증 Intrapartum Group B streptococcus infection
(분만 중 그룹 B 연쇄구균 감염증)

병태 & 증상

Intrapartum Group B streptococcus infection

➡ Intrapartum
➡ Th2 cell ↓
➡ complement production ↓
➡ normal flora: Group B streptococcus (GBS) 형질전환
➡ GBS: ScpB-lmb mutation
➡ GBS gene transcription ↑
➡ C5a peptidase & hyaluronate lyase & laminin binding protein 생산
➡ microvascular invasion
➡ chorioamniotics / endometritis / urinary tract infection
➡ GBS bacteremia
➡ blood-brain barrier (BBB) / Lung
➡ hyaluronate lyase & laminin binding protein 분비
➡ BBB damage
➡ 투과성 증가
➡ T cell 유입
➡ T cell: cytokine
➡ neuron: intracellular lactate ↑
➡ neuron damage / pneumonia
➡ 분만 힘주기 & 분만 호흡: 실패

처방 목표 GBS gene transcription 억제 / intracellular lactate 교정 / T cell 이동 억제 / 뇌실질 T cell apoptosis 유도 / 분만 힘주기 촉진 / 분만 호흡 촉진

처방 구성 生竹茹 二分 / 石膏 二分 / 桂枝 一分 / 甘草 七分 / 白薇 一分, 有熱者 倍白薇 , 煩 喘 者 加 柏實 一 分 。

처방 약리

백미 atratoside, 약리추측 ➡ GBS gene transcription (-) modulator

계지 cinnamic acid ➡ lactate oxidizer
➡ pyruvate 전환 촉진

감초 glycyrrhetinic acid
➡ 11-beta-hydroxysteroid dehydrogenase1 (HSD11B1) inhibitor

➡ glucocorticoid 작용
➡ IκBα 생성
➡ NF-κB 억제
➡ T cell 이동 억제됨

석고 CaSO4 ➡ Calcium Mediated T-Cell Apoptosis 유도

죽여 Tyrosine ➡ Dopamine / Norepinephrine / Epinephrine biosynthesis
➡ 분만 힘주기 촉진

백실 약리 추측 ➡ neuromuscular junction: nicotinic Rc agonist
➡ 근수축 강화

지실작약산 (枳實芍藥散)

원문 産 後 腹 痛， 煩 滿 不 得 臥，枳實芍藥散 主之。

원문 해설 산 후에 복통이 있고 괴로운 팽만감으로 눕지 못하는 경우에는 지실작약산을 쓴다.

적응증 Retained placenta (잔존태반)

병태 & 증상

Retained placenta

➡ postpartum
➡ uterus contraction ↓
➡ placenta separation 실패
➡ chorionic villi: ischemia
➡ chorionic villi: superoxide ↑
➡ superoxide mediated matrix metalloproteinase 발현 ↑
➡ uterine basal lamina: 분해됨
➡ chorionic villi: uterine muscles 침투
➡ retained placenta

처방 목표 chorionic villi superoxide 제거 / matrix metalloproteinase 차단

처방 구성 枳實(燒令黑, 勿太過) / 芍藥 等分 。

처방 약리

작약 paeoniflorin ➡ superoxide scavenger

지실 auraptene ➡ matrix metalloproteinase (MMP) blocker

지실치자시탕 (枳實梔子豉湯)

원문 大 病 差 後 , 勞 復 者 , 枳實梔子豉湯 主之 。, 若 有 宿 食 者 , 內 大黃 如 博棋 子 五 六 枚

원문 해설 큰 병이 나은 후에 노동을 하는 경우에는 지실치자시탕을 쓴다. 만약 변비가 있는 경우에는 (세포증식에 의한 수분 손실) 바둑알 크기만 한 대황 5~6개를 추가한다.

적응증 Macrophage foam cell formation (동맥경화증 단계 중 거품세포 생성)

병태 & 증상

Macrophage foam cell formation

➡ blood stream: LDL ▶ Monocyte ROS burst & other free radical 접촉
➡ free radical: LDL 공격
➡ LDL 자체 항산화 인자(carotenoid/ α-tocopherol/ cryptoxanthin/ ubiquinol-10) 고갈
➡ LDL: FUFAs lipid peroxidation
➡ ox-LDL 생성
➡ ox-LDL: 혈관내피 ox-LDL Rc 부착
➡ 혈관 내피 밑으로 이동
paraoxonase1: ox-LDL 환원 ➡ 혈류로 방출
대식세포에 탐식, paraoxonase2: ox-LDL 환원 ➡ 혈류로 방출
➡ paraoxonase1 & paraoxonase2 고갈
➡ ox-LDL 탐식한 대식세포 (Mp foam cell): cholesterol crystal 전환
➡ Mp foam cell formation
➡ Mp foam cell: matrix metalloproteinase(MMP) 분비

➡ matrix 분해
➡ 평활근 유도
➡ dying Mp & 지단백: 평활근 endocytosis
➡ 평활근내 ox-LDL ↑
➡ 평활근 괴사
➡ lipid core: tissue factor ↑
➡ 평활근 종양화 ↑

처방 목표 LDL 자체의 항산화인자 보충 / 혈관내피의 nitric oxide 생성 촉진: ox-LDL 부착 억제 / matrix 분해 억제 / 평활근 종양화 억제

처방 구성 枳實 三枚 (炙) / 梔子 十四個 / 香豉 一升

처방 약리

치자 crocin ➡ Low-Density Lipoprotein (LDL) antioxidant

향시 L-arginine ➡ nitric oxide synthesis 촉진

지실 auraptene ➡ matrix metalloproteinase (MMP) blocker

대황 emodin ➡ tyrosine kinase blocker
➡ 평활근 성장 억제

지실해백계지탕 (枳實薤白桂枝湯)

원문 胸痹 心中痞, 留 氣結 在 胸, 胸滿, 脅下 逆 搶 心, 枳實薤白桂枝湯 主之。; 人參湯 亦 主之。

원문 해설 가슴부위에 마비감이 있고 심장이 저리며 심박동이 불안정하면서 그득해지고 저리는 기운이 겨드랑이까지 뻗치는 경우에는 지실해백계지탕을 쓴다. 인삼탕도 쓸 수 있다.

적응증 Unstable angina (불안정형 협심증)

병태 & 증상

Unstable angina

➡ coronary artery: unstable fibrous cap
➡ 성분: collagen/ SMC/ proteoglycan/ cholesterol monohydrate crystal / lipid
➡ smooth muscle cell: VEGF autocrine
➡ smooth muscle cell: proliferation
➡ fibrous cap 내부: 활발한 염증 발생
➡ macrophage 유도: matrix metalloproteinase(MMP) 분비
➡ 신생혈관 출혈: smooth muscle cell 괴사 --> lipid 유출
➡ fibrous cap 내부: lipid
➡ fibrous cap 내부: 압력 증가
➡ fibrous cap: expansion
➡ coronary artery: 내강 좁아짐 (완전경색)
➡ myocardiocyte ischemia
➡ TCA cycle ↓
➡ myocardiocyte: lactate ↑
➡ unstable angina: chest pain, pulmonary edema, pain radiation
➡ 허혈부위 심근세포: 섬유아세포로 분화됨

처방 목표 VEGF Rc 차단 / matrix metalloproteinase 차단 / TCA cycle 촉진 / lactate 교정 / 심근세포의 섬유아세포로 분화 억제

처방 구성 枳實 四枚 / 厚朴 四兩 / 薤白 半斤 / 桂枝 一兩 / 栝蔞實 一枚

처방 약리

후박 honokiol ➡ VEGF receptor blocker

지실 auraptene ➡ matrix metalloproteinase blocker

해백 vitamin B1
➡ Pyruvate dehydrogenase & Oxoglutarate dehydrogenase의 coenzymes
➡ TCA cycle 활성화

계지 cinnamic acid ➡ lactate oxidizer
➡ pyruvate 전환 촉진

과루실 cucurbitacin

➡ endothelium의 fibroblast로 분화에 필요한 actin cytoskeleton을 붕괴시킴

➡ 심근세포의 섬유아세포로 분화 억제

진무탕 (真武湯)

원문 太陽病 發汗，汗出 不解，其人 仍 發熱，心下 悸，頭眩, 身 瞤動，振振 欲 擗地 者, 真武湯 主 之。少陰病，二 三 日 不 已，至 四 五 日，腹痛，小便 不利，四肢 沉重 疼痛，自下利 者，此 為 有 水氣，其 人 或 咳, 或 小便利，或下利，或 嘔 者, 真武湯 主 之。若 欬 者，加 五味子 半斤，細辛 一兩，乾薑一兩。若 小便利 者，去 茯苓。若 下利 者, 去 芍藥，加 乾薑 二兩。若 嘔者，去 附子，加 生薑，足 前 為 半斤。

원문 해설 림프절 감염병에서 IL-1 매개 면역반응이 끝난 후에도 증상이 낫지 않고 오히려 발열하며 동계가 있으면서 어지럽고 근육이 흔들리며 몸이 비틀거려 쓰러질 것 같은 경우에는 진무탕을 쓴다. 항체매개 감염병이 2~3일이 지나도 낫지 않고 4~5일이 되어 복통이 있고, 소변이 불편하고 팔다리가 무거우면서 쑤시고, 설사하는 것은 정맥울혈이 있는 것으로 혹 기침하거나, 혹 빈뇨가 있거나, 혹 설사하거나, 혹 구역하는 경우에는 진무탕을 쓴다. 만약 기침이 있으면 오미자 / 세신 / 건강을 추가한다. 만약 빈뇨가 있으면 복령을 뺀다. 만약 설사가 있으면 작약을 빼고 건강을 추가한다. 만약 구역이 있으면 포부자를 빼고 생강을 추가한다.

적응증 c-ANCA associated vasculitis (항호중구 세포질항체-매개 혈관염), c-ANCA: Classical antineutrophil cytoplasmic antibodies

병태 & 증상

c-ANCA associated vasculitis

➡ virus & bacteria infection: IL-1 ↑

➡ neutrophil 활성화: 세포막에 proteinase 3 발현

➡ medium-size vessel: c-ANCA bind <u>proteinase 3 expressed neutrophil</u>

➡ c-ANCA * neutrophil complex

➡ complement 유도

➡ vascular endothelial cell: <u>superoxide & H2O2</u> mediated <u>VCAM-1</u> 발현

➡ neutrophil adhesion
➡ neutrophil elastase 분비
➡ medium-size vessel: vasculitis
➡ thrombus formation
➡ 침범 조직
: Heart / Kidney / Gastrointestinal / Lung / Nerves system / Arthritis / Trachea

처방 목표 vascular endothelial cell: superoxide 제거 / vascular endothelial cell: H2O2 제거 / vascular endothelial cell: VCAM-1 차단 / neutrophil elastase 분비 억제 / thrombus 제거

처방 구성 茯苓 / 芍藥 / 生薑 各 三兩 / 白朮 二兩 / 炮附子 一枚

처방 약리

작약 paeoniflorin ➡ superoxide scavenger

생강 gingerol ➡ H2O2 scavenger

백출 atractylon ➡ vascular cell adhesion molecule-1 (VCAM-1) blocker

포부자 aconitine
➡ 약리추측: neutrophil` Voltage-gated proton channels blocker
(식균작용에 의해 증가된 세포내 proton을 세포외로 방출시키는 채널)
➡ Voltage-gated proton channels 차단
➡ 호중구내 수소이온 축적
➡ neutrophil 대사 억제
➡ elastase 분비

복령 pachymic acid ➡ glycoprotein IIb/IIIa (gpIIb/IIIa) (-) modulator
➡ thrombus formation 억제

천웅산 (天雄散)

원문 天雄散 方: 男子 平人, 脈 虛 弱 細 微 者, 喜 盜 汗 也。人年 五六十, 其病脈大者, 痹 俠 背 行, 若 腸鳴, 馬刀 俠癭, 皆為 勞得之。脈 沉 小 遲, 名 脫

氣, 其人 疾 行 則 喘喝 手足 逆寒, 腹滿, 甚 則 溏泄, 食 不 消化 也。脈 弦 而 大, 弦 則 為 減, 大 則 為 芤, 減 則 為 寒, 芤 則 為 虛, 虛寒 相搏, 此 名 為 革, 婦人 則 半產 漏下, 男子 則 亡血 失精。

원문 해설 평소 건강한 남성이 잠잘 때 식은땀이 나면서 맥이 약하고 가는 경우. 50~60세가 되어 맥이 크고, 저린 증상이 등까지 뻗쳐 있는데, 배에서 소리가 나고, 혹 같은 멍울이 생기는 것은 피로가 원인이다. 맥이 가라앉고 약간 더딘 경우를 탈기라고 하는데, 그 병에 걸리면 호흡곤란과 갈증이 생기고 손발이 심하게 차가워지며, 복부팽만감이 있고 설사를 하며 소화를 못 시킨다. 맥이 팽팽하면서 큰 경우에, 누르면 팽팽함이 줄고, 큰 진동이 비워지면 세포허혈이 있는 것으로써 혁(위독함)이라 부르며, 부인의 경우에 유산이나 대하증, 남자의 경우 실혈 때에 생긴다.

적응증 bone marrow EBV-mediated neutrophilia (호중구증가증)

병태 & 증상

bone marrow EBV-mediated neutrophilia

➡ overwork
➡ cortisol 지속
➡ bone marrow lymphocyte: latent Epstein-Barr virus ▶ reactivation
➡ EBV infected lymphocyte: IL-1 autocrine ▶ sweating
➡ IL-1: immature neutrophil ▶ proliferation
➡ circulating neutrophil pool ↑
➡ IL-1 mediated VCAM-1 발현 ↑
➡ IL-1: tissue macrophage 활성화 ▶ neutrophil 유도
➡ circulating neutrophil: 조직 이동 ▶ 폐 / 위장관 / 간 / 비장 / 피부
➡ neutrohil elastase: 폐 ▶ aveolar-capillary barrier 손상
▶ 폐포내 삼출물 유입: thirsty
▶ 급성호흡곤란증 후군 ▶ severe hypoxemia: dyspnoea
▶ lactic acidosis: cold hands and feet

위장관 ▶ gastrointestinal inflammation
: abdominal distension, diarrhea

간 ▶ hepatitis
비장 ▶ splenitis
피부 ▶ hump

처방 구성 VCAM-1 차단 / neutrohil elastase 분비 억제 / lactic acidosis 교정

처방 구성 炮天雄 三兩 / 白朮 八兩 / 桂枝 六兩 / 龍骨 三兩
처방 약리

백출 atractylon ➡ vascular cell adhesion molecule-1 (VCAM-1) blocker

포천웅 (포부자): aconitine

➡ 약리추측: neutrophil` Voltage-gated proton channels blocker
(식균작용에 의해 증가된 세포내 proton을 세포외로 방출시키는 채널)
➡ Voltage-gated proton channels 차단
➡ 호중구내 수소이온 축적
➡ neutrophil 대사 억제
➡ elastase 분비 억제

계지 cinnamic acid ➡ lactate oxidizer
➡ Cori cycle: pyruvate 전환 촉진

용골 CaCO3 ➡ NaHCO3 공급원 ➡ 산증 교정

초석반석탕 (硝石礬石散)

원문 黃家 日晡 所 發熱，而 反 惡寒，此 為 女勞 得 之 ；膀胱 急，少腹 滿, 身 盡 黃，額 上 黑，足 下 熱，因 作 黑 疸，其 腹 脹 如 水 狀, 大便 必 黑，時 溏，此 女勞 之 病，非水 也, 腹 滿 者 難 治, 硝石礬石散 主之 。病 隨 大小便 去, 小便 正 黃，大便 正 黑，是 候 也 。

원문 해설 황달이 생기면 해질 무렵에 발열하는데, 반대로 오한이 생기는 것은 여로달이라 한다: 방광이 땅기고 아랫배에 팽만감이 있으며 몸 전체가 누렇고, 이마 위로는 검으며 발바닥은 열이 나게 된다. 검은색 황달이 있으면 뱃속에 수분정체가 있는 것처럼 팽창감이 있고 대변이 까맣게 되며 때때로 묽어지는데 여로달이라 한다 이 병은 수분정체가 아니며, 복부에 팽만감이 있는 경우는 치료하기 힘들며 초석반석산을 쓴다. 병변은 대소변으로 제거되며 소변은 완전히 누렇고, 대변은 완전히 까매진다.

적응증 Bilirubin encephalopathy (빌리루빈 뇌병증)

병태 & 증상

Bilirubin encephalopathy

➡ intravascular hemolysis, reticuloendothelial hemolysis
➡ hyperbilirubinemia
➡ serum albumin: bilirubin 결합
➡ serum albumin 〈 bilirubin
➡ blood: free bilirubin 출현
➡ blood brain-barrier: free bilirubin 통과
➡ 뇌기저핵 (담창구 / 시상하핵 / 해마), 뇌간: free bilirubin 축적
➡ glia cell: TNF-α 분비 ▶ chills
➡ neuron: free bilirubin 흡수 ▶ 핵농축 (pyknosis)
➡ 뇌세포부종
➡ neuron degeneration

처방 목표 blood: free bilirubin 제거 / 뇌기저핵, 뇌간: free bilirubin 제거

처방 구성 硝石 / 礬石 (燒) 等 分

초석 Sodium Sulfate ➡ zwitterion (양쪽성 이온)
➡ 강한 산도: 음이온 흡착, 약한 산도: 양이온 흡착
➡ blood: free bilirubin 흡착

반석 KAl(SO4)2·12H2O (aluminium potassium sulfate = Alum)
➡ astringent (수렴제)
➡ 뇌세포내 수분 수렴

촉칠산 (蜀漆散)

원문 瘧 多 寒 者，名 曰 牝瘧，蜀漆散 主之。

원문 해설 학질 증상이 있는데, 오한이 많은 경우는 암컷모기에 물려서 생긴 것으로 촉칠산을 쓴다.

적응증 Plasmodium malariae & vivas & ovale malaria
(사일열원충 & 삼일열원충 & 난형열원충)

병태 & 증상

Plasmodium malariae & vivas & ovale malaria

➡ liver stage: sporozoite
➡ bloodstream stage: merozoite
➡ erythrocyte stage: ring trophozoite
➡ monocyte CD36: ring collagen 부착
➡ monocyte phagocytosis: ring-stage-infected erythrocyte
➡ ring-stage-infected erythrocyte: schizont 증식 (48~72 hours)
➡ monocyte: TNF-α 분비 ▶ chill
➡ severe fever: 39-41℃
➡ excessive sweating: 알카리 소실
➡ 대사성 산증

처방 목표 erythrocyte stage: ring trophozoite 형성 억제 / severe fever 교정 / 알카리 보충

처방 구성 蜀漆 / 雲母 / 龍骨 等分

처방 약리

촉칠 halofuginone ➡ ring-collagen synthesis inhibitor

운모 sheat silicate ➡ Heat absorber

용골 $CaCO_3$ ➡ $NaHCO_3$ 공급원 ➡ 산증 교정

치자감초시탕 (梔子甘草豉湯)

원문 發汗 吐 下後, 虛煩 不 得眠, 若 劇 者, 必 反覆 顚倒, 心中懊憹, 若 少氣 者, 梔子甘草豉湯 主之。

원문 해설 IL-1 매개 감염증이나 기관지와 식도 상피 감염 또는, 위장관 MALT 감염 후 몸이 괴로워지면서 불면증이 생기고, 심한 경우에는 계속 반복되고 악화되어, 심장이 괴롭고 갑갑해지며, 호흡이 짧아지는 경우에는 치자감초시탕을 쓴다.

적응증 Coronary arteris spasm & Myocardial ischemia
(관상동맥 경련 & 심근허혈)

병태 & 증상

➡ blood stream: LDL ▶ Monocyte ROS burst & other free radical 접촉
➡ free radical: LDL 공격
➡ LDL 자체 항산화 인자(carotenoid/ α-tocopherol/ cryptoxanthin/ ubiquinol-10) 고갈
➡ LDL: FUFAs lipid peroxidation
➡ ox-LDL 생성
➡ 관상동맥 혈관내피: ox-LDL Rc 부착
➡ 관상동맥 혈관내피: nitric oxide 분사
➡ ox-LDL을 떨어뜨림
➡ nitric oxide 고갈
➡ 관상동맥 혈관 확장력 ↓
➡ 협심증
➡ 심근세포 허혈
➡ Na+/ K+ pump activity 감소
➡ 심근 수축력 : shortness of breath

처방 목표 LDL 자체의 항산화 인자를 보충해줌 / nitric oxide의 원료인 arginine을 보충해줌 / 심근세포의 Na+/ K+pump 활성화

처방 구성 梔子 十四個 / 炙甘草 二兩 / 香豉 四合

처방 약리

치자 crocin ➡ Low-Density Lipoprotein (LDL) antioxidant
향시 L-arginine ➡ nitric oxide synthesis 촉진

구감초 18β-24-Hydroxyglycyrrhetinic acid
➡ HSD11B2 inhibitor
➡ cortisol 분해 억제
➡ mineralocorticoid receptors 자극 지속
➡ 심근세포 Na+/ K+ pumps 전사 활성화

치자건강탕 (梔子乾薑湯)

원문 傷寒, 醫 以 丸藥 大 下 之, 身熱 不去, 微 煩 者, 梔子乾薑湯 主之。

원문 해설 세포병변성 감염병을 의사가 환약을 써서 위장관 점막림프절의 림프구 배출을 심하게 일으킨 뒤, 열이 생겨서 지속되고 약간 괴로운 증상이 있는 경우에는 치자건강탕을 쓴다.

적응증 위장관 점막손상 후 LDL 산화

병태 & 증상

위장관 점막상피 손상

➡ 호중구 유입: 점막상피 necrotic cell debris 탐식
➡ neutrophil phagocytosis
➡ HClO 분비 via H2O2
➡ 점막상피 손상
➡ 지용성 비타민 흡수 저하됨
➡ LDL 자체의 항산화 인자(carotenoid/ α-tocopherol) 고갈
➡ 혈 중 ox-LDL
➡ 관상동맥 내피에 부착
➡ 대식세포 탐식: fever
➡ 관상동맥내피에서 ox-LDL을 떼어내려고 동맥 이완 반복됨
➡ vasospasm: agony

처방 목표 HClO 분비 억제 / LDL 자체의 항산화 인자(carotenoid/ α-tocopherol) 보충

처방 구성 梔子 十四個 / 乾薑 二兩

처방 약리

건강 shogaol ➡ neutrophil H2O2 scavenger
➡ HClO 분비 억제

치자 crocin ➡ Low-Density Lipoprotein (LDL) antioxidant

치자대황탕 (梔子大黃湯)

원문 酒 黃疸 , 心中 懊憹 或 熱痛 , 梔子大黃湯 主之 。

원문 해설 알코올성 황달이 있고, 가슴속이 심하게 괴로우며 열통이 있는 경우에는 치자대황탕을 쓴다.

적응증 Liver cirrhosis (간경변)

병태 & 증상

Alcoholic cirrhosis

➡ alcohol
➡ gut permeability
➡ portal circulation: G- bacteria ` LPS & endotoxin 유입
➡ Kupffer cell 활성화
➡ matrix metalloproteinase (MMP) 분비
➡ latent TGF-β ▶ active TGF-β 전환
➡ active TGF-β

➡ alcohol
➡ hepatocyte: alcohol detoxifying ▶ O2 소모
➡ liver acinus: hypoxia
➡ sinusoidal endothelium: endothelin-1 분비
➡ quiescent hepatic stellate cell (HSC) ▶ fibrogenic HSC 전환
➡ fibrogenic HSC tyrosine kinase Rc: active TGF-β 부착
➡ fibrogenic HSC: proliferation
➡ macrofibril 생성
➡ cirrhosis
➡ unconjugated bilirubin 역류: jaundice

처방 목표 matrix metalloproteinase 차단 / liver acinus: hypoxia 개선 / tyrosine kinase Rc 차단 / unconjugated bilirubin 해독

처방 구성 梔子 十四枚 / 大黃 一兩 / 枳實 五枚 / 豉 一升

처방 약리

지실 auraptene ➡ matrix metalloproteinase (MMP) blocker

향시 L-arginine ➡ nitric oxide synthesis 촉진
➡ liver acinus: hypoxia 개선

대황 emodin ➡ tyrosine kinase Rc blocker

치자 crocin ➡ unconjugated bilirubin antioxidant

치자생강시탕 (梔子生薑豉湯)

원문 發汗 吐 下後 , 虛煩 不 得眠 , 若 劇 者 , 必 反覆 顚倒 , 心中懊憹, 若 嘔 者, 梔子生薑豉湯 主之 。

원문 해설 IL-1 매개 감염증이나 기관지와 식도 상피 감염 또는, 위장관 MALT 감염 후 몸이 괴로워지면서 불면증이 생기고, 심한 경우에는 계속 반복되고 악화되어, 심장이 괴롭고 갑갑해지는데, 구역까지 있는 경우에는 치자생강시탕을 쓴다.

적응증 Coronary arteris spasm & Myocardial referfusion
(관상동맥 경련 & 심근재관류)

병태 & 증상

➡ blood stream: LDL ▶ Monocyte ROS burst & other free radical 접촉
➡ free radical: LDL 공격
➡ LDL 자체 항산화 인자(carotenoid/ α-tocopherol/ cryptoxanthin/ ubiquinol-10) 고갈
➡ LDL: FUFAs lipid peroxidation
➡ ox-LDL 생성
➡ 관상동맥 혈관내피: ox-LDL Rc 통해 부착
➡ 관상동맥 혈관내피: nitric oxide 분사
➡ ox-LDL을 떨어뜨림
➡ nitric oxide 고갈: 뇌혈류 ↓ : insomnia
➡ 관상동맥 혈관 확장력 ↓

➡ vasospasm: agony
➡ 재관류
➡ 심근세포: hydrogen peroxide ↑
➡ myocarditis
➡ 손상 부위로 정상 심근세포 이동: free sulfate ↑ : nausea

처방 목표 LDL 자체의 항산화 인자를 보충해줌 / nitric oxide의 원료인 arginine을 보충해줌 / hydrogen peroxide 제거

처방 구성 梔子 十四個 / 生薑 五兩 / 香豉 四合

처방 구성

치자 crocin ➡ Low-Density Lipoprotein (LDL) antioxidant

향시 L-arginine ➡ nitric oxide synthesis 촉진

생강 gingerol ➡ hydrogen peroxide scavenger

치자시탕 (梔子豉湯)

원문 發汗 吐 下後，虛煩 不得眠，若 劇 者, 必 反覆 顚倒，心中懊憹, 梔子豉湯 主之。發汗，若 下之, 而 煩熱, 胸中 窒 者, 梔子豉湯 主之。傷寒 五 六 日, 大 下 之 後, 身熱 不去, 心 中 結痛 者, 未 欲解 也, 梔子豉湯 主之。

원문 해설 IL-1 매개 감염증이나 기관지와 식도 상피 감염 또는, 위장관 MALT 감염 후 몸이 괴로워지면서 불면증이 생기고, 심한 경우에는 계속 반복되고 악화되어, 심장이 괴롭고 갑갑해지는 경우에는 치자시탕을 쓴다. IL-1 매개 감염증에서 증상이 풀린 뒤에 괴로운 열이 생기고, 심장이 막힌 듯한 경우에는 치자시탕을 쓴다. 세포병변성 감염병이 5~6일 지나서, 위장관 점막림프절 림프구 배출 후에, 열이 지속되고 심장에 뭉친 듯한 통증이 풀리지 않는 경우에는 치자시탕을 쓴다.

적응증 Coronary arteris spasm (관상동맥 경련)

병태 & 증상

Coronary arteris spasm

➡ blood stream: LDL ▶ Monocyte ROS burst & other free radical 접촉
➡ free radical: LDL 공격
➡ LDL 자체 항산화 인자(carotenoid/ α-tocopherol/ cryptoxanthin/ ubiquinol-10) 고갈
➡ LDL: FUFAs lipid peroxidation
➡ ox-LDL 생성
➡ ox-LDL: 관상동맥 혈관내피 ox-LDL Rc 부착
➡ 대식세포 탐식: fever
➡ 관상동맥 혈관내피: nitric oxide 분사
➡ ox-LDL을 떨어뜨림
➡ nitric oxide 고갈
➡ 관상동맥 혈관 확장력 ↓
➡ vasospasm: agony
➡ 협심증

처방 목표 LDL 자체의 항산화 인자를 보충해줌 / nitric oxide의 원료인 arginine을 보충해줌

처방 구성 梔子 十四個 / 香豉 四合

처방 약리

치자 crocin ➡ Low-Density Lipoprotein (LDL) antioxidant

향시 L-arginine ➡ nitric oxide synthesis 촉진

치자후박탕 (梔子厚朴湯)

원문 傷寒, 下 後, 心煩, 腹滿, 臥起 不安 者, 梔子厚朴湯 主之 。

원문 해설 세포병변성 감염병에서 위장관 점막림프절 림프구 배출후에, 심장부위가 괴롭고, 복부팽만감이 있으며, 눕거나 앉거나 편하지 않은 경우에는 치자탕을 쓴다.

적응증 Atheroma formation (죽종 형성)

병태 & 증상

Atheroma formation

➡ blood stream: LDL ▶ Monocyte ROS burst & other free radical 접촉
➡ free radical: LDL 공격
➡ LDL 자체 항산화 인자(carotenoid/ α-tocopherol/ cryptoxanthin/ ubiquinol-10) 고갈
➡ LDL: FUFAs lipid peroxidation
➡ ox-LDL 생성
➡ ox-LDL: 혈관내피 ox-LDL Rc 부착
➡ 혈관 내피 밑으로 이동
 # paraoxonase1: ox-LDL 환원-> 혈류로 방출
 # 대식세포에 탐식, paraoxonase2: ox-LDL 환원-> 혈류로 방출
➡ paraoxonase1 & paraoxonase2 고갈
➡ ox-LDL 탐식한 대식세포 (Mp foam cell): cholesterol crystal 전환
➡ Mp foam cell formation
➡ Mp foam cell: cholesterol crystal 축적
➡ Mp foam cell: MMP 분비
➡ 혈관내피속 matrix 분해
➡ 평활근세포 이동
➡ 이동된 평활근세포: cholesterol crystal & 대식세포의 분해소체 ▶ endocytosis
➡ cholesterol crystal ▶ free cholesterol 전환: 자체 활용함
➡ cholesterol crystal & 대식세포의 분해소체가 현저히 많아지면 평활근세포 증식함
➡ 신생혈관 생성
➡ 평활근세포 증식
➡ Atheroma formation
➡ 주로 복부대동맥에서 발생됨: agony & indigestion

처방 목표 대식세포내 ox-LDL를 환원 시킴 / 혈관내피속 matrix 분해 억제 시킴 / 평활근 세포 증식 억제

처방 구성 梔子 十四個 / 厚朴 四兩 (炙) / 枳實 四枚 (炙)

처방 약리

치자 crocin ➡ Low-Density Lipoprotein (LDL) antioxidant
➡ 대식세포내 ox-LDL 환원

지실 auraptene ➡ matrix metalloproteinases (MMPs) blocker

➡ 혈관내피속 matrix 분해 억제

후박 honokiol ➡ VEGF receptor blocker
➡ 평활근 세포 증식 억제

택사탕 (澤瀉湯)

원문 心 下 有 支飮，其人 苦 冒 眩，澤瀉湯 主之。

원문 해설 체액이 증가해서 (고혈압) 머리가 무겁고 어지러운 경우에는 택사탕을 쓴다.

적응증 Hypertension

병태 & 증상

Hypertension

➡ stress & overwork
➡ corticosteroids ↑
➡ angiotensinogen levels ↑
➡ angiotensin II persistence in blood
➡ vascular smooth muscle: type 1 ANG II receptor
➡ vascular smooth muscle: contraction
➡ vascular smooth muscle: NADH / NADPH oxidase ↑
➡ redox-sensitive transcription 활성화
➡ vascular smooth muscle: VCAM-1 발현
➡ leukocyte & monocyte adhesion
➡ inflammation
➡ 혈관 내강 좁아짐
➡ 세소동맥경화증
➡ 조직 허혈, 특히 뇌허혈: heavy head, dizziness

처방 목표 type 1 ANG II receptor 차단 / VCAM-1 발현 억제

처방 구성 澤瀉 五兩 / 白朮 二兩

처방 약리

택사 alisol ➡ angiotensin II receptor blocker

백출 atractylon ➡ vascular cell adhesion molecule-1 (VCAM-1) blocker

택칠탕 (澤漆湯)

원문 咳 而 脈浮 者 , 厚朴麻黃湯 主之, 脈沈 者 , 澤漆湯 主之 。

원문 해설 기침하며 맥이 뜨는 경우에는 후박마황탕을 쓰고, 맥이 가라앉는 경우에는 택칠탕을 쓴다.

적응증 Respiratory syncytial virus (RSV) bronchiolitis
(호흡기 세포융합 바이러스 세기관지염)

병태 & 증상

RSV bronchiolitis

➡ bronchiol epithelium: RSV entry
➡ RSV F protein: bronchiol epithelium TLR4 손상
➡ TLR4-mediated immune response 불활성화
➡ RSV infected bronchiol epithelium & normal bronchiol epithelium
➡ syncytium formation
➡ normal bronchiol epithelium: necrosis
➡ peribronchiolar inflammation: cytokine
➡ lymphocyte & plasma cell & macrophage 유도
➡ submucosal edema
➡ mucus plugging
➡ alveolar macrophage: RSV phagocytosis
➡ extracellular peroxynitrite ($ONOO^-$) ↑
➡ bronchiol epithelium: membrane protein ▶ nitrotyrosine 변성
➡ bronchiol epithelium: loss
➡ air trapping: obstruction
➡ alveolar cell: oxygen ↓

➡ hypoxemia: blood lactate ↑

처방 목표 bronchiol epithelium: RSV entry 차단 / bronchiol epithelium: immune response 활성화 / normal bronchiol epithelium 증식 & 상환 촉진 / lymphocyte & plasma cell & macrophage 유도 억제 / extracellular peroxynitrite ($ONOO^-$) 제거 / mucus plugging 제거 / blood lactate 교정

처방 구성 半夏 半升 / 紫參 五兩 (一作 紫菀) / 澤漆 三斤 / 生薑 五兩 / 白前 五兩 / 甘草 三兩 / 黃芩 三兩 / 人參 三兩 / 桂枝 三兩

처방 약리

택칠 quercetin ➡ β-defensin (+) modulator
➡ β-defensin: 점막세포에서 분비하는 항균, 항바이러스 펩타이드
➡ respiratory syncytial virus envelope 분해
➡ RSV: bronchiol epithelium 침입 억제

백전 pregnane glycoside ➡ PXR ligand
➡ detoxification protein 전사 촉진
➡ immune response 활성화
➡ RSV 복제 억제

인삼 panax ginsenoside
➡ Transforming growth factor β (TGF-β) (+) modulator
➡ bronchiol epithelium: proliferation 촉진

반하 triterpenoid (C30H48O7S)
➡ Rho GTPase family transcription promotor
➡ focal adhesion 생성
➡ bronchiol epithelium 상환 촉진

생강 gingerol ➡ hydrogen peroxide scavenger
➡ focal adhesion kinase 활성화
➡ bronchiol epithelium 입체적 이동 촉진

감초 glycyrrhetinic acid
➡ 11-beta-hydroxysteroid dehydrogenase1 (HSD11B1) inhibitor

➡ glucocorticoid 작용
➡ IκBα 생성
➡ NF-κB 억제
➡ lymphocyte & plasma cell & macrophage: cytokine 생성 억제
➡ 이동 억제

자삼 gallic acid ➡ mucus astringent

황금 baicalin ➡ peroxynitrite ($ONOO^-$) scavenger

계지 cinnamic acid ➡ lactate oxidizer
➡ pyruvate 전환
➡ Cori cycle 촉진

토과근산 (土瓜根散)

원문 帶下 經水 不利，少腹 滿痛，經 一 月 再 見 者，土瓜根散 主之。

원문 해설 대하증이 있고 생리가 정상적이지 않으면서 아랫배가 그득하게 아프며 생리가 한 달에 두 번 보이는 경우에는 토과근산을 쓴다.

적응증 Endometriosis (자궁내막증식증)

병태 & 증상

Endometriosis

➡ endometrial gland cell & stroma cell: pelvic cavity 이동
➡ mense with heparin
➡ 탈락
➡ pelvic cavity: erythrocyte fluid 유출
➡ hemosiderin-laden macrophage 출현
➡ hemosiderin-laden macrophage: growth factor 분비
➡ stroma cell: stromal fibroblast 전환
➡ stromal fibroblast: collagen 분비

➡ 골반 섬유화
➡ 골반 & 하부생식기 근육, 자궁천골인대, 난소인대 유착
: leukorrhea, dysmenorrhea
➡ 인대, 근육: stimulation ▶ 세포내 대사 ↑
➡ 인대, 근육세포: superoxide & lactate ↑
➡ necrotic nodules 형성

처방 목표 골반강 적혈구 제거 촉진 / stromal fibroblast: collagen 합성 억제 / 인대, 근육세포: superoxide 제거 / 인대, 근육세포: lactate 제거

처방 구성 土瓜根 三兩 / 芍藥 三兩 / 桂枝 三兩 / 蟅蟲 三兩

처방 약리

자충 ESW extraction ➡ erythrocyte C3b receptor (+) modulator
➡ 백혈구 식균 촉진

토과근 (과루근) trichosanthin ➡ ribosome inactivating protein
➡ collagen 생성 억제

작약 paeoniflorin ➡ superoxide scavenger

계지 cinnamic acid ➡ lactate oxidizer
➡ pyruvate 전환 촉진

통맥사역가저담즙탕 (通脈四逆加豬膽汁湯)

원문 吐 已 下 斷, 汗出 而 厥, 四肢 拘急 不 解, 脈 微 欲 絕 者, 通脈四逆加豬膽汁湯 主之。

원문 해설 구토와 설사가 모두 나와서 그쳤는데 땀이 나오면서 몸 상태가 이상하며 손발이 땅기고 불편한 것이 낫지 않고 맥이 끊어지려는 경우에는 통맥사역가저담즙탕을 쓴다.

적응증 Systemic lupus erythematosis-associated nervous syetem dysfunction
(전신성 홍반 루푸스에 의한 신경계 손상)

병태 & 증상

Systemic lupus erythematosis

➡ Type IV & V collagen autoantibody
➡ basement membrane & interstitial tissue: autoantibody 부착
➡ antibody-dependent cell-mediated cytotoxicity (ADCC)
➡ macrophage 유도
➡ IL-8 분비
➡ neutrophil phagocytosis
➡ HClO 분비 via H2O2
➡ 결합조직 구성 세포: Na+/ K+ pumps 손상
➡ connective tissue disease & collagen vascular disease 발생
➡ 모세혈관 퇴행 및 소실 / 피부괴사 / 위장관 허혈 / 폐간질 염증 / 신경계 손상
➡ 신경계 손상: 운동신경 손상 ▶ paralysis
교감신경 손상 ▶ IL-1 : sweating
위장관 부교감신경 손상: vomit, diarrhea, paralytic ileus

처방 목표 macrophage IL-8 분비 억제 / HClO 분비 억제 / 결합조직 구성 세포: Na+/ K+ pumps 활성화 / paralytic ileus 개선

처방 구성 炙甘草 二兩 / 乾薑 三兩 / 豬膽汁 半合 / 附子 大者 一枚

처방 약리

부자 hypaconitine

➡ 약리 추측: macrophage` Voltage-gated proton channels blocker
(식균작용에 의해 증가된 세포내 proton을 세포외로 방출시키는 채널)
➡ proton 방출 억제
➡ 세포내 pH ↓
➡ macrophage 대사 억제
➡ IL-8 분비 억제

건강 shogaol ➡ neutrophil H2O2 scavenger
➡ HClO 분비 억제

구감초 18β-24-Hydroxyglycyrrhetinic acid
➡ HSD11B2 inhibitor
➡ cortisol 분해 억제

➡ mineralocorticoid receptors 자극 지속

➡ Na+/ K+ pumps 전사 활성화

돼지 담즙 장운동 촉진시킴

통맥사역탕 (通脈四逆湯)

원문 少陰病, 下利 清穀, 裡寒 外熱, 手足 厥逆, 脈 微 欲 絕, 身 反 不惡寒, 其人 面色赤, 或 腹痛, 或 乾嘔, 或 咽痛, 或 利 止 脈 不 出 者, 通脈四逆湯 主之。

원문 해설 항체매개 감염증으로 소화되지 않은 음식을 설사하고 속은 춥고 겉은 열나며, 손발이 극도로 차갑고 맥이 약해서 끊어질 것 같은데 반대로 오한은 없다. 또, 얼굴이 붉고, 혹은 복통이 있거나, 혹은 마른 구역이 있거나, 혹은 인후통이있거나, 혹은 설사는 그쳤으나 맥이 원래대로 돌아오지 않는 경우에는 통맥사역탕을 쓴다.

적응증 Systemic lupus erythematosis (전신홍반성 낭창)

병태 & 증상

Systemic lupus erythematosis

➡ Type IV & V collagen autoantibody

➡ basement membrane & interstitial tissue: autoantibody 부착

➡ antibody-dependent cell-mediated cytotoxicity (ADCC)

➡ macrophage 유도

➡ IL-8 분비

➡ neutrophil phagocytosis

➡ HClO 분비 via H2O2

➡ 결합조직 구성 세포: Na+/ K+ pumps 손상

➡ connective tissue disease & collagen vascular disease 발생

➡ 모세혈관 퇴행 및 소실 / 피부괴사 / 위장관 허혈 / 폐간질 염증 / 신경계 손상

처방 목표 macrophage IL-8 분비 억제 / HClO 분비 억제 / 결합조직 구성 세포: Na+/K+ pumps 활성화

처방 구성 炙甘草 二兩 / 附子 大者 一枚 / 乾薑 三兩

처방 약리

부자 hypaconitine

➡ 약리 추측: macrophage` Voltage-gated proton channels blocker

(식균작용에 의해 증가된 세포내 proton을 세포외로 방출시키는 채널)

➡ proton 방출 억제

➡ 세포내 pH ↓

➡ macrophage 대사 억제

➡ IL-8 분비 억제

건강 shogaol ➡ neutrophil H2O2 scavenger

➡ HClO 분비 억제

구감초 18β-24-Hydroxyglycyrrhetinic acid

➡ HSD11B2 inhibitor

➡ cortisol 분해 억제

➡ mineralocorticoid receptors 자극 지속

➡ Na+/ K+ pumps 전사 활성화

팔미신기환 (八味腎氣丸)

원문 虛勞 腰痛，少腹 拘急，小便 不利 者，八味腎氣丸 主之。

원문 해설 과로로 인해 요통이 있으며, 아랫배가 쥐어짜듯이 당기고, 소변이 불편한 경우에는 팔미신기환을 쓴다.

적응증 Endothelin-1 mediated Renal failure

병태 & 증상

Endothelin-1 mediated Renal failure

➡ overwork

➡ cortisol ↑

➡ angiotensin II ↑

➡ renal artery endothelium: angiotensin II type 1 Rc 자극

➡ renal artery endothelium: endothelin-1 생산
➡ renal artery: strong, long-lasting constriction
➡ monocyte: endothelin receptor subtype A
➡ monocyte 활성화: ROS burst
➡ renal artery: vasculitis
➡ tubular endothelium: ischemia
➡ tubular endothelium: lactate ↑ ▶ ATP ↓
➡ tubular endothelium: reperfusion
➡ tubular endothelium: reactive oxygen species ↑
➡ ERK (extracellular signal-regulated kinases) 1/2 phosphorylation
➡ caspase 3 활성화
➡ tubular endothelium: apoptosis
➡ erythropoietin ↓
➡ erythrocyte 생산 ↓
➡ systemic hypoxia
➡ tubular endothelium: reactive oxygen species ↑
➡ renal parenchyma: neutrophil 유도
➡ neutrophil elastase 분비
➡ renal parenchyma: injury

처방 목표 renal artery endothelium: angiotensin II type 1 Rc 차단 / vasculitis 억제 / tubular endothelium: lactate 교정 / tubular endothelium: ATP 생산 촉진 / tubular endothelium: manganese superoxide dismutase & glutathione peroxidase 전사 촉진 / ERK 1/2 phosphorylation 억제 / erythrocyte 생산 촉진 / renal parenchyma: neutrophil elastase 분비 억제

처방 구성 乾地黃 八兩 / 山藥 四兩 / 山茱萸 四兩 / 澤瀉 三兩 / 牡丹皮 三兩 / 茯苓 三兩 / 桂枝 一兩 / 炮附子 一兩

처방 약리

택사 alisol ➡ angiotensin II receptor blocker

복령 pachymic acid ➡ glycoprotein IIb/IIIa (gpIIb/IIIa) (-) modulator
➡ thrombus formation 억제

계지 cinnamic acid ➡ lactate oxidizer

➡ pyruvate 전환

산약 diosgenin ➡ GLUT1 (+) modulator (GLUT1: glucose transporters)
➡ glucose 유입 촉진
➡ ATP 증가

목단피 β-Sitosterol
➡ manganese superoxide dismutase & glutathione peroxidase (+) modulator
➡ tubular endothelium: reactive oxygen species 제거

산수유 ursolic acid ➡ ERK (extracellular signal-regulated kinases) blocker

건지황 catalpol, 약리 추측 ➡ CD133+ CFU-S (+) modulator
➡ hematopoietic stem cell 분화 촉진
➡ erythrocyte 생성 촉진

포부자 aconitine
➡ 약리추측: neutrophil` Voltage-gated proton channels blocker
(식균작용에 의해 증가된 세포내 proton을 세포외로 방출시키는 채널)
➡ Voltage-gated proton channels 차단
➡ 호중구내 수소이온 축적
➡ neutrophil 대사 억제
➡ elastase 분비 억제

포탄산 (蒲灰散)

원문 小便 不利，蒲灰散 主之 ； 滑石白魚散，茯苓戎鹽湯 并 主之 。

원문 해설 소변이 불편한 경우에는 포탄산, 활석백어산, 복령융염탕을 병용하여 쓴다.

적응증 Pyelonephritis (신우신염)

병태 & 증상

Pyelonephritis

➡ kidney pyelum: E. coli / Enterococcus faecalis / streptococcus infection

➡ E. coli / Enterococcus faecalis / streptococcus
: HMG-CoA reductase gene 활성화

➡ isopentenyl pyrophosphate (IPP) & dimethylallyl pyrophosphate (DMAPP) 생성

➡ cholesterol biosynthesis

➡ cell growth

➡ pyelonephritis

➡ 혈장단백 유출

처방 목표 HMG-CoA reductase 억제 / 혈장단백 유출 억제

처방 구성 蒲灰 七分 / 滑石 三分

처방 약리

창포 (부들) asarone ➡ HMG-CoA reductase blocker

활석 $Mg_3(Si_4O_{10})(OH)_2$ ➡ ammonia absorbent
➡ 혈장단백 흡착

풍인탕 (風引湯)

원문 風引湯, 除熱癱癎

원문 해설 풍인탕은 간질을 치료한다.

적응증 Epilepsy (뇌전증)

병태 & 증상

Epilepsy

➡ viral infection

➡ virus antigen & metabolic glutamate receptor (mGluR)
▶ molecular mimic response
➡ peripheral blood: mGluR specific T cell 출현
➡ hepatocyte: glutamate receptor ▶ autoantigen 전환
▶ glutamate 대사 감소 ▶ hyperammonemia
➡ blood-brain barrier: leakage

➡ T cell 유입
➡ B cell 유도: mGluR autoantibody 생성
➡ GABAergic neuron & neuroglial cell: metabolic glutamate receptor (mGluR)
▶ antibody 부착
➡ GABAergic neuron & neuroglial cell: glutamate 흡수 감소
➡ GABAergic neuron & neuroglial cell: GABA 생성 감소
➡ synapse: glutamate ↑
➡ postsynaptic neuron: glutamate cytotoxicity ▶ apoptosis

➡ hippocampus: 흥분 전도 감소
➡ hippocampus: 흥분성 신경세포 유입
➡ hippocampal neuron: granular cell 흥분성 ↑
➡ granular cell 흥분 신호 ▶ mossy fiber ▶ CA3 흥분성 ↑ ▶ seizure

➡ blood-brain barrier: adhesion molecule 발현
➡ neutrophil 유입
➡ neutrophil phagocytosis
➡ HClO 분비 via H2O2
➡ astrocyte damage
➡ glutamate uptake 감소: glutamate cytotoxicity
➡ hippocampal neuron: 흥분 전도 ↑
➡ hippocampal neuron: 세포질 lactate ↑ ▶ 세포내 산증 ▶ ATP 고갈
▶ ion pump 손상 ▶ 세포외액 유입 ▶ 뇌세포부종
➡ hippocampal neuron: apoptosis
➡ hippocampal sclerosis
➡ hippocampus: brain-derived neurotrophic factor (BDNF) 축적
➡ hippocampal neurons: tyrosine kinase B receptors 자극
➡ hippocampal neurons: hyperexcitability
➡ hippocampal neurons: long-term potentiation
➡ excitatory synaptic transmission ↑

➡ epilepsy
➡ metabolic acidosis

처방 목표 hyperammonemia 교정 / T cell apoptosis 유도 / B cell 유도: mGluR autoantibody 생성 억제 / glutamate 생성 억제 / HClO 분비 억제 / hippocampal neuron: 세포질 lactate 교정 / hippocampal neuron: 뇌세포부종 교정 / hippocampal neurons: tyrosine kinase B receptors 차단 / hippocampal neurons: long-term potentiation 억제 / metabolic acidosis 교정

처방 구성 大黃 四兩 / 乾薑 四兩 / 龍骨 四兩 / 桂枝 三兩 / 甘草 二兩 / 牡蠣 二兩 / 寒水石 / 滑石 / 赤石脂 / 白石脂 / 紫石英 / 石膏 各 六兩

처방 약리

활석 Talc, $Mg_3(Si_4O_{10})(OH)_2$ ➡ ammonia absorbent
➡ hyperammonemia 교정

석고 $CaSO_4$ ➡ calcium mediated T-cell apoptosis 유도

감초 glycyrrhetinic acid
➡ 11-beta-hydroxysteroid dehydrogenase1 (HSD11B1) inhibitor
➡ glucocorticoid 작용
➡ $I\kappa B\alpha$ 생성
➡ NF-κB 억제
➡ 항체 생성 억제

자석영 플루오르화칼슘 (CaF_2) ➡ phosphate binder
➡ phosphate-activated glutaminase inhibitor
➡ glutamate 합성 억제

건강 shogaol ➡ neutrophil H_2O_2 scavenger
➡ HClO 분비 억제

계지 cinnamic acid ➡ lactate oxidizer
➡ pyruvate 전환

모려NaCl ➡ 세포외액 삼투압 상승 ➡ 뇌세포 부종 억제

백석지 Halloysite ➡ (Al,Mg)2(Si4O10)(OH)2·nH2O
➡ Water absorbent
➡ 뇌세포 부종 억제

대황 emodin ➡ tyrosine kinase blocker

적석지 풍화가 진행되어 K이온이 제거된 후 양이온 교환 능력이 커진 갈색 점토 광물
: Vermiculite ➡ Al2O3, 2SiO2·4H2O
➡ Cation absorbent
➡ 뇌세포외액 Na, K 흡착
➡ hippocampal neurons: long-term potentiation 억제

용골 CaCO3 ➡ NaHCO3 공급원 ➡ 산증 교정

한수석 Calcite ➡ CaCO3 ➡ NaHCO3 공급원 ➡ 산증 교정

하어혈탕 (下瘀血湯)

원문 産 婦 腹痛 `法 當 以 枳實芍藥散 , 假令 不愈 者 , 此為 腹 中 有 瘀血 著 臍 下, 宜 下瘀血湯 主之 , 亦 主 經水 不利 。

원문 해설 산 후에 복통이 있으면 꼭 지실작약산을 쓰고, 낫지 않으면 탯줄이 있던 자리에 혈종이 있는 것이므로 하어혈탕을 쓰며 또, 산 후에 생리불순이 있는 경우에도 쓴다.

적응증 Placenta accreta (태반유착)

병태 & 증상

Placenta accreta

➡ retained placenta
➡ 구성 세포: chorionic villi
➡ ischemia
➡ chorionic villi: estrogen receptor 발현 ↑

➡ estrogen signal: tyrosine kinase Rc 발현 ↑
➡ growth factor: autocrine
➡ tyrosine kinase Rc 자극
➡ chorionic villi: proliferation
➡ uterine myometrium: hemorrhage
➡ hematoma 생성

처방 목표 estrogen receptor 차단 / tyrosine kinase 차단 / hematoma 제거

처방 구성 大黃 二兩 / 桃仁 二十枚 / 蟅蟲 二十枚 (熬 `去 足)

처방 약리

도인 amygdalin

➡ 체내 활성 성분: thiocyanate (amygdalin metabolite)
➡ 4S estrogen receptor (ER) ▶ 5S estrogen receptor 전환 억제
(4S monomer: estrogen 저친화성, 5S dimer: estrogen 고친화성)

대황 emodin ➡ tyrosine kinase blocker

자충 ESW extraction, 약리 추측 ➡ Erythrocyte C3b receptor (+) modulator
➡ 백혈구 hematoma 식균 촉진

활석대자탕 (滑石代赭湯)

원문 百合病 下 之 後 者 , 滑石代赭湯 主之 。

원문 해설 백합병에서 소변으로 바이러스가 배출되고 있다면(붉은 소변) 활석대자탕을 쓴다.

적응증 Bornavirus blood-borne infection

병태 & 증상

Bornavirus blood-borne infection

➡ peripheral blood: bornavirus RNA
➡ erythrocyte heme: bornavirus RNA 부착

➡ nervous site: 이동
➡ axoplasmic transport

처방 목표 bornavirus RNA 흡착 제거 / erythrocyte heme: bornavirus RNA 부착 억제 / axoplasmic transport 억제

처방 구성 百合 七枚 / 滑石 三兩 / 代赭石 大一枚

처방 약리

활석 Mg3(Si4O10)(OH)2 ➡ ammonia & Nucleic acid absorbent
➡ bornavirus RNA 흡착

대자석 삼산화이철 (Fe2O3) ➡ erythrocyte heme: bornavirus RNA 부착 억제

백합 colchicine ➡ microtubule polymerization inhibitor
➡ axoplasmic transport 억제됨

활석백어산 (滑石白魚散)

원문 小便 不利 , 蒲灰散 主之 ; 滑石白魚散 , 茯苓戎鹽湯 并 主之 。

원문 해설 소변이 불편한 경우에는 포탄산, 활석백어산, 복령융염탕을 병용하여 쓴다.

적응증 Kidney stones (콩팥 결석)

병태 & 증상

Kidney stones

➡ calcium diets ↓
➡ GI tract: free oxalate 흡수 ↑
➡ urinary tract: oxalate 배설 ↑
➡ urine calcium + oxalate
➡ calcium oxalate 형성

➡ collecting duct 손상
➡ 혈장단백 유출

처방 목표 calcium oxalate 형성 억제 / 혈장단백 유출 억제

처방 구성 滑石 二分 / 燒亂髮 二分 / 白魚 三分

처방 약리

소난발 (사람 머리털 태운 것): keratin ➡ calcium chelater

백어 (옷좀) cellulase ➡ oxalate binder

활석 $Mg_3(Si_4O_{10})(OH)_2$ ➡ ammonia absorbent
➡ 혈장단백 흡착

황금가반하생강탕 (黃芩加半夏生薑湯)

원문 太陽 與 少陽 合病, 自下利 者, 與 黃芩湯 ; 若 嘔 者, 黃芩加半夏生薑湯 主之。

원문 해설 림프절 & 비장 공통 면역반응을 유발하는 감염증으로 설사하는 경우는 황금탕을 쓰고 구역까지 있는 경우에는 황금가반하생강탕을 쓴다.

적응증 Typhoid fever

병태 & 증상

Salmonella typhi

➡ small intestine mucosal epithelium: Salmonella typhi 부착
➡ Salmonella typhi: SopE, SopE2, SopB 분비
➡ mucosal epithelium: Rho GTPases 활성화
➡ actin cytoskeleton 재배열
➡ tight junction 분리: neusea
➡ Salmonella typhi: intracellular infection
➡ Salmonella: SopB 생성

➡ inositol phosphatase 활성화
➡ GTP binding protein 활성화
➡ adenylate cyclase 지속적인 활성
➡ c-AMP ↑
➡ chloride channel 활성 지속
➡ Cl^- secretion ↑
➡ Na+/ K+ pump 손상
➡ 세포간질: Na+, H2O secretion ↑
➡ exhaustive diarrhea
➡ macrophage: Salmonella typhi 식균
➡ extracellular peroxynitrite ($ONOO^-$) ↑
➡ enteritis

처방 목표 tight junction 회복 / GTP binding protein 생성에 필요한 $O2^-$ 제거 / cAMP 농도를 지속시켜서 Cl^- secretion 억제시킴 / mucosal epithelium: Na+/ K+ pump 활성화 / extracellular peroxynitrite ($ONOO^-$) 제거

처방 구성 黃芩 三兩 / 芍藥 三兩 / 炙甘草 三兩 / 大棗 十二枚 / 半夏 半升 / 生薑 一兩

처방 약리

반하 triterpenoid (C30H48O7S)
➡ Rho GTPase family transcription promotor
➡ actin cytoskeleton 복구

생강 gingerol ➡ hydrogen peroxide scavenger
➡ focal adhesion kinase 활성화
➡ actin cytoskeleton 결집 촉진
➡ tight junction 회복

작약 paeoniflorin ➡ superoxide scavenger

대조 cAMP ➡ 세포질 granule-membrane protein: phospholylation 억제
➡ Cl^- secretion 억제

구감초 18β-24-Hydroxyglycyrrhetinic acid

➡ HSD11B2 inhibitor
➡ cortisol 분해 억제
➡ mineralocorticoid receptors 자극 지속
➡ Na+/ K+ pumps 전사 활성화

황금 baicalin ➡ peroxynitrite ($ONOO^-$) scavenger

황금탕 (黃芩湯)

원문 太陽 與 少陽 合病 , 自下利 者, 黃芩湯 主之 。

원문 해설 림프절 & 비장의 면역반응을 동시에 유발하는 감염증으로 설사하는 경우에는 황금탕을 쓴다.

적응증 Cholera

병태 & 증상

Vibrio cholerae

➡ small intestine mucosal epithelium: Vibrio cholerae infection
➡ cholera toxin
➡ GTP binding protein ▶ GDP 전환: 방해
➡ adenylate cyclase 지속적인 활성
➡ cAMP ↑
➡ chloride channel 활성 지속
➡ Cl^- secretion ↑
➡ Na+/ K+ pump 손상
➡ 세포간질: Na+, H2O secretion ↑
➡ exhaustive diarrhea
➡ macrophage: Vibrio cholerae 식균
➡ extracellular peroxynitrite ($ONOO^-$) ↑
➡ enteritis

처방 목표 GTP binding protein 생성에 필요한 $O2^-$ 제거 / cAMP 농도를 지속시켜서 Cl^-

secretion 억제시킴 / mucosal epithelium: Na+/ K+ pump 활성화 / extracellular peroxynitrite ($ONOO^-$) 제거

처방 구성 黃芩 三兩 / 芍藥 二兩 / 炙甘草 二兩 / 大棗 十二枚

처방 약리

작약 paeoniflorin ➡ superoxide scavenger

대조 cAMP ➡ 세포질 granule-membrane protein: phospholylation 억제
➡ Cl^- secretion 억제

구감초 18β-24-Hydroxyglycyrrhetinic acid
➡ HSD11B2 inhibitor
➡ cortisol 분해 억제
➡ mineralocorticoid receptors 자극 지속
➡ Na+/ K+ pumps 전사 활성화

황금 baicalin ➡ peroxynitrite ($ONOO^-$) scavenger

황기건중탕 (黃耆建中湯)

원문 虛勞 裡急 `諸 不足 , 黃耆建中湯 主之 。, 餘 依 上 法 , 氣短 胸滿 者 加 生薑, 腹滿 者 去 棗 , 加 茯苓 一兩半, 及 療 肺虛 損 不足 , 補氣 加 半夏 三兩 。

원문 해설 심한 육체노동 후 몸 전체가 땅기고, 전신에 허혈감이 있을 경우에는 황기건중탕을 쓴다. 위의 방법대로 한 후에 호흡이 힘들고 심장부위가 갑갑해지면 생강을 배로 쓰고 복부팽만감이 있으면 대조를 빼고 복령을 1량반 가하고 치료를 계속 한 후에도 폐에 저산소증이 발생되면 반하 3량을 가한다.

적응증 Skeletal smooth muscle capillaritis
-mediated disseminated intravascular coagulation
(골격평활근 모세혈관염-매개 파종성 혈관내응고증)

병태 & 증상

Overwork

➡ skeletal smooth muscle contraction
➡ capillary contriction ↑ in smooth muscle
➡ capillary leak
➡ capillary subendothelial tissue: thromboplastin 분비
➡ thrombin formation
➡ capillaritis: fibrin 형성
➡ ischemic myonecrosis
➡ capillary leak 많을 경우: thromboplastin ↑
➡ 혈류 유입
➡ thrombus formation
➡ disseminated intravascular coagulation

처방 목표 fibrin 제거 / ischemic myonecrosis 억제 / thrombus 억제 / 혈관내피세포 heparan sulfate 합성을 증가시킴

처방 구성 桂枝 三兩 / 炙甘草 三兩 / 大棗 十二枚 / 芍藥 六兩 / 生薑 三兩 / 膠飴 一升 / 黃耆 一兩半 / 茯苓 一兩 / 半夏 三兩

처방 약리

황기 astragaloside ➡ Tissue plasminogen activator (+) modulator
➡ fibrin 용해

계지 cinnamic acid ➡ lactate oxidizer
➡ pyruvate 전환 촉진

생강 gingerol ➡ hydrogen peroxide scavenger
➡ 허혈 근육세포의 hydrogen peroxide 제거

작약 paeoniflorin ➡ superoxide scavenger
➡ 허혈 근육세포의 superoxide 제거

구감초 18β-24-Hydroxyglycyrrhetinic acid

➡ HSD11B2 inhibitor
➡ cortisol 분해 억제
➡ mineralocorticoid receptors 자극 지속
➡ 허혈 근육세포 Na+/ K+ pumps 전사 활성화

대조 c-AMP ➡ Protein kinase A avtivator
➡ 허혈 근육세포의 ATP 생산 촉진

복령 pachymic acid ➡ glycoprotein IIb/IIIa (gpIIb/IIIa) (-) modulator
➡ thrombus formation 억제

반하 triterpenoid (C30H48O7S)
➡ Rho GTPase family transcription promotor
➡ heparan sulfate 합성 촉진
➡ heparin 유사작용
➡ thrombus 분해

황기계지오물탕 (黃耆桂枝五物湯)

원문 血痹 陰陽 俱 微 , 寸口 關上 微 , 尺中 小緊 , 外證 身體 不仁 , 如 風痹狀, 黃耆桂枝五物湯 主之 。

원문 해설 감염증과 영양결핍이 동반된 듯한 마비감이 약간 있고, 촌구맥과 관상맥이 약하며, 척 중맥은 약간 급하고, 전신 움직임이 힘들어 보이며, 중풍 같은 마비감이 있는 경우에는, 황기계지오물탕을 쓴다.

적응증 Axon terminal capillaritis (축삭종말 모세혈관염)

병태 & 증상

Axon terminal capillaritis

➡ axon terminal: capillary congestion
➡ capillaritis

➡ fibrin formation
➡ neuron ischemia
➡ neuritis
➡ axon terminal: acetylcholine 분비 ↓
➡ skeletal muscle fiber: 자극 감소
➡ skeletal muscle fiber: total enzyme 감소
➡ lactate dehydrogenase ↓ / superoxide dismutase ↓ / glutathione ↓ / c-AMP↓
➡ lactate ↑ / superoxide ↑ / hydrogen peroxide ↑ / glucolysis ↓
➡ ATP ↓
➡ skeletal muscle fiber: 수축 실패
➡ paralysis

처방 목표 fibrin 제거 / lactate 교정 / superoxide 제거 / hydrogen peroxide 제거 / c-AMP 보충

처방 구성 黃耆 三兩 / 芍藥 三兩 / 桂枝 三兩 / 生薑 六兩 / 大棗 十二枚

처방 약리

황기 astragaloside ➡ Tissue plasminogen activator (+) modulator
➡ fibrin 용해

계지 cinnamic acid ➡ lactate oxidizer
➡ pyruvate 전환 촉진

작약 paeoniflorin ➡ superoxide scavenger

생강 gingerol ➡ hydrogen peroxide scavenger

대조 c-AMP ➡ Protein kinase A avtivator
➡ ATP 생산 촉진

황기작약계지고주탕 (黃耆芍藥桂枝苦酒湯)

원문 黃汗之為病, 身體腫,一作 重。發熱汗出而渴, 狀如風水汗沾衣, 色正黃如柏汁,脈自沉, 何從得之? 師曰 : 以汗入水中浴,水從汗孔入得之,宜耆芍桂酒湯主之。

원문 해설 누런땀이 있고, 전신이 부은 것처럼 보이는 것을 중이라고 부른다. 열나고 땀을 흘리면 갈증이 나며, 피부에 수분이 고인 것처럼 보이고, 옷이 땀에 젖으면 황백껍질 같이 누렇게 되고, 맥은 가라 앉아 있는 경우는 무슨 병이 걸린 겁니까? 선생이 답하기를: 땀 흘릴 때 물에 들어가서 땀관을 따라 물이 스며들어서 생긴 병으로 황기작약계지고주탕을 쓴다.

적응증 Chromohidrosis (색깔 땀 분비증)

병태 & 증상

Chromohidrosis

➡ sweat pore: open
➡ 물속에 들어감
➡ eccrine duct: 물유입
➡ eccrine duct capillary: congestion
➡ capillaritis
➡ fibrin formation
➡ eccrine sweat gland: ischemia
➡ 분비세포: 재관류 손상 ▶ lactate & superoxide ↑
➡ eccrine sweat gland: 땀분비 정지
➡ apocrine sweat gland: 땀분비 대체됨
➡ apocrine sweat: lipofusin 색소 함유
➡ yellow sweat

처방 목표 fibrin 용해 / lactate 교정 / superoxide 제거 / 분비세포로 glycogen 유입 촉진

처방 구성 黃耆 五兩 / 芍藥 三兩 / 桂枝 三兩 / 苦酒 一升

처방 약리

황기 astragaloside ➡ Tissue plasminogen activator (+) modulator

➡ fibrin 용해

계지 cinnamic acid ➡ lactate oxidizer
➡ pyruvate 전환 촉진

작약 paeoniflorin ➡ superoxide scavenger

식초 분비세포로 glycogen 유입 촉진 & 미각성 발한 유도

황련아교탕 (黃連阿膠湯)

원문 少陰病，得 之 二 三 日 以 上，心中煩，不 得 臥，黃連阿膠湯 主之。

원문 해설 항체매개독성병이 생긴지 2~3일이 지나서, 심장부위에 괴로운 증상이 생기고, 누워도 편하지 않는 경우에는 황련아교탕을 쓴다.

적응증 Bacterial endocarditis (세균성 심내막염)

병태 & 증상

Bacterial endocarditis

➡ bacteria infection: Streptococci / Staphylococci
➡ bacteremia
➡ heart endocardium valve: Streptococci / Staphylococci infection
➡ heart valve (주로, mitral valve): bacteria colony 형성
➡ Streptococci / Staphylococci 대사 ↑: superoxide ↑
➡ macrophage: Streptococci / Staphylococci 식균 ▶ NO 증가
➡ extracellular peroxynitrite ($ONOO^-$) 생성
➡ valve collagen: destruction
➡ valvulitis
➡ 좌심실 혈액: 좌심방으로 역류

처방 목표 heart valve: bacteria colony 항균 / superoxide 제거 / extracellular peroxynitrite ($ONOO^-$) 제거 / valve collagen 합성 / 좌심방 혈류 유입 억제

처방 구성 黃連 四兩 / 黃芩 二兩 / 芍藥 二兩 / 雞子黃 二枚 / 阿膠 三兩

처방 약리

황련 berberine ➡ sortase inhibitor
➡ Streptococci / Staphylococci: peptidoglycan 합성 억제
➡ 삼투압성 용균 유도

작약 paeoniflorin ➡ superoxide scavenger

황금 baicalin ➡ peroxynitrite ($ONOO^-$) scavenger
➡ macrophage 식균 후 판막 손상 억제

아교 Glycine / Proline / Hydroxyproline / Alanine
➡ collagen 주요 아미노산
➡ collagen 합성 촉진

계자황 (계란노른자) lecithin ➡ acetylcholine 생성
➡ M2 muscarinic Rc 자극
➡ cAMP ↓
➡ heart rate ↓
➡ 좌심방 혈류 유입 감소

황련탕 (黃連湯)

원문 傷寒, 胸中 有熱, 胃中 有 邪氣 , 腹中痛, 欲 嘔吐 者, 黃連湯 主之 。

원문 해설 세포병변성 감염병으로 가슴부위에 열감이 있고, 위장 독소로 인한 복통과 구토가 있는 경우에는 황련탕을 쓴다.

적응증 Group A streptococcus (GAS) infection (그룹 A 연쇄상구균감염증)

병태 & 증상

Group A streptococcus (GAS) infection

➡ 인두 점막: Group A streptococcus 감염
➡ 인두 점막세포 손상
➡ streptococcal pyrogenic exotoxin (SPE) 전파: vomiting, stomachache
➡ GAS bacteremia
➡ 심근: colony 형성 ▶ heart hot flashes
➡ 심근 대사 촉진: lactate ↑
➡ ATP 생성 ↓
➡ 심근: Na+/ K+ pump 약화
➡ 심근 손상
➡ 호중구 유도
➡ GAS phagocytosis
➡ HClO 분비 via H2O2
➡ GAS 살균되지 않고 오히려 GAS gene expression 활성화되어 생존력
➡ GAS phagocytosis macrophage: GAS Streptolysin O
➡ macrophage: mitochondrial depolarization
➡ macrophage apoptosis

처방 목표 Group A streptococcus 살균 / 인두 점막세포 상환 촉진 / 심근 lactate 교정 / 심근 Na+/ K+ pump 활성화 / 심근세포 증식 촉진 / HClO 분비 억제

처방 구성 黃連 二兩 / 炙甘草 三兩 / 乾薑 三兩 / 桂枝 三兩 / 人參 二兩 / 半夏 半升 / 大棗 十二枚

처방 약리

황련 berberine ➡ sortase inhibitor
➡ Group A streptococcus: peptidoglycan 합성 억제
➡ 삼투압성 용균 유도

반하 triterpenoid (C30H48O7S)
➡ Rho GTPase family transcription promotor
➡ focal adhesion 생성
➡ tissue damage: 상피세포 이동 촉진

계지 cinnamic acid ➡ lactate oxidizer
➡ pyruvate 전환

구감초 18β-24-Hydroxyglycyrrhetinic acid ➡ HSD11B2 inhibitor
➡ cortisol 분해 억제
➡ mineralocorticoid receptors 자극 지속
➡ 심근세포 Na+/ K+ pumps 전사 활성화

인삼 panax ginsenoside
➡ Transforming growth factor β (TGF-β) (+) modulator
➡ myocardiocyte & tissue damage: proliferation 촉진

대조 c-AMP ➡ protein kinase A avtivator
➡ ATP 생산 촉진
➡ cell cycle ↑

건강 shogaol ➡ neutrophil H2O2 scavenger
➡ HClO 분비 억제

황토탕 (黃土湯)

원문 下血, 先 便 後 血, 此 遠 血 也, 黃土湯 主之, 亦 主 吐血 衄血 。

원문 해설 하혈이 있는데, 변을 보고 나중에 하혈이 있다면, 먼쪽 혈관에서 출혈이 있는 것이므로 황토탕을 쓴다. 황토탕은 토혈과 코피가 있는 경우도 치료한다.

적응증 Immune thrombocytopenic purpura (면역성 혈소판감소 자반증)

병태 & 증상

Immune thrombocytopenic purpura

➡ virus infection: Ex. parvovirus B19
➡ antibody 출현
➡ platelet membrane: glycoproteins IIb-IIIa or Ib-IX ▶ cross reaction
➡ antibody coated thrombocyte 출현
➡ neutrophil FcR: antibody coated thrombocyte 식균
➡ neutrophil cathepsis 분비

➡ platelet apoptosis
➡ thrombocytopenia
➡ nitric oxide ↑
➡ peroxynitrite 생성
➡ vascular endothelium: VCAM-1 발현
➡ leukocyte 부착 & 침윤
➡ leukocyte: cytokine 분비
➡ subendothelial collagen 손상
➡ hemorrhage & hematoma

처방 목표 neutrophil cathepsis 분비 / thrombocyte 생성 촉진 / peroxynitrite 제거 / vascular endothelium: VCAM-1 차단 / leukocyte: cytokine 생성 억제 / subendothelial collagen 생성 / 지혈

처방 구성 甘草 / 乾地黃 / 白朮 / 炮附子 / 阿膠 / 黃芩 各 三兩 / 灶中黃土 半斤

처방 약리

포부자 aconitine
➡ 약리추측: neutrophil` Voltage-gated proton channels blocker
(식균작용에 의해 증가된 세포내 proton을 세포외로 방출시키는 채널)
➡ Voltage-gated proton channels 차단
➡ 호중구내 수소이온 축적
➡ neutrophil 대사 억제
➡ cathepsis 분비 억제

건지황 catalpol, 약리 추측 ➡ CD133+ CFU-S (+) modulator
➡ hematopoietic stem cell 분화 촉진
➡ thrombocyte 생성 촉진

황금 baicalin ➡ peroxynitrite ($ONOO^-$) scavenger

백출 atractylon ➡ vascular cell adhesion molecule-1 (VCAM-1) blocker

감초 glycyrrhetinic acid
➡ 11-beta-hydroxysteroid dehydrogenase1 (HSD11B1) inhibitor
➡ glucocorticoid 작용

➡ IκBα 생성
➡ NF-κB 억제
➡ leukocyte cytokine 생성 억제

아교 Glycine / Proline / Hydroxyproline / Alanine
➡ collagen biosynthesis 촉진

조 중황토 SiO_2 ➡ subendothelial collagen absorbent
➡ 지혈 작용
: 아궁이 밑에서 오랫동안 가열된 누런 진흙으로, 10년 이상 된 아궁이 바닥을 30㎠ 깊이로 파내면 나오는 자줏빛 진흙

후박대황탕 (厚朴大黃湯)

원문 支 飮 胸 滿 者，厚朴大黃湯 主之。

원문 해설 삼출액으로 인해 흉부가 그득해지는 경우에는 대황탕을 쓴다.

적응증 Lung adenocarcinoma & Large cell lung carcinoma (폐선암 & 대세포폐암)

병태 & 증상

Lung adenocarcinoma & Large cell lung carcinoma

➡ bronchial epithelium: c-myc change
➡ oncogenesis
➡ carcinoma cell 분화
➡ 주요 발생부위: 폐포 & 폐표면
➡ EGF receptor tyrosine kinase ↑ ▶ 증식
VEGF 발현 ▶ angiogenesis ▶ 성장
matrix metalloproteinase 분비 ▶ 침윤
➡ pleural invasion
➡ pleural effusion (흉막 삼출)

처방 목표 tyrosine kinase Rc 차단 / VEGF Rc 차단 / matrix metalloproteinase 차단

처방 구성 厚朴 一尺 / 大黃 六兩 / 枳實 四枚

대황 emodin ➡ tyrosine kinase blocker

후박 honokiol ➡ VEGF receptor blocker

지실 auraptene ➡ matrix metalloproteinase (MMP) blocker

후박마황탕 (厚朴麻黃湯)

원문 咳 而 脈 浮 者， 厚朴麻黃湯 主之。

원문 해설 기침하며 맥이 뜨는 경우에는 후박마황탕을 쓴다.

적응증 Emphysema (폐기종)

병태 & 증상

Emphysema

➡ lobule (폐소엽) bronchiol epithelium: chronic infection
➡ dendritic cell: antigen 제시
➡ immature T cell: antigen 전달 받음
➡ immature T cell: T-helper type 2 (Th2) cells 분화
➡ Th2 cells: chemokine 분비
➡ eosinophil 유도
➡ eosinophil granule 활성화
: degranulation & eosinophil peroxidase (EPO) 활성화
➡ EPO generated hydroxyl radical 생성
➡ extracellular matrix: hydroxyl radical 유출
➡ bronchiolitis
➡ Th2 cells: CXCR3 분비
➡ neutrophil 유도
➡ neutrophil: 폐포 간질 침윤
➡ neutrophil phagocytosis

➡ HClO 분비 via H2O2
➡ 폐포 간질: chronic inflammation
➡ alveolar-capillary barrier 손상
➡ 폐포 간질: erythrocyte 유입
➡ Met hemoglobin 형성 ▶ 혈관 수축
➡ alveolitis
➡ 폐포 간질 fibroblast: VEGF 생성
➡ fibroblast: 세포외기질 생성 증가
➡ interstitial fibrosis
➡ 폐포 세포 이탈
➡ 폐포 탄력성 저하
➡ 폐포 늘어짐
➡ emphysema
➡ alveolar-capillary gas exchange ↓

처방 목표 Th2 cells apoptosis 유도 / eosinophil degranulation & eosinophil peroxidase (EPO) 억제 / hydroxyl radical 제거 / HClO 분비 억제 / Met hemoglobin 환원 / 폐포 세포 상환 촉진 / VEGF Rc 차단 / alveolar-capillary gas exchange 촉진

처방 구성 厚朴 五兩 / 麻黃 四兩 / 石膏 如 雞子大 / 杏仁 半升 / 半夏 半升 / 乾薑 二兩 / 細辛 二兩 / 五味子 半升 / 小麥 一升

처방 약리

석고 CaSO4 ➡ calcium mediated T cell apoptosis 유도

마황 ephedrine ➡ Epinephrine receptors agonist
➡ adenylate cyclase 활성화
➡ cAMP ↑
➡ eosinophil degranulation 억제

행인 benzoic acid ➡ hydroxyl radical scavenger

건강 shogaol ➡ neutrophil H2O2 scavenger
➡ HClO 분비 억제

세신 eugenol ➡ MetHb reducer

반하 triterpenoid (C30H48O7S)

➡ Rho GTPase family transcription promotor

➡ focal adhesion 생성

➡ 폐포 세포 상환 촉진

후박 honokiol ➡ VEGF receptor blocker

소맥 Vitamin B6 (Pyridoxine) ➡ γ-Aminobutyric acid (GABA) biosynthesis

➡ airway smooth muscle 이완

➡ 폐포 호흡량 증가

오미자 schizandrin ➡ acetylcholinesterase inhibitor

➡ 횡격막근 수축 강화

➡ 폐포 환기 증가

후박삼물탕 (厚朴三物湯)

원문 腹中痛 而 閉 者，厚朴三物湯 主之。

원문 해설 배가 아프고 막히는 감이 있는 경우에는 후박삼물탕을 쓴다.

적응증 Adenomatous polyp (선종성 용종)

병태 & 증상

Adenomatous polyp

➡ high fat diets

➡ bile acids 분비 ↑

➡ colon mucosa: deoxycholic acid (DCA) & lithocholic acid (LCA) 접촉 ↑

➡ DCA & LCA mediated cytotoxicity

➡ adenomatous polyposis coli (APC) gene: mutation

➡ colon mucosa: cancerous cell 전환

➡ colon mucosa: EGF receptor tyrosine kinase ↑ ▶ 증식

VEGF 발현 ▶ angiogenesis ▶ 성장

matrix metalloproteinase 분비 ▶ 침윤

➡ adenomatous polyp 형성

처방 목표 tyrosine kinase Rc 차단 / VEGF Rc 차단 / matrix metalloproteinase 차단

처방 구성 厚朴 八兩 / 大黃 四兩 / 枳實 五枚

대황 emodin ➡ tyrosine kinase blocker

후박 honokiol ➡ VEGF receptor blocker

지실 auraptene ➡ matrix metalloproteinase (MMP) blocker

후박생강반하감초인삼탕 (厚朴生薑半夏甘草人參湯)

원문 發汗 後, 腹 脹滿 者, 厚朴生薑半夏甘草人參湯 主之。

원문 해설 IL-1 매개 감염증을 앓은 후 복부에 터질 듯한 팽만감이 생긴 경우에는 후박생강반하감초인삼탕을 쓴다.

적응증 Pancreatic ductal adenocarcinoma (췌장암)

병태 & 증상

Pancreatic ductal adenocarcinoma

➡ duct cell: proliferation
➡ NF-kB pathway: anti-apoptosis gene ↑
➡ KRAS mutation
➡ INK4A gene loss: p53 protein 생산 안됨
➡ duct cell: neogenesis
➡ heparanase 분비
➡ duct cell: heparan sulfate 분해
➡ TGF-β 분리됨: TGF-β mediated cell apoptosis 실패
➡ pancreatic ductal adenocarcinoma 지속

➡ 세포질내: hydrogen peroxide ↑
➡ VEGF expression ↑ : angiogenesis
➡ pancreatic ductal adenocarcinoma 성장

처방 목표 NF-kB 억제 / heparan sulfate 생성 / TGF-β 전사 촉진 / hydrogen peroxide 제거 / VEGF Rc 차단

처방 구성 厚朴 半斤 (炙) / 生薑 半斤 / 半夏 半升 / 甘草 二兩 / 人參 一兩

처방 약리

감초 glycyrrhetinic acid

➡ 11-beta-hydroxysteroid dehydrogenase1 (HSD11B1) inhibitor
➡ glucocorticoid 작용
➡ IκBα 생성
➡ NF-κB 억제

반하 triterpenoid (C30H48O7S)

➡ Rho GTPase family transcription promotor
➡ heparan sulfate 합성 촉진

인삼 panax ginsenoside

➡ Transforming growth factor β (TGF-β) (+) modulator

생강 gingerol ➡ hydrogen peroxide scavenger

후박 honokiol ➡ VEGF receptor blocker

후박칠물탕 (厚朴七物湯)

원문 病 腹 滿 , 發熱 十日 , 脈 浮 而 數 , 飲 食 如 故 , 厚朴七物湯 主之 。

원문 해설 복부팽만감이 있고 10일 동안 발열이 있으며 맥이 떠있고 잦으면서 식사는 여전한 경우에는 후박칠물탕을 쓴다.

적응증 Gastrointestinal leiomyosarcoma (위장관 평활근육종)

병태 & 증상

Gastrointestinal leiomyosarcoma

➡ gastrointestinal smooth muscle cell: Epstein-Barr virus (EBV) latent infection
➡ EBV infected smooth muscle cell: c-kit 돌연변이
➡ receptor tyrosine kinase 과발현
➡ GI smooth muscle cell: hyperplasia --〉 IL-1: fever
➡ 돌연변이 smooth muscle cell: hypoxia
➡ H2O2 ↑ ▶ JNK 활성화 ▶ Src gene 활성화 ▶ EGF Rc 과발현 ▶ cell mitosis
➡ Hypoxia-inducible factor-1α (HIF-1α) 활성화
▶ glycolytic enzyme 증가 ▶ 세포질 lactate ↑ ▶ growth factor 반응 ↑
▶ 분화촉진

➡ Hypoxia-inducible factor-1α (HIF-1α) 활성화
▶ VEGF 발현 ▶ phospholipase C ↑ : endoplasmic reticulum ▶ Ca2+ 분비
▶ 세포 대사 ↑ ▶ angiogenesis

➡ Hypoxia-inducible factor-1α (HIF-1α) 활성화
▶ erythropoietin 생산 ▶ autocrine ▶ NF-κB 활성화 ▶ MMP 분비 ▶ 기질 분해

➡ leiomyosarcoma ▶ heparanase 분비 ▶ heparan sulfate 분해 ▶ 기질과 분리
▶ 전이 ▶ sulfate ion : vommiting

처방 목표 leiomyosarcoma 성장 억제 / H2O2 제거 / 세포질 lactate 교정 / VEGF Rc 차단 / endoplasmic reticulum ▶ Ca2+ 분비 억제 / NF-κB 억제 / MMP 차단 / heparan sulfate 생성

처방 구성 厚朴 半斤 / 甘草 三兩 / 大黃 三兩 / 大棗 十枚 / 枳實 五枚 / 桂枝 二兩 / 生薑 五兩 / 嘔 者 加 半夏 五合 / 下利 去 大黃 / 寒多 者 加 生薑 至 半斤

처방 약리

대황 emodin ➡ tyrosine kinase blocker

생강 gingerol ➡ hydrogen peroxide scavenger
계지 cinnamic acid ➡ lactate oxidizer
➡ pyruvate 전환

후박 honokiol ➡ VEGF receptor blocker

대조 cAMP ➡ 세포질 granule-membrane protein: phospholylation 억제
➡ endoplasmic reticulum ▶ Ca2+ 분비 억제

감초 glycyrrhetinic acid
➡ 11-beta-hydroxysteroid dehydrogenase1 (HSD11B1) inhibitor
➡ glucocorticoid 작용
➡ IκBα 생성
➡ NF-κB 억제

지실 auraptene ➡ matrix metalloproteinase (MMP) blocker

반하 triterpenoid (C30H48O7S)
➡ Rho GTPase family transcription promotor
➡ heparan sulfate 합성 촉진

후씨흑산 (侯氏黑散)

원문 侯氏黑散:治 大風 四肢 煩 重, 心中 惡寒 不足 者 。, 上 十 四 味 , 杵 為 散 , 酒 服 方 寸 匕 , 日 一服 , 初服 二十日 , 溫酒 調 服 , 禁 一切 魚肉 大蒜 , 常 宜 冷食 , 六十日 止 , 即 藥 積 在 腹 中 不 下 也 。熱食 即 下矣 , 冷食 自 能 助 藥力 。

원문 해설 후씨흑산은 뇌경색(중풍)으로 인해 팔다리가 무겁고 괴로워지는 것을 치료한다.

적응증 Cerebral infarction (뇌경색)

병태 & 증상

Cerebral infarction

➡ brain blood vessel atherothrombotic or embolic
➡ 폐색 부위 속목동맥 / 앞대뇌동맥 / 중간대뇌동맥 / 후대뇌동맥 (후두 뇌경색, 시상 뇌경색) / 기저동맥 (중뇌 뇌경색, 뇌교 경색) / 소뇌 뇌경색 / 측부 연수 뇌경색

➡ **허혈부위 혈관내피세포** oxidative stress ▶ VCAM-1 발현 ▶ monocyte 부착
▶ 모세혈관 폐쇄 ▶ erythrocyte 정체
▶ 적혈구 골격단백질 불안정화
▶ deformity erythrocyte 생성
▶ met-hemoglobin 생성
▶ nitric oxide 소진
▶ 혈관평활근: oxidative stress
▶ α-adrenergic Rc Ca channel 자극
▶ 혈관평활근 경련
▶ 허혈 ↑

➡ **완전 뇌세포 허혈** 세포질 lactate ↑ ▶ 세포내 산증 ▶ ATP 고갈
▶ ion pump 손상 ▶ 세포외액 유입 ▶ 뇌세포부종
▶ calcium influx
▶ 세포막 PIP2 ▶ β-amyloid 분비 ▶ β-amyloid plaque 생성
▶ 신경 퇴행

➡ **허혈 주변부 뇌세포** calcium influx ▶ Phospholipases A2 activation
▶ arachidonic acid 대사 증가
▶ cyclooxygenase-2 mediated prostaglandins 생성
▶ neutrophil 유도
▶ neutrophil phagocytosis
▶ HClO 분비 via H2O2
▶ neuroinflammation

➡ **재관류** monocyte 활성화 ▶ NOS (nitric oxide synthase) 촉진
▶ peroxynitrite ($ONOO^-$) 생성
▶ 뇌실질 손상

처방목표 thrombus 제거 / VCAM-1 차단 / 적혈구 골격단백질 유지 / met-hemoglobin 환원 / α-adrenergic Rc 차단 / 세포질 lactate 제거 / 뇌세포부종 억제 / β-amyloid plaque 제거 / Phospholipases A2 억제 / cyclooxygenase-2 억제 / HClO 분비 억제 / peroxynitrite ($ONOO^-$) 제거 / neuron 재생

처방 구성 菊花 四十分 / 白朮 十分 / 細辛 三分 / 茯苓 三分 / 牡蠣 三分 / 桔梗 八分 / 防風 十分 / 人參 三分 / 礬石 三分 / 黃芩 五分 / 當歸 三分 / 乾薑 三分 / 芎藭 三分 / 桂枝 三分

처방 약리

복령 pachymic acid ➡ glycoprotein IIb/IIIa (gpIIb/IIIa) (-) modulator
➡ thrombus formation 억제

백출 atractylon ➡ vascular cell adhesion molecule-1 (VCAM-1) blocker

당귀 decurcin ➡ erythrocyte protein kinase C inhibitor
➡ adducin-spectrin-actin complex 유지시킴

세신 eugenol ➡ Met-hemoglobin reducer

천궁 cnidilide ➡ α-adrenergic receptor blocker

계지 cinnamic acid ➡ lactate oxidizer
➡ pyruvate 전환

모려 NaCl ➡ 세포외액 삼투압 증가 ➡ 뇌세포액 세포외로 방출 ➡ 뇌세포 부종 교정

반석 KAl(SO4)2·12H2O (aluminium potassium sulfate = Alum)
➡ astringent (수렴제)
➡ 뇌세포내 수분 수렴

길경 platycodin, 약리 추측 ➡ toll like receptor (TLR) activator
➡ microglia 식균작용 증가
➡ β-amyloid plaque 식균

감국 apigenin, 약리추측 ➡ Phospholipases A2 blocker

방풍 deltoin ➡ cyclooxygenase-2 blocker

건강 shogaol ➡ neutrophil H2O2 scavenger
➡ HClO 분비 억제

황금 baicalin ➡ peroxynitrite ($ONOO^-$) scavenger

인삼 panax ginsenoside
➡ Transforming growth factor β (TGF-β) (+) modulator
➡ SVZ neuronal progenitors: TGF-β (+) modulation
➡ neuron proliferation 촉진

| INDEX |

A

Adenomatous polyp (선종성 용종) : 후박삼물탕 ·513

Adenovirus infection : 건강부자탕 ·179

Airway remodeling-mediated Asthma (기도 개형-매개 천식) : 계지가행자탕 ·197

Alcoholic cirrhosis (알코올성 간경변) : 치자대황탕 ·476

Amebic liver abscess (아메바성 간농양) : 삼물황금탕 ·375

Angina (협심증) : 인삼탕 / 지실해백계지탕 ·436 / 466

Appendicitis (충수염) : 의이부자패장산 ·433

Asthma (천식) : 계지가행자탕 / 마황행인감초석고탕 ·197 / 298

Atheroma formation (죽종 형성) : 치자 후박탕 ·479

Atherosclerosis (죽상동맥경화증) : 지실치자시탕 / 치자 후박탕 ·465 / 479

Atrial fibrilation (심방세동) : 복령계지백출감초탕 ·350

Autoimmune enteropathy (자가면역성 장병증) : 계지가대황탕 / 계지가작약탕 ·188 / 194

Autoimmune hemolytic anemia (자가면역 용혈성빈혈) : 당귀사역탕 ·247

Autoimmune hemolytic anemia-mediated pancreatitis
(자가면역 용혈성빈혈-매개 췌장염) : 당귀사역가오수유생강탕 ·244

Autoimmune response-mediated Methemoglobinemia : 계지거작약가마황세신부자탕 ·203

Axon terminal capillaritis (축삭종말 모세혈관염) : 황기계지오물탕 ·502

B

Bacterial endocarditis (세균성 심내막염) : 황련아교탕 ·505

Bacterial pharyngitis (인두염) : 길경탕 ·242

Barrett`s esophagus (바렛 식도) : 대황감초탕 ·267

Basilar artery hemorrhage-mediated Insomnia
(뇌저동맥 출혈에 의한 불면증) : 산조인탕 ·372

B cell MALT lymphoma : 대승기탕 / 대황황련사심탕 / 소승기탕 / 조위승기탕
(점막림프조직 B세포 림프종) ·256 / 275 / 387 / 455

Behcet's Disease : 대반하탕/ 반하후박탕/ 복령음/ 부자경미탕/ 소반하가복령탕/ 소반하탕
(베체트병) ·255 / 316 / 354 / 359 / 385/ 386

Beriberi (각기병) : 반석탕 ·309

Bilirubin encephalopathy (빌리루빈 뇌병증) : 초석반석탕 ·471

Bipolar affective disorder (양극성 정동장애) : 감맥대조탕 ·172

Bone marrow EBV-mediated neutrophilia : 천웅산 ·469

Bornavirus infection : 과루모려산/ 백합계자탕/ 백합세방/ 백합지모탕/ 백합지황탕 / 백합활석산/ 활석대자탕 ·469
Botulism (보툴리누스 독소증) : 갈근황금황련탕 ·169
Bronchiectasis (기관지 확장증) : 조협환 ·456

C

c-ANCA associated vasculitis (항호중구 세포질항체-매개 혈관염) : 진무탕 ·468
Cardiac toxicity : 계지가계탕 / 계지거작약가부자탕 / 계지거작약탕 ·187 / 205 / 208
Cardiomyopathy : 계지감초탕 ·200
Capillaritis(모세혈관염) : 계지가황기탕 / 황기건중탕 / 황기계지오물탕 ·195 / 500 / 502
Cerebral infarction (뇌경색) : 후씨흑산 ·517
Cerebral venous sinus thrombosis (뇌 정맥동 혈전증) : 방기지황탕 ·319
Cervical cancer (자궁암) : 도핵승기탕 ·276
Chagas disease (샤가스 병) : 구감초탕 ·234
Chlamydia : 낭아탕 ·244
Cholecystitis (담낭염) : 부자사심탕 ·360
Cholera : 황금탕 ·499
Chromohidrosis (색깔 땀 분비증) : 황기작약계지고주탕 ·504
Chronic left heart failure-mediated alveolar-capillary barrier damage (만성좌심부전-매개 폐포-모세혈관 장벽 손상) : 령감오미강신탕 ·284
Chronic left heart failure-mediated alveolar carcinoma (만성좌심부전-매개 폐포암) : 령감오미가강신반행대황탕 ·282
Chronic left heart failure-mediated alveolitis (폐포염) : 령감오미가강신반하행인탕 ·280
Chronic right heart failure-mediated systemic congestion (만성우심부전-매개 전신울혈) : 방기복령탕 ·318
Chylothorax (유미흉증) : 귤지강탕 ·238
Clostridial necrotic enteritis (클로스트리디움균 괴사성장염) : 이중환 ·434
Coronary arteris spasm (관상동맥 경련) : 치자시탕 ·478
Coronary arteris spasm & Myocardial ischemia (관상동맥 경련 & 심근허혈) : 치자감초시탕 ·473
Coronary arteris spasm & Myocardial referfusion (관상동맥 경련 & 심근재관류) : 치자생강시탕 ·477
Colon cancer (대장암) : 마자인환 ·286
Common cold : 계지탕 ·222
Complement-mediated vasculitis (보체-매개 혈관염) : 적환 ·453
COPD-mediated hyponatremia (만성폐쇄성 폐질환-매개 저나트륨혈증) : 문합탕 ·308

Coxsackie B4 virus-mediated Type 1 diabetes : 백호가인삼탕 ·339
Coxsackie virus-mediated polymyositis & polyarthritis (다발성근염 & 다발성관절염) : 감초부자탕 ·175
Crohn's disease : 백두옹가감초아교탕 / 백두옹탕 ·324 / 326
Cytomegalovirus inclusion colitis (봉입체 대장염) : 적석지우여량탕 ·452
Cytomegalovirus infection in 인후상피 & 기관지상피 & 식도상피 : 과체산 ·228
Cytomegalovirus-mediated placental villitis (태반 융모세포염) : 건강인삼반하환 ·180

D

Decompensated heart failure (보상기전 실패 심부전) : 복령택사탕 ·356
Deep venous thrombosis in pregnancy (임신부 심부정맥혈전증) : 규자복령산 ·237
Distal extrahepatic cholangiocarcinoma (원위부 간외담관암) : 대황부자탕 ·269
Diverticulitis (게실염) : 대황목단탕 ·268
Duodenal ulcer (십이지장궤양) : 생강사심탕 ·377

E

Early autoimmune response : 마황부자감초탕 / 마황세신부자탕 ·289 / 290
EBV infection : 계지가부자탕 / 천웅산 ·190 / 469
Eccrine sweat gland capillaritis (에크린분비선 모세혈관염) : 계지가황기탕 ·195
Emphysema (폐기종) : 후박마황탕 ·511
Encephalopathy (뇌병증) : 분돈탕 / 초석반석탕 ·363 / 471
Endometrial adenocarcinoma (자궁내막선종) : 저당환 ·446
Endometrioma in uterine serosa & ovary (자궁장막 & 난소에 발생된 자궁내막종) : 저당탕 ·445
Endometriosis (자궁내막증식증) : 토과근산 ·484
Endometrium grandular polyp (자궁내막 용종) : 반석환 ·310
Endothelin-1 mediated Renal failure : 팔미신기환 ·488
Enterovirus-mediated Meningoencephalitis(장바이러스-매개 뇌수막염) : 갈근가반하탕 ·166
Eosinophilic gastroenteritis (호산구성 위장관염) : 반하마황환 ·312
Epilepsy (뇌전증) : 풍인탕 ·491
Epinephrine-mediated encephalopathy (에피네프린-매개 뇌병증) : 분돈탕 ·363
Erysipelas (단독) : 배농탕 ·323
Esophageal adenocarcinoma (식도선암) : 삼물비급환 ·373
Esophageal varices bleeding (식도정맥류 출혈) : 백엽탕 ·328
Esophagitis (식도염) : 반하건강산 ·311

F

Free bile acids-mediated glomerulonephritis
(자유담즙산-매개 사구체신염) : 인진오령산 ·437

Free conjugated bilirubin-mediated renal failure
(유리형 결합빌리루빈-매개 신부전) : 저고발전 ·444

G

Gastric adenocarcinoma (위암) : 소함흉탕 ·394

Gastric ulcer (위궤양) : 반하사심탕 ·313

Gastrointestinal leiomyosarcoma (위장관 평활근육종) : 후박칠물탕 ·515

Gastrointestinal stromal tumor (위장관 간질세포암) : 삼물비급환 ·373

Glomerulonephritis (사구체신염)
: 감강영출탕 / 복령융염탕 / 오령산 / 인진오령산 / 저령탕 ·170 / 353 / 413 / 437 / 449

Glomerulosclerosis (사구체 경화증) : 괄루구맥환 ·231

Group A streptococcus (GAS) infection (그룹 A 연쇄상구균감염증) : 황련탕 ·506

H

Hashimoto's thyroiditis (하시모토 갑상선염) : 사역산 ·368

Heat shock protein-resistant viral infection : 계지이마황일탕 ·215

Heat shock protein & IFN-a resistant viral infection : 마황탕 ·296

Helicobacter pylori-mediated stomach bleeding : 사심탕 ·366

Hemolytic anemia (용혈성빈혈) : 당귀사역탕 / 당귀사역가오수유생강탕
/ 마황연교적소두탕 / 적두당귀산 ·247 / 244 / 294 / 450

Henoch-Schonlein purpura
(헤노호-쉐라인 자반증에 연관된 대장염) : 백통탕 ·332

Henoch-Schonlein purpura-associated colitis & paralytic ileus
(헤노호-쉐라인 자반증에 연관된 대장염 & 장마비) : 백통가저담즙탕 ·330

Hepatocellular carcinoma (간암) : 대시호탕 ·258

Herpesvirus vagus neuritis (헤르페스 미주신경염) : 생강반하탕 ·376

Human T-Lymphotropic Virus (HTLV) infection : 작약감초부자탕 ·441

Hypernatremia : 계지가용골모려탕 / 계지거작약가촉칠모려용골구역탕 ·192 / 206

Hypersensitivity pneumonitis (과민성 폐렴) : 월비가반하탕 ·422

Hypertension : 택사탕 ·481

Hyperthermia (악성고열증) : 일물과체산 ·440

Hypoglycemia (저혈당) : 소건중탕 ·384

Hyponatremia : 계지감초용골모려탕 / 문합탕 ·198 / 308

I

IFN-a mediated Meningoencephalitis : 계지가갈근탕 ·186

IFN-a resistant viral infection : 계지마황각반탕 ·210

IFN-γ resistant viral infection : 대청룡탕 ·261

IgA nephropathy (IgA 신병증) : 저령산 ·448

IL-1 deficiency-mediated viral infection : 계지이월비일탕 ·216

IL-1 mediated arthritis : 두풍마산 ·279

IL-1 mediated Cardiac toxicity : 계지거작약가부자탕 / 계지거작약탕 ·205 / 208

IL-1 mediated Type 1 diabetes : 백호탕 ·341

Immune complex-mediated glomerulonephritis (면역복합체-매개 사구체신염) : 오령산 ·413

Immune complexes-mediated Rapidly progressive glomerulonephritis (면역복합체 매개-급속진행성 사구체신염) : 복령융염탕 ·353

Immune complexes-mediated vasculitis : 마황가출탕 (면역복합체-매개 혈관염) ·287

Immune thrombocytopenic purpura (면역성 혈소판감소 자반증) : 황토탕 ·508

Impetigo (농가진) : 배농산 ·322

Inclusion body myositis (봉입체 근염) : 작약감초탕 ·443

Infectious mononucleosis (전염성 단핵구증) : 마황승마탕 ·291

Influenza myositis (인플루엔자 근염) : 계지부자탕 ·213

Insomnia (불면증) : 산조인탕 ·372

Intestine MALT lymphoma-complicated perforation (소장 점막림프종에 의한 천공) : 대함흉탕 ·263

Intracerebral hemorrhage (뇌출혈) : 속명탕 ·395

Intrahepatic cholangiocarcinoma (간내담도암) : 인진호탕 ·439

Intrapartum Group B streptococcus infection (분만 중 그룹 B 연쇄구균 감염증) : 죽피대환 ·462

Intussusception (장 중첩) : 대건 중탕 ·254

Isonatremic dehydration (등장성 탈수) : 문합산 ·307

K

Kaposi sarcoma : 대황자충환 (카포시 육종) ·271

Kawasaki disease : 계지거계가복령백출탕 ·201

Kidney stones (콩팥 결석) : 활석백어산 ·496

Klatskin tumor (간문부 담관암) : 대황초석탕 ·317

L

Lactacidemia-mediated cardiomyopathy (지방산혈증-매개 심근병증) : 계지감초탕 ·200
Laryngitis (후두염) : 고주탕 ·224
Left heart failure-mediated pleural effusion
(좌심부전-매개 흉막삼출) : 목방기탕거석고가복령망초탕 ·305
left heart failure-mediated pulmonary venous congestion : 목방기탕 ·304
Lipacidemia-mediated Cardiac toxicity (지방산혈증-매개 심장독성) : 계지가계탕 ·187
Liver cirrhosis (간경변) : 시호계지건강탕 / 치자대황탕 ·404 / 476
Liver clonorchiasis (간흡충증) : 오두적석지환 ·410
Lung abscess (폐농양) : 정력대조사폐탕 ·454
Lung adenocarcinoma & Large cell lung carcinoma (폐선암 & 대세포폐암)
: 후박대황탕 ·510
Lymphatic filariasis (림프사상충증) : 모려택사탕 ·302

M

Macrophage foam cell formation (동맥경화증 단계 중 거품세포 생성) : 지실치자시탕 ·465
Malaria : 별갑전환 / 촉칠산 ·343 / 472
Malnutrition-mediated disease (영양실조-매개 질병) : 서여환 ·379
Meningoencephalitis (뇌수막염) : 갈근가반하탕 / 갈근탕 / 계지가갈근탕 ·166 / 167 / 186
Mesenteric lymphoma (장간막 림프종) : 기초역황환 ·241
Mesenteritis-mediated volvulus (장간막염-매개 장꼬임증) : 오두계지탕 ·408
Methemoglobinemia : 계지거작약가마황세신부자탕 ·203
Mononucleosis (단핵구증) : 죽엽탕 ·460
Mosquito-borne encephalitis virus & Enterovirus-mediated Meningoencephalitis
(모기-매개 뇌염바이러스 & 장바이러스-매개 뇌수막염) : 갈근탕 ·167
Multiple sclerosis (다발성경화증) : 귤피죽여탕 ·239
Myelitis (척수염) : 귤피탕 ·240
Myocardial infarction (심근경색) : 과루해백백주탕 ·227
Myocardial infarction & micro-emboli (심근경색 & 미세혈전) : 과루해백반하탕 ·226
Myocarditis (심근염) : 복령사역탕 / 복령감초탕 ·352 / 347
Myoglobin-mediated renal failure : 백출부자탕 ·329
Myositis (근육염) : 계지부자탕 / 작약감초탕 ·213 / 443

O

Osteoarthritis (퇴행성 관절염) : 오두탕 ·411
Ovarian cancer (난소암) : 대황감수탕 ·266

P

p-ANCA associated vasculitis (핵주위 항호중구 세포질항체-매개 혈관염) : 부자탕 ·362

p-ANCA mediated crescentic glomerulonephritis
(핵주위 항호중구 세포질 항체-매개 반월상 사구체신염) : 감강영출탕 ·170

Pancreatic ductal adenocarcinoma (췌장암) : 후박생강반하감초인삼탕 ·514

Pancreatitis (췌장염) : 오수유탕 / 당귀사역가오수유생강탕 ·415 / 244

Pathogenic E. coli infection : 육물황금탕 ·430

Peptic ulcer-complicated perforation (소화성궤양에 합병된 천공) : 감초사심탕 ·176

Perforation (천공) : 감초사심탕 / 대함흉탕 ·176 / 263

Peritonitis (복막염) : 대함흉환 ·264

Pharyngitis (인두염) : 감초탕 / 길경탕 ·178 / 242

Picornavirus infection : 소건 중탕 ·384

Placenta accreta (태반유착) : 하어혈탕 ·494

Placental villitis (태반 융모세포염) : 건강인삼반하환 ·180

Plasmodium falciparum malaria (열대열원충 말라리아) : 별갑전환 ·343

Plasmodium malariae & vivas & ovale malaria
(사일열원충 & 삼일열원충 & 난형열원충) : 촉칠산 ·472

Pneumonia complications-mediated hypoxemia
(폐렴합병증-매개 저산소혈증) : 계령오미감초탕 ·185

Poliomyelitis (회백수염, 소아마비) : 괄루계지탕 ·229

Polyarthritis (다발성관절염) : 감초부자탕 ·175

Polyclonal IgM cold agglutinins - mediated hemolytic anemia
(다클론IgM 한냉응집소-매개 용혈성빈혈) : 적두당귀산 ·450

Polymyositis (다발성근염) : 감초부자탕 / 사역탕 ·175 / 370

Polymyositis-associated gastrointestinal myositis
(다발성근염에 연관된 위장관근염) : 사역가인삼탕 ·367

Portal vein thrombosis (간문맥 혈전증) : 선복화탕 ·383

Postherpetic neuralgia (대상포진 후 신경통) : 의이부자산 ·432

Postpartum Crohn's disease (산 후 크론병) : 백두옹가감초아교탕 ·324

Postpartum mononucleosis (산 후 단핵구증) : 죽엽탕 ·460

Post-perforation peritonitis (천공 후 복막염) : 대함흉환 ·264

Pregnancy essential supplements (임신 필수보충제) : 당귀산 ·248

Pregnancy hypertention (임신고혈압) : 당귀작약산 ·251

Pregnancy trichomonasis (임신부 트리코모나스증) : 당귀패모고삼환 ·253

Pulmonary tuberculosis (폐결핵) : 맥문동탕 ·301

Pyelonephritis (신우신염) : 포탄산 ·490

R

Rapid hyponatremia (급속 저나트륨혈증) : 계지감초용골모려탕 ·198
Reactive arthritis (반응성 관절염) : 마황행인의이감초탕 ·299
Renal failure : 백출부자탕 / 저고발전 / 팔미신기환 ·329 / 444 / 488
Retained placenta (잔존태반) : 지실작약산 ·464
Rheumatic myocarditis (류마티스 심근염) : 복령감초탕 ·347
Rheumatic valvulitis (류마티스 판막염) : 복령행인감초탕 ·358
Rheumatoid arthritis (류마티스 관절염) : 계지작약지모탕 ·321
Right heart failure-mediated venous congestion (우심부전-매개 정맥울혈) : 방기황기탕 ·217
Rotavirus enteritis (로타바이러스 장염) : 계지인삼탕 ·490
RSV bronchiolitis (호흡기 세포융합 바이러스 세기관지염) : 택칠탕 ·482

S

Secondary tuberculosis (이차성 결핵) : 죽엽석고탕 ·458
Sjogren's syndrome (쇼그렌증 후군) : 감초건강탕 ·173
Small cell lung carcinoma (소세포폐암) : 삼물비급환 ·373

Skeletal smooth muscle capillaritis-mediated disseminated intravascular coagulation (골격평활근 모세혈관염-매개 파종성 혈관내응고증) : 황기건 중탕 ·500
Soft palate ulcer (연구개염) : 반하산급탕 ·315
Spherocytosis (원형적혈구증) : 당귀생강양육탕 ·250
Squamous cell carcinoma (편평세포암) : 주마탕 ·457
Staphylococcal food poisoning (포도구균 식 중독) : 건강황금황련인삼탕 ·181
Streptococcal rheumatic myocarditis (연쇄구균 류마티스 심근염) : 복령감초탕 ·347
Systemic lupus erythematosis (전신홍반성 루푸스) : 통맥사역탕 ·487
Systemic lupus erythematosis-associated nervous syetem dysfunction (전신성 홍반 루푸스에 의한 신경계 손상) : 통맥사역가저담즙탕 ·485

T

Tetanus (파상풍) : 왕불류행산 ·419
Toxoplasmosis (톡소플라즈마증) : 승마별갑탕 ·398
Type B hepatitis-mediated immune complex disease : 시호계지탕 ·406
Type 1 diabetes : 백호가인삼탕 / 백호탕 ·339 / 341
Type I hypersensitive reaction: eosinophil-mediated late phase reaction : 월비가출탕 ·426
Type I hypersensitive reaction: first sensitization : 감초마황탕 ·174

Type I hypersensitive reaction : neutrophil mediated late phase reaction : 월비가부자탕 · 424
Type I hypersensitive reaction : second sensitization: 월비탕 · 428
Typhoid fever : 황금가반하생강탕 · 497
Tuberculosis (결핵) : 맥문동탕 / 죽엽석고탕 · 301 / 458
Tuberculous endometritis (결핵성 자궁내막염) : 온경탕 · 416

U

Ulcerative colitis (궤양성대장염) : 도화탕 · 278
Unstable angina (불안정형 협심증) : 지실해백계지탕 · 466
Unstable angina-mediated coronary calcification (불안정형 협심증-매개 관상동맥 석회화) : 인삼탕 · 436
Uterine bleeding (자궁출혈) : 교애탕 · 233
Uterine myoma (자궁근종) : 계지복령환 · 211

V

Vasculitis (혈관염) : 마황가출탕 / 부자탕 / 적환 / 진무탕 · 287 / 362 / 453 / 468
Ventricular tachycardia (심실빈맥) : 복령계지감초대조탕 · 349
Viral fulminant hepatitis (바이러스성 전격성간염) : 시호가용골모려탕 · 402
Viral hepatitis (type A, B) (바이러스성 간염) : 소시호탕 · 388
Viral hepatitis (type C) : 시호가망초탕 · 400
Viral myocarditis (바이러스성 심근염) : 복령사역탕 · 352
Viral pharyngitis : 감초탕 · 178
Viral pneumonia (바이러스성 폐렴) : 소청룡탕 · 392
Viral thyroiditis (바이러스성 갑상선염) : 백호가계지탕 · 338
Volvulus (장꼬임증) : 대오두전 · 260

W

Warm autoantibody-mediated hemolytic anemia (온난자가항체-매개 용혈성빈혈) : 마황연교적소두탕 · 294

내과적 분류

1. 호흡기-알러지 작용약

감초탕 : Viral pharyngitis (바이러스성 인두염) ·178
계지탕 : Common cold ·222
고주탕 : Laryngitis (후두염) ·224
마황행인감초석고탕 : Asthma (천식) ·298
소청룡탕 : Viral pneumonia (바이러스성 폐렴) ·392
월비가반하탕 : Hypersensitivity pneumonitis (과민성 폐렴) ·422
월비탕 : Type I hypersensitive reaction: second sensitization (I형 과민반응) ·428
정력대조사폐탕 : Lung abscess (폐농양) ·454
택칠탕 : RSV (Respiratory Syncytial Virus) bronchiolitis (호흡기 세포융합 바이러스에 의한 세기관지염) ·482
후박마황탕 : Emphysema (폐기종) ·511

2. 소화기 작용약

당귀사역가오수유생강탕 : Autoimmune hemolytic anemia-mediated pancreatitis (자가면역성 용혈에 의한 췌장염) ·244
대건 중탕 : Intussusception (장 중첩) ·254
대반하탕 : Pyloric stenosis in Behcet's Disease (베체트 유문협착증) ·255
대오두전 : Volvulus (장꼬임증) ·260
대함흉탕 : Intestine MALT lymphoma-complicated perforation (소장 점막림프종에 의한 천공) ·263
대함흉환 : Post-perforation peritonitis (천공 후 복막염) ·264
대황목단탕 : Diverticulitis (게실염) ·268
도화탕 : Ulcerative colitis (궤양성 대장염) ·278
반하건강산 : Cytomegalovirus esophagitis (사이토메갈로 바이러스에 의한 식도염) ·311
반하사심탕 : Gastric ulcer (위궤양) ·313
백두옹탕 : Crohn's disease (크론병) ·326
부자사심탕 : Cholecystitis (담낭염) ·360
삼물황금탕 : Amebic liver abscess (아메바성 간농양) ·375
생강사심탕 : Duodenal ulcer (십이지장궤양) ·377
소반하탕 : Esophagitis in Behcet's Disease (베체트 식도염) ·386
소시호탕 : Viral hepatitis (type A,B) (바이러스성 간염) ·388
시호가망초탕 : Type C hepatitis (C형 간염) ·400
시호가용골모려탕 : Viral fulminant hepatitis (바이러스 전격성간염) ·402

시호계지건강탕 : Liver cirrhosis (간경변) ·404
시호계지탕 : Type B hepatitis-mediated immune complex disease (B형 바이러스성간염에 의한 면역복합체 질환) ·406
오수유탕 : Pancreatitis (췌장염) ·415
의이부자패장산 : Appendicitis (충수염) ·433
후박삼물탕 : Adenomatous polyp (선종성 용종) ·513

3. 순환기 작용약

당귀사역탕 : Autoimmune hemolytic anemia (자가면역 용혈성빈혈) ·247
당귀생강양육탕 : Spherocytosis (원형적혈구증) ·250
목방기탕 : left heart failure-mediated pulmonary venous congestion (좌심부전에 의한 폐정맥 울혈) ·304
목방기탕거석고가복령망초탕 : Left heart failure-mediated pleural effusion (좌심부전-매개 흉막삼출) ·305
반하탕 : Inferior pharyngeal stenosis in Behcet's Disease (베체트 하인두 협착증) ·316
방기복령탕 : Chronic right heart failure-mediated systemic congestion (만성우심부전-매개 전신울혈) ·318
방기황기탕 : Right heart failure-mediated venous congestion (우심부전-매개 정맥울혈) ·319
복령계지감초대조탕 : Ventricular tachycardia (심실빈맥) ·349
복령계지백출감초탕 : Atrial fibrilation (심방세동) ·350
복령사역탕 : Viral myocarditis (바이러스성 심근염) ·352
부자탕 : p-ANCA associated vasculitis (핵주위 항호중구 세포질 항체-매개 혈관염) ·362
소반하가복령탕 : Superior vena cava thrombosis in Behcet's Disease (베체트 상대정맥 혈전증) ·385
지실치자시탕 : Macrophage foam cell formation(동맥경화증 단계 중 거품세포 생성) ·465
지실해백계지탕 : Unstable angina (불안정형 협심증) ·466
치자시탕 : Coronary arteris spasm (관상동맥 경련) ·478
택사탕 : Hypertension (고혈압) ·481
통맥사역탕 : Systemic lupus erythematosis (전신성 홍반성 루푸스) ·487
황토탕 : Immune thrombocytopenic purpura (면역성 혈소판감소 자반증) ·508

4. 신장 작용약

괄루구맥환 : Glomerulosclerosis (사구체 경화증) ·231
오령산 : Immune complex-mediated glomerulonephriti (면역복합체에 의한 사구체신염) ·413
인진오령산 : Free bile acids-mediated glomerulonephritis (자유담즙산-매개 사구체신염) ·437
저령산 : IgA nephropathy (IgA 신병증) ·448
저령탕 : anti-GBM glomerulonephritis (항-사구체기저막 사구체신염) ·449
팔미신기환 : Endothelin-1 mediated Renal failure ·488
포탄산 : Pyelonephritis (신우신염) ·490

5. 내분비 작용약

백호가계지탕 : Viral thyroiditis (바이러스성 갑상선염) ·338
백호가인삼탕 : Coxsackie B4 virus-mediated Type 1 diabetes ·339
백호탕 : IL-1 mediated Type 1 diabetes ·341
소건 중탕 : Picornavirus infection / Hypoglycemia (저혈당) ·384

6. 산부인과 작용약

건강인삼반하환 : Cytomegalovirus-mediated placental villitis (태반 융모세포염) ·180
계지복령환 : Uterine myoma (자궁근종) ·211
교애탕 : Uterine bleeding (자궁출혈) ·233
낭아탕 : Chlamydia ·244
당귀산 : Pregnancy essential supplements (임신 필수보충제) ·248
당귀작약산 : Pregnancy hypertention (임신 고혈압) ·251
당귀패모고삼환 : Pregnancy trichomonasis (임신부 트리코모나스증) ·253
대황감수탕 : Ovarian cancer (난소암) ·266
도핵승기탕 : Cervical cancer (자궁암) ·276
반석환 : Endometrium grandular polyp (자궁내막 용종) ·310
백두옹가감초아교탕 : Postpartum Crohn's disease (산 후 크론병) ·324
온경탕 : Tuberculous endometritis (결핵성 자궁내막염) ·416
죽피대환 : Intrapartum Group B streptococcus infection (분만 중 그룹 B 연쇄구균 감염증) ·462
지실작약산 : Retained placenta (잔존태반) ·464
토과근산 : Endometriosis (자궁내막증식증) ·484
하어혈탕 : Placenta accreta (태반유착) ·494

7. 류마티스 작용약

계지작약지모탕 : Rheumatoid arthritis (류마티스 관절염) ·219
복령감초탕 : Streptococcal rheumatic myocarditis (연쇄구균 류마티스 심근염) ·347
복령행인감초탕 : Rheumatic valvulitis (류마티스 판막염) ·358

8. 뇌-신경 작용약

귤피죽여탕 : Multiple sclerosis (다발성 경화증) ·239
귤피탕 : Myelitis (척수염) ·240
생강반하탕 : Herpesvirus vagus neuritis (헤르페스에 의한 미주신경염) ·376
산조인탕 : basilar artery hemorrhage-mediated Insomnia
(뇌저동맥 출혈에 의한 불면증) ·372
속명탕 : Intracerebral hemorrhage (뇌출혈) ·395
의이부자산 : Postherpetic neuralgia (대상포진 후 신경통) ·432
풍인탕 : Epilepsy (뇌전증) ·491
후씨흑산 : Cerebral infarction (뇌경색) ·517

9. 근골격계 작용약

오두탕 : Osteoarthritis (퇴행성 관절염) ·411
작약감초탕 : Inclusion body myositis (봉입체 근염) ·443

10. 종양 작용약

기초역황환 : Mesenteric lymphoma (장간막 림프종) ·241
대승기탕 : Diffuse large B cell lymphoma of small intestine MALT
(소장 점막림프조직의 미만성 B세포 림프종) ·256
대시호탕 : Hepatocellular carcinoma (간암) ·258
대황감수탕 : Ovarian cancer (난소암) ·266
대황감초탕 : Barrett`s esophagus (바렛 식도) ·267
대황부자탕 : Distal extrahepatic cholangiocarcinoma (원위부 간외담관암) ·269
대황자충환 : Kaposi sarcoma (카포시 육종) ·271
대황초석탕 : Klatskin tumor (간문부 담관암) ·274
대황황련사심탕 : Gastric MALT lympoma (위장 점막림프종) ·275
도핵승기탕 : Cervical cancer (자궁암) ·276
마자인환 : Colon cancer (대장암) ·286

삼물비급환 : Esophageal adenocarcinoma & Small cell lung carcinoma & Gastrointestinal stromal tumor (식도암 / 소세포폐암 / 위장관간질 종양) ·373
소승기탕 : Diffuse large B cell lymphoma of gastric MALT (위장 점막림프조직의 미만성 B세포 림프종) ·387
소함흉탕 : Gastric adenocarcinoma (위암) ·394
인진호탕 : Intrahepatic cholangiocarcinoma (간내담도암) ·439
저당탕 : Endometrioma in uterine serosa & ovary (자궁장막 & 난소에 발생된 자궁내막종) ·445
저당환 : Endometrial adenocarcinoma (자궁내막선종) ·446
조위승기탕 : Small intestine MALT lymphoma (소장 점막림프조직 림프종) ·455
주마탕 : Squamous cell carcinoma (편평세포암) ·457
후박대황탕 : Lung adenocarcinoma & Large cell lung carcinoma (폐선암 & 대세포폐암) ·510
후박생강반하감초인삼탕 : Pancreatic ductal adenocarcinoma (췌장암) ·514

11. 감염

건강황금황련인삼탕 : Staphylococcal food poisoning (포도구균 식중독) ·181
구감초탕 : Chagas disease (샤가스 병) ·234
길경탕 : Bacterial pharyngitis (세균성 인두염) ·242
마황행인의이감초탕 : Reactive arthritis (반응성 관절염) ·299
맥문동탕 : Pulmonary tuberculosis (폐결핵) ·301
배농산 : Impetigo (농가진) ·322
배농탕 : Erysipelas (단독) ·323
별갑전환 : Plasmodium falciparum malaria (열대열원충 말라리아) ·343
오두적석지환 : Liver clonorchiasis (간흡충증) ·410
왕불류행산 : Tetanus (파상풍) ·419
육물황금탕 : Pathogenic E. coli infection (병원성 대장균 감염증) ·430
이중환 : Clostridial necrotic enteritis (클로스트리디움균 괴사성 장염) ·434
죽엽석고탕 : Secondary tuberculosis (이차성 결핵) ·458
황금가반하생강탕 : Typhoid fever (장티푸스) ·497
황금탕 : Cholera ·499
황련아교탕 : Bacterial endocarditis (세균성 심내막염) ·505
황련탕 : Group A streptococcus (그룹 A 연쇄상구균) infection ·506

약리 분류

1. 산화-환원제

계지 : 젖산 산화제 ·28
작약 : 슈퍼옥사이드 (superoxide) 환원제 ·119
생강 : 과산화수소 (hydrogen-peroxide) 환원제 ·87
건강 : 호중구내 과산화수소 (hydrogen-peroxide) 환원제 ·23
세신 : Met-hemoglobin 환원제 ·93
인진호 : Chenodeoxycholic acid (CDCA) 환원제 ·116
치자 : Low-Density Lipoprotein (LDL) 환원제
& conjugated-bilirubin 산화제 ·143
행인 : 하이드록시 라디칼 (hydroxyl radical) 환원제 ·153
황금 : 활성질소 (peroxynitrite, $ONOO^-$) 환원제 ·157

2. 리셉터 자극-차단제

갈근 : Ionotropic glutamate receptor 차단제 ·18
감수 : Aldosterone receptor 차단제 ·19
도인 : 4S estrogen receptor (ER) 차단제 ·52
마황 : Epinephrine receptors 자극제 ·55
백출 : vascular cell adhesion molecule-1 (VCAM-1) 차단제 ·72
복령 : glycoprotein IIb/IIIa (gpIIb/IIIa) 차단제 ·74
소엽 : Estrogen receptor alpha (ERα) 자극제 ·95
오수유 : Low-affinity Cholecystokinin (CCK) receptor 차단제 ·105
택사 : Angiotensin II receptor 차단제 ·114
천궁 : α-adrenergic receptor 차단제 ·137
후박 : VEGF receptor 차단제 ·163
황백 : Monocyte / Macrophage / Neutrophil CD14 차단제 ·162

3. 채널 차단제

부자 : 대식세포 Voltage-gated proton channels 차단제 ·78
상백피 : Capsaicin sensitive channel 차단제 ·85
촉초 : Potassium leak channel 차단제 ·140
포부자 : 호중구 Voltage-gated proton channels 차단제 ·150

4. 효소 촉진-억제제

감초 : 11-beta-hydroxysteroid dehydrogenase1 (HSD11B1) 억제제 · 20
구운 감초 : 11-beta-hydroxysteroid dehydrogenase2 (HSD11B2) 억제제 · 36
국화 : Phospholipases A2 억제제 · 41
귤피 : Proteolysis 촉진제 · 43
당귀 : 적혈구 PKC (protein kinase C) 억제제 · 46
대추 : Protein kinase A 촉진제 · 48
대황 : Tyrosine kinase 억제제 · 50
맹충 : Thrombin esterase 억제제 · 59
방풍 : Cyclooxygenase-2 억제제 · 68
오미자 : Acetylcholinesterase 억제제 · 104
제조 (굼벵이) : fibrinolytic serine protease · 127
지실 : Matrix metalloproteinases (MMPs) 억제제 · 133
파두 : Squamous cell PKC 촉진제 · 146
황련 : Sortase 억제제 · 160

5. 전사 촉진-억제제

고삼 : Protozoa tyrosinase transcription 억제제 · 32
건지황 : CD133+ CFU-GEMM 증식 촉진제 · 25
길경: Toll like receptor 전사 촉진제 · 44
맥문동 : M. tuberculosis SigF 전사 억제제 · 58
목단피 : antioxidant enzyme 전사 촉진제 · 61
반하 : Rho GTPase family 전사 촉진제 · 65
방기 : Prostaglandin I2 전사 촉진제 · 66
산약 : Glucose transporters 전사 촉진제 · 82
산조인 : serotonin / norepinephrine 전사 촉진제 · 83
생지황 : CD133+ circulating endothelial progenitor cell 증식 촉진제 · 89
시호 : Small interfering RNA (siRNA) 전사 촉진제 · 97
의이인 : Major histocompatibility complex (MHC) 전사 억제제 · 112
인삼 : Transforming growth factor beta (TGF-β) 전사 촉진제 · 113
저령 : Mesangial cell proliferation 억제제 · 122
죽엽 : β-amyloid gene expression 전사 억제제 · 130
지모 : nestin 전사 촉진제 · 131
황기 : Tissue plasminogen activator 전사 촉진제 · 159

6. 세포내 단백질 타겟

과루근 : Ribosome inactivating protein ·33

과루실 : Endothelium actin 분해제 ·34

백두옹 : 소장세포 NF-kB 억제제 ·69

산수유 : ERK (extracellular signal-regulated kinases) 억제제 ·80

7. 기타

경미 : magnesium ▶ DNA 복제 조효소 ·27

망초 : Sodium Sulfate (Na2SO4)
▶ Intraluminal distention pressure 상승제 ·57

모려 : NaCl ▶ Saline solution ·60

반석 : KAl(SO4)2·12H2O (Alum) ▶ astringent (수렴제) ·64

부소맥 : Vitamin B6 ▶ γ-gamma-aminobutyric acid (GABA)
& dopamine 생합성 촉진 ·78

석고 : CaSO4 ▶ T cell apoptosis 촉진제 ·90

아교 : Glycine / Proline / Hydroxyproline / Alanine
▶ Collagen 생합성 촉진 ·101

용골 : CaCO3 & Ca3(PO4)2 ▶ acidosis 교정 ·107

이근백피 : Potassium citrate
▶ extracellular Ca2+ influx inhibitor
& endoplasmic reticulum (ER) Ca2+ release inhibitor ·113

적석지 : Al2O3, 2SiO2·4H2O ▶ 양이온 흡착제 ·123

정력자 : helveticoside ▶ 강심배당체 ·126

죽여 : Tyrosine ▶ Dopamine / Norepinephrine / Epinephrine 생합성 ·129

초목 : xanthoxin ▶ 경련독 ·139

해백 (부추) : vitamin B1
▶ Pyruvate dehydrogenase
& Oxoglutarate dehydrogenase 조효소 ·151

향시 : L-arginine ▶ nitric oxide 합성 ·154

활석 : Mg3(Si4O10)(OH)2 ▶ Nitrogen group & Nucleic acid 흡착제 ·155